48.00 cs

MANAGING
CONDUCT AND DATA
QUALITY
OF TOXICOLOGY STUDIES

MANAGING
CONDUCT AND DATA
QUALITY
OF TOXICOLOGY STUDIES

Sharing Perspectives 266562
Expanding Horizons

Conference Proceedings
Raleigh, North Carolina
November 18–20, 1985

RA1199
M35
1986

Organizing/Editorial Committee:

Industry:

B. Kristin Hoover, ARCO Chemical Company
Judith K. Baldwin, Exxon Corporation
Arthur F. Uelner, Monsanto Company

National Insitute of Environmental Health Sciences/
National Toxicology Program

Carrie E. Whitmire
Christine L. Davies
Douglas W. Bristol

Sponsors:

National Institute of Environmental Health Sciences/
National Toxicology Program
American Industrial Health Council
American Petroleum Institute
Chemical Manufacturers Association
National Agricultural Chemical Association

PRINCETON SCIENTIFIC PUBLISHING CO., INC.

Printed and bound in the United States of America.

PRINCETON SCIENTIFIC PUBLISHING CO., INC.
P.O. Box 2155
Princeton, New Jersey 08543
Tel.: 609/683-4750

LIBRARY OF CONGRESS CATALOG CARD NUMBER: 85-63837
ISBN 0-911131-93-0

Cover Art: Adapted from an illustration by Alfred C. Laoang. See page 339.

DEDICATION

This book is dedicated to those engaged in the management and conduct of toxicology studies. We are indebted to those managers, scientists and support personnel who have inspired us by their efforts and high standards. We challenge ourselves, our colleagues and those who will come after us to maintain quality on a daily basis to assure accurate toxicology information.

ACKNOWLEDGEMENT

The Organizing/Editorial Committee acknowledges the support of their respective managements and staff for help in bringing the conference and this publication to fruition. Additionally, certain individuals deserve mention because without their insight and special contributions, this effort would not have been possible: Frances K. Abram (Monsanto), Loretta Brammell (NIEHS), Eugene C. Capaldi (ARCO Chemical Company), Scot Eustis (NIEHS), Nancy Mitchell (NIEHS), Dennis Poller (Exxon Corporation), Kent Shillam (Huntingdon Research Center, UK), Carl Umland (Exxon Chemical Americas).

PREFACE

Recognizing that both the National Toxicology Program (NTP) and industry share mutual concerns for managing the quality of toxicology studies, representatives of the American Industrial Health Council (AIHC) and NTP endorsed the concept of a joint conference on this subject. A committee, composed of three representatives from the NTP and three from the AIHC, was formed to plan and conduct the conference.

The charge to the committee was to bring together all interested parties involved in the conduct of toxicology studies, including top-level managers, scientists from various disciplines, quality assurance (QA) professionals and technical staff, to discuss the broad range of factors which affect the quality of toxicology studies. The conference title, objectives and program were developed to achieve the desired focus on quality. The objectives were to:

- Review and exchange current concepts and strategies to improve the quality of toxicology studies.
- Present and discuss QA programs utilized by government and industry.
- Provide a forum for the exchange of ideas between government and industry to strengthen common commitment to quality.
- Publish conference proceedings.

Funding for the conference was provided by the National Institute of Environmental Health Sciences/National Toxicology Program, American Industrial Health Council, American Petroleum Institute, Chemical Manufacturers Association, and National Agricultural Chemicals Association. The conference, held in Raleigh, North Carolina, on November 18–20, 1985, was international in scope and attracted over 600 attendees.

During the two-and-one-half-day conference, individuals at all levels, representing government, industry and academia, openly discussed managing the quality of toxicology studies. Formal discussion sessions involving speaker and audience dialogue, as well as informal discussions, were characterized by an enthusiasm not easily captured by mere reiteration of the manuscripts and transcripts from the conference. Luncheons with assigned seating were an integral part of the conference and provided additional opportunities for exchange of ideas. Speakers representing industry and government summarized the essential topics and issues dealt with during the conference. The conference ended on a high note of cooperation and strengthened the common commitment to quality.

With the publication of this book, the organizing committee completes the last of its four objectives. However, it was recognized by participants that this unique conference represented only one step towards continuing, cooperative efforts to improve the quality of all aspects of toxicology studies. The wide variety of topics and issues identified during the conference present a challenge to continue the effort through existing and new forums. The committee analyzed the response to a questionnaire distributed during the conference, presentations, dialogue and informal discussion. Topics for future consideration were grouped into the categories below.

- Education—Stratified training programs should be offered as integral parts of academic training and as continuing education programs for the various types and levels of professionals responsible for the quality of toxicology studies. Programs that are available need to be identified and the information disseminated. Topics suggested for development in training programs are specific audit techniques, computerized data systems and auditing of interdisciplinary data essential to toxicology.
- Regulation—A variety of regulatory issues were discussed which can be summarized as four major areas for future clarification. Annual publication of results from regulatory inspections of toxicology studies should be explored, with citations listed by kind, number and study type, so that managers and scientists are alerted to priority areas for improvement. The impact of the regulatory Memoranda of Understanding on the acceptability of test data should be assessed. Industry and the regulatory agencies should establish mechanisms to discuss appropriate methods for test substance characterization. A more detailed understanding of international requirements for toxicology study quality needs to be promoted.
- Public Interest—Suggestions on three topics of particular interest to the public's perception of science issues were made. A regular television program would allow scientists to discuss current issues in a public forum. Dissemination of information on ethical practices, as exemplified by existing codes of ethics, would inform the public about the high standards followed by those responsible for the quality of toxicology studies. Greater use of data quality indicators would serve the public through improvement of toxicology data bases used to make decisions.
- Resource Development—The committee recommends that professional societies and those who sponsor, conduct and audit toxicology studies need to explore possibilities for cooperative monitoring, sharing generic findings and further development of Quality Assurance programs.
- Continued Dialogue—A number of topics and issues suitable for future workshops and conferences were clearly identified. These include:
  - impact of animal health, environmental parameters and laboratory design on study quality;
  - development of minimum validity criteria;
  - impact of error on study interpretation;
  - methods for evaluation of studies conducted before and after implementation of GLP regulations;
  - clarification of the study director's role;
  - definition of goals for scientific and GLP compliance inspections and audits;
  - identification of acceptable quality levels for statistical based auditing;
  - storage and timely retrieval of toxicology data.

The spirit of commitment which prevailed during the conference is captured by these published proceedings. We hope that this book represents the first of many cooperative steps taken to better manage the conduct and data quality of toxicology studies.

TABLE OF CONTENTS

CHAPTER III Tools of Quality—Prestudy Organization

CHAPTER IV Animal Quality

CHAPTER V Study Conduct Quality

CHAPTER VI Quality of Pathology

CHAPTER VII International Regulatory Aspects of Quality

CHAPTER VIII Joint Conference Summation

Industrial View

Government View

Chapter I
QUALITY—MANAGEMENT
PERSPECTIVES

QUALITY MANAGEMENT PERSPECTIVES

David P. Rall
National Institute of Environmental Health Sciences
Research Triangle Park, North Carolina

OPENING REMARKS

This is clearly a relevant meeting in today's times of concern about the role of science in American society. What impresses me about the need for this conference is the fact that society now must use the results of enormously complex scientific studies to make certain important decisions. However, long-term chronic toxicity studies, complex environmental monitoring studies, and large-scale epidemiological studies generate so much data and take so long to perform that the old concept of a single scientist in one laboratory looking at his few animals next door is simply outdated. We need major and better tools to monitor the quality of toxicology studies which assure us at their end that the data are what those responsible for their conduct say they are. It seems to me that the added utilization of resources, cost, and time of doing this additional monitoring is one of the best investments we can make.

This conference represents the best form of cooperation between the private and public sectors. In conducting large-scale studies we both have the same ends in mind. We want a good, credible study that will convince all those who see it.

It gives me great pleasure to introduce Frank Press, who I think is one of the most accomplished scientist-administrators in the country today. As you know, since 1981, Dr. Press has been President of the National Academy of Sciences.

1

QUALITY MANAGEMENT
PERSPECTIVES

OPENING REMARKS

THE IMPORTANCE OF QUALITY IN TOXICOLOGY RESEARCH

Frank Press
National Academy of Sciences
Washington, DC

I'm delighted to be here on several grounds. Most obviously, because this is an impressive conference on an important issue. Judging by the programs and the abstracts, you are in for a rich three days. Second, this conference embodies the sort of cooperative spirit being sought among academia, government and industry. Indeed, that is the spirit which I, through the National Research Council, have sought to foster. That you were able to accomplish it is a tribute to the organizers and, indeed, to all of you. Third, I'm especially pleased to respond to an invitation from David Rall, and to have an opportunity to salute him for his enormous accomplishments reflected in the high quality of his Institute and, more subtly, in much of the work you will hear discussed at this conference. David Rall has been a ceaseless champion of scientific excellence, of rational decision-making, of dedication to training young men and women for toxicological research.

As you know, I'm a geophysicist, not a toxicologist. And just as you won't lecture me on wave mechanics, so I won't presume to lecture you on dose-response curves and the like. However, I suspect that quality assurance in both geophysics and toxicology does share a few things. Both our sciences are, of course, subject to Murphy's Law: If anything can go wrong, it will. But we also share some other rules. For example, Patrick's Theorem: If the experiment works, you must be using the wrong equipment. Or Horner's Five Thumb Postulate: Experience varies directly with the equipment ruined. Or Skinner's Constant, which is the quantity that when multiplied by, divided into, added to or subtracted from the answer you got, gives you the answer you really wanted.

But even if we are scientific brothers under the skin, I come to you more as someone who has worked both sides of the policy house, so to speak. And it is from that vantage that I want to talk about three perspectives which I think pertinent to this conference. These three perspectives involve history, science and the future.

First, the historical perspective. As you know, toxic substances as a national concern and toxicology as a science are both relatively new. The toxics problem didn't really gain any force until the 1970s. And even as late as 1974, an EPA analysis of federal laws dealing with the environment did not include a separate chapter on toxic substances. Now, of course, the world has turned upside down,

1. Address correspondence to: Dr. Frank Press, National Academy of Sciences, 2101 Constitution Avenue, N.W., Washington, DC 20418.
2. Key words: quality, regulation, research, risk, toxicology.

3

and toxic substances are thought by many to be our number-one environmental issue.

Similarly, toxicology remains a precocious, even a hothouse, science. Precocious because it is young, but is still being asked to carry enormous burdens; hothouse because its rapid growth has been forced by the urgent need to assess the risks of the chemical ambiance we have created for ourselves.

Overall, then, an important historical perspective is the forced march imposed upon both the issue of toxic substances and the relevant science. Since World War II, the history of federal policy vis-a-vis toxic substances has been one of a slow realization of the problem, followed by massive concern and legislation. A product of that history is the complex federal apparatus for dealing with the issue. As many of you already know, there are some 25 federal statutes regarding one or another aspect of regulating toxic substances. And six different agencies administer those statutes.

These 25 laws were written at different times, by different committees, reflecting different constituencies, philosophies and rationales. Considering that, we can't expect the laws to be consistent. And, of course, they are not. We find, for example, that the toxic substances in consumer goods fall under different laws, criteria and agencies than do the same substances in drinking water.

Yet, as inconsistent as they may be, these 25 or so laws are tied together by a common dilemma—what has been called the low-exposure dilemma. The dilemma is that we now know that certain toxic substances may cause harm at low doses—doses we couldn't even measure a few years ago. At the same time, many of these low-dose dangers are of enormous economic importance. And eliminating them exacts costs, including the very large economic, social and even psychic costs of banning toxics and thereby forcing companies, perhaps industries, to shut down.

That is the low-exposure dilemma, one that forces enormous pressures upon toxicological science, and one that demands that the science be first-rate, that judgments rest upon sound data. The dilemma will certainly not go away. Rather, it will become more acute. Science will march on, and our measurement capabilities will become ever more impressive. Injuries masked by long latencies will emerge. Increasingly, we will be caught between living with the possibility of harm owing to low exposures to certain chemicals or exacting enormous costs for their removal.

It is that dilemma which has, in part, led the government and the Congress to take such intense interest in your work. For example, rarely has a federal research program been subject to greater scrutiny than has the National Toxicology Program, most recently in the form of a favorable review by the General Accounting Office. Similarly, agencies have moved to improve their programs, notably the criteria for Good Laboratory Practices, of both the Food and Drug Administration and the Environmental Protection Agency.

These reviews and procedural maneuvers are important in stabilizing governmental and public confidence. But what remains supremely critical is the underlying science base. Without that, the best policies will fail. That leads to my second perspective, the scientific one. And that perspective has two parts. One is the relation of science to law; the second is the science itself.

On the first point, that of science and law, we have had a series of what have been called "science-forcing" laws. That is, we've had laws which triggered regulatory actions based on scientific information which, almost without exception, was incomplete. Such science-forcing laws include the Clean Air Act Amendments of 1970 and the Federal Water Pollution Control Act Amendments of 1972.

Some have called this legislated confrontation of science and law a "shotgun wedding." It's a wedding that has had a number of offspring, including a sharper attention to the processes of risk assessment and management. Another is occasional, sometimes painful, reminders of the chronic frictions that appear, owing to the enormous gulf in professional training and outlook between law and science. The British physicist John Ziman once pointed out that, "in science, as in law, we are almost always dealing with theories that are disputable, and that can be challenged by an appeal to evidence for or against them." Ziman added that, in science, when evidence conflicts, scientists repeat the experiment. But that option is generally not available in law, where legal disputes must be settled yes or no.

Learning how to deal with this cultural gulf is not easy. We are still learning how. But I think we have come to appreciate that, in regulatory action, science shares the stage with many other actors. We've come to appreciate the messiness of decision-making when the values of different worlds conflict. And we've seen some of the misbegotten costs of that forced wedding of science and law. We've had examples of blinkered analyses, incomplete data and limited scientific judgments too quickly turned into public policy, with enormous costs in money and public trust.

Mistakes have been made. Yet, I think that there is a growing appreciation by all sides of the impossibility of offering up firm answers in the face of insufficient data, forced extrapolations from animal to man or from high to very low doses and limited if not absent epidemiology. All of you have accepted as a fact of life that regulatory action will be taken in the face of incomplete information.

That seemingly gloomy acceptance is lightened by the widening powers of biological science. While uncertainty will be timeless, it will narrow, thanks to what *The Washington Post* once called "The Era of Biology." Everywhere we look, we see in basic biology a torrent of insights, new tools and remarkable applications. The sometimes startling advances of what we conveniently label biotechnology are universal in their effects. The ability to piece out specific genes, to copy them and to reproduce them in abundance opens the way not only to new commerce; it also offers a lever for probing the response of living cells and organs to outside intrusions, including toxic substances. Monoclonal antibodies are offering an unprecedented ability to detect molecular faults on cell surfaces.

That work joined with other achievements, notably in biochemistry, is sparking the entry of powerful new techniques for tracking the molecular and genetic passage of chemicals strange to the body. In helping us to understand what

5

happens to chemicals as they are metabolized, that work is beginning to impose a logic on the ocean of chemicals that surround us. Slowly, insights into the fate of these chemicals in the human body are focusing attention from that diversity to a relatively narrow range of highly reactive metabolites.

That work is very important. It both enlarges the power of toxicological science and narrows the cone of uncertainties. Yet, as all of you know, we remain, in many ways, desperately ignorant. Sometime ago, my institution prepared a briefing for the President's Science Advisor on the human health effects of hazardous chemical exposures. That report listed six areas where research is needed if scientific uncertainties are to be reduced, public confidence increased and the costs of imposing controls on hazardous chemicals justified.

Those areas are:

- Improving our abilities to extrapolate from high to low doses and from animals to humans;
- Improving our abilities to predict effects of exposures of chemical mixtures—from the workplace, hazardous waste sites and the like;
- Improving our abilities to predict reproductive and developmental effects of exposure to chemicals;
- Much better definition of the various stages of a cancer, so as to be able to identify potential cancer-causing chemicals;
- Making much better use of existing federal data to evaluate the impacts of chemical exposures on human populations; and
- Developing sensitive detectors, or markers, of both exposure to chemicals and their preclinical effects.

On the last point, biological markers, I'm pleased to announce that the National Institute of Environmental Health Sciences, together with the EPA, has funded a three-year study of biological markers by the National Research Council.

You'll quickly recognize that these six research priorities all relate to the theme of this conference. Each promises to improve your abilities to make supportable scientific judgments. And each demands ever more exacting science, more exacting data and more exacting interpretation. I'm sure you all have your own horror stories of good data badly interpreted. I'll tell you mine. Through great effort and patience, a researcher has trained a caterpillar to jump over a little fence whenever he says "jump." He then wonders how the caterpillar can jump so well. So he pulls off the front legs. But the caterpillar still makes the jump—not well, but he does it. Then the researcher pulls off the middle two legs, and again the caterpillar makes the jump. Finally, the last two legs are pulled off, and sure enough, when the scientist gives the command to jump, the caterpillar doesn't. The researcher then draws his conclusion: Pulling off the hind legs has made the caterpillar deaf.

I'll remind you of what I said earlier: That the daily pressures all of you live under will not go away; rather, they'll worsen. Quality assurance will be critical to dealing with these pressures.

Thus, our abilities to assess public health issues are trivialized if the data are inadequate owing to poor records. And just as a good study resting on poor data is a poor study, so a badly designed study is a bad study no matter how well it is conducted. The immediate issue is to design studies that are scientifically valid and that rest on believable data. And validity includes publishing results that are consistent with the data and that can stand up against careful audits of the underlying experiments.

All of you know the reasons for exercising such extraordinary care. The first is that experimental results can, at sometimes startling speed, be translated into public policy, and we have to be absolutely sure that any actions are consistent with the facts. A second reason is cheapness. While toxicological work is very expensive in both time and resources, the additional costs involved in high quality control are a lot less than repeating the experiment or correcting errors after the fact.

I say all this as someone who has observed the close links between toxicological science and public policy. And I say it as someone who has some appreciation for your difficulties. I realize that, even with the greatest of care and dedication, it is extraordinarily difficult to do reliable studies. The length of the studies, the thousands of data points that must be taken, the pileup of an avalanche of experimental material and the fact that fallible humans do them all argue against perfect studies. Mistakes happen. But they can be reduced; we can learn from errors; we can be tough both on our data and on our interpretations of what they tell us.

That said, let me finish up with my third, and final, perspective: that on future needs. I have two issues I'd like you to think about. One has to do with a common theme these days, that of conduits for transferring information, and the second with risk assessments. Both, again, tie into your theme. Information transfer is as vital in quality assurance as it is in all scientific endeavors. Similarly, while the problems of risk assessments can trigger a timeless debate, we know that these assessments are vitiated by poor data inadequately analyzed.

On the first issue, that of information transfer, we already see the seemingly instantaneous transfer of information across disciplinary lines. For example, in oncogene work, we see virtually seamless lines of communication between molecular and cellular biology, pharmacology, biochemistry and virology. The same thing has happened in other fields, such as work on the mechanisms underlying atherosclerosis or, more recently, parasitology. Moving away from the basic level, similar mechanisms for transferring information exist between science and technology, between research and commercial application. They are becoming more and more effective with time.

This conference is an important contributor to information transfer in toxicology. But I wonder if more of a continuing, even stronger, effort isn't needed. As Donald Kennedy, then Commissioner of the Food and Drug Administration, once commented, biology departments have competed with each other in their neglect of toxicology. You'll have to tell me if that neglect continues. I suspect it does.

The really tricky part of setting up communication lines is that we know the receiver, but not all of the senders. That is, we know that the receivers are those doing toxicological science. The information senders are likely to come from any corner of the scientific and technical community. We may see new tools emerging from wholly unsuspected directions, as did, for example, the use of nuclear magnetic resonance in diagnosis. We may see distant sciences offering telling insights, for example, recent work by physicists expanding our understanding of how signals move across cellular membranes.

The point is how to assure that the communication channels of toxicology are multiple and broad-banded. Can the crosstalk between basic science and toxicology be heightened? What can and should drive the crosstalk? In many areas—computer architectures, biochemical engineering, new materials—the drivers are obvious. They include international competition, national security, a healthy U.S. economy and the like. Those same goals are important in toxicology. But, as yet, they don't have the same force. The upshot is still fairly weak mechanisms for assuring that the triumphs of biology are rapidly turned toward public protection. Dealing with that issue—creating better mechanisms for information transfer—is, then, an important agenda item for toxicology.

The second issue is risk assessment. As you well know, that topic is as controversial as it is necessary. Risk assessments remain formal ways of forcing facts, experiments, observations and experience into decisions. They are not science as I understand it, but they certainly are science-based. That is not to denigrate risk assessments nor to deny their need. It simply recognizes them as forcing functions for uncertainties.

Our present unhappiness with risk assessments is neither procedural nor organizational; it is scientific. The organization which I chair, the National Research Council, last year issued a report entitled *Risk Assessment in the Federal Government: Managing the Process*. That report pointed out that "the basic problem with risk assessment is not its administrative setting, but rather the sparseness and uncertainty of the scientific knowledge of the health hazards assessed."

In short, risk assessments will be as good as you can make them. They will be as good as the underlying science that you use. They will be as good as the data you use and the interpretations you put upon them.

That this conference is being held argues for better risk assessments. That it brings together people from the universities, from the government and from industry argues for major advances in toxicological studies, studies that will advance both the underlying science and the public interest.

QUALITY AND THE
NATIONAL TOXICOLOGY PROGRAM

Ernest E. McConnell
National Institute of Environmental Health Sciences
Research Triangle Park, North Carolina

ABSTRACT

Studies conducted under the auspices of the National Toxicology Program (NTP) are often some of the most essential data used by regulatory agencies in determining the potential health hazard of a given chemical. In this way, these studies become the interface between science and regulatory decision-making. In the long run, the NTP studies promote a cleaner environment and affect human health. In addition, NTP studies are often viewed as the standard for the conduct of toxicological investigations.

Therefore, it is a primary responsibility of NTP to assure that these studies are conducted in such a way that the results are valid. The only way to assure this is through a definitive quality assurance program that begins at the time of chemical selection and which is then followed throughout the study until and after the results are published.

Creating an atmosphere for study quality and implementing it are complex exercises requiring the expertise of many disciplines, not of just toxicology *per se*. The goal of this conference is to describe the various aspects of quality of toxicology and to demonstrate that they can be managed and coordinated effectively.

INTRODUCTION

Studies conducted under the auspices of the National Toxicology Program are designed primarily to determine if a given chemical causes or represents a potential health hazard (hazard is a qualitative term relative to a specific health effect). NTP studies often constitute some of the most essential data used by regulatory agencies as part of the "Weight of Evidence" in their decision making. Therefore, the accurate establishment of the hazards associated with exposure to a chemical is extremely important and represents the first and one of the most important criteria in establishing risk (risk is the summation of

1. Address correspondence to: Ernest E. McConnell, N.I.E.H.S., P.O. Box 12233, Research Triangle Park, NC 27709.
2. Key words: exposure, hazard, quality, risk.
3. Abbreviation: NTP, National Toxicology Program.

hazard plus exposure). In this way, NTP studies become the interface between science and regulatory decision-making. For this reason, it is imperative that the toxicology studies conducted by the NTP be of the highest quality.

IMPORTANCE OF MANAGEMENT'S ROLE

Achieving quality in toxicology studies is a complex and often difficult exercise to accomplish. Management, in this case that provided by the NTP to the contractor laboratories, is of prime importance in establishing the overall quality of a study. If management does not give the impetus to the staff who are responsible for carrying out the various aspects of the study, then the quality will never be of the level required. In this sense, quality within the NTP to a certain extent has to involve a "top-down" philosophy (Figure 1). This does not negate the need for staff at all levels to also stimulate management to the value of quality.

One important aspect of this "top-down" philosophy is that the principal scientists involved in all aspects of the study need to be inured with the concept that quality is one of the most important, if not the most important, aspect of the study. To assure quality, one of the first requirements is to have people managing the study who have the technical expertise and background to appreciate the necessity for quality in a study. This means that the study (chemical) manager needs to have a broad enough background to understand the input of the various disciplines other than classic toxicology, such as chemistry and pathology. He or she needs to have enough working knowledge of these areas to know when a given area is deficient. More importantly, this person has to have the ability and incentive to discuss with discipline leaders the findings in this area and the way in which they impact on the study as a whole.

Quality has to be an integral part of the study from beginning to end. This entails an in-depth knowledge of the chemical prior to the start of the study to make sure that one is asking the right questions about a given chemical. Second, the quality of the experimental design must be such that the protocol is designed to answer these scientific questions in an effective manner. Next, the in-life phase of the study must be conducted according to the protocol. The next critical step is the quality of the pathology. It must be of such quality that it is beyond question. Finally, the data from the study as a whole must be recorded

"TOP-DOWN"

MANAGEMENT
↓
STUDY MANAGER
↓
LABORATORY STAFF
(Professional and Technical)

FIGURE 1. The quality of NTP studies is directly influenced by management.

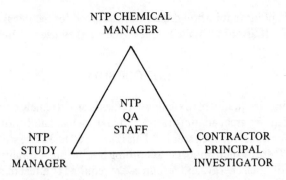

NTP CHEMICAL
MANAGER

NTP
QA
STAFF

NTP
STUDY
MANAGER

CONTRACTOR
PRINCIPAL
INVESTIGATOR

FIGURE 2. The NTP quality assurance staff coordinate and direct the QA activities between the government and the contractor laboratory.

in such a way that all the pieces can be put back together retrospectively. All of these steps are required to assure that the study was carried out in a proper manner. There is no substitute for continual scrutiny of a study (from beginning to end) if one is to have confidence in the data from that study.

While the above ensures that the quality of the study is of such a nature that it will withstand close scrutiny, this does not mean that the interpretation of the study is not debatable. The interpretation of the study, that is, whether a chemical caused a given effect or not, is obviously dependent upon the study's quality. Suffice it to say that reasonable people can differ in their interpretation of data but that the interpretation of the data will always be in question if the quality of the data is suspect.

One issue that should not be overlooked is the value of the NTP staff who are responsible for the quality of data as a whole (Figure 2). In addition to having knowledge of the various disciplines that are critical in these studies, the quality staff also need to be aware of technical procedures for data tracking, good laboratory practices, various regulations, and have a close working relationship with other federal agencies that use data generated by the NTP.

An important aspect of a study that the NTP Quality Assurance staff are intimately involved with is identifying flaws in a given study and, in concert with other members of the staff, reviewing these flaws to determine how they impact on the results of the study as a whole and the interpretation of the study. Most experienced toxicologists would agree that there is no such thing as a perfect study. This is particularly true with long-term studies. In fact, the potential for error is directly proportional to the length of the study and is impacted additionally by the study's complexity. Therefore, one has to admit that errors will be made; the important point is being able to determine the seriousness of those errors.

One of the hardest, yet one of the most important tasks that the NTP staff have to achieve is knowing when to make higher management aware that a study is deficient in a given area or is not achieving the goals that were outlined prior to the start of the study. It is only human nature to continue with a study beyond the point that it should have been stopped for technical reasons. These are difficult decisions to make but nevertheless they need to be made.

CONCLUSION

Managing the quality of toxicology studies is an extremely complex issue and one that requires great administrative and management ability on the part of the people responsible for such studies. This is no small task. The studies conducted by the NTP are of such import that nothing but the finest quality will suffice. A great deal of time, energy, and resources are required to effect this quality, but in my opinion these are resources well spent.

IMPLEMENTATION OF GLP COMPLIANCE IN A GOVERNMENT OFFICE

Sidney Green
Division of Toxicology
Food and Drug Administration
Washington, DC

ABSTRACT

The implementation of Good Laboratory Practices in a government office is discussed. Early attitudes are summarized. The 1980 inspection and its aftermath are described. Changes in attitudes and actions and their role in the outcome of a subsequent inspection are discussed.

INTRODUCTION

Ostensibly, the implementation of Good Laboratory Practices (GLPs) in a government office should be very similar to implementation elsewhere. Yet there are peculiarities associated with management and employees in a government setting that are reflected in the ways in which these individuals respond to such a change as initiation of GLPs. Admittedly, some of these attitudes are similar to those in nongovernmental organizations. Regardless of the contrasting initial responses of various organizations, the process leading to ultimate acceptance and compliance with GLPs is probably the same.

At the outset, I believe that there are a number of things that need to be said about our experience in implementing GLPs. To speak bluntly, we probably exercised rather poor judgment in our initial reactions to the regulation. We can now state that, in all likelihood, this poor judgment was a reflection of our attitude toward the regulation. That attitude and rather poor judgment had a large part to play in delaying our eventual acceptance and compliance with the act. In what follows, I will discuss some of these attitudes, how they resulted in a less than desirable outcome, the measures taken to correct the situation and, finally, the benefits of those corrective actions.

1. Address correspondence to: Dr. Sidney Green, Food and Drug Administration, HFF 160, 200 C Street SW, Washington, DC 20204.
2. Key words: compliance, monitoring, observation, regulation.
3. Abbreviations: GLP, Good Laboratory Practice; QAU, Quality Assurance Unit; SOP, Standard Operating Procedure.

EARLY ATTITUDES OF INVESTIGATORS

I would like to begin by providing what I consider the bench scientist's view of the GLP regulations when first applied at the Center. To do that, let me dwell for a moment on the "personality," if you will, of scientists, particularly those of us who conduct laboratory studies. As you know, scientists are rather strong-willed and independent in thought; some would even call them opinionated. Most are not easily dictated to and most accept major changes somewhat reluctantly. These comments are not meant to cast bench scientists in a negative light, but are made in recognition of some characteristics which have made scientists major contributors to our present way of life.

Given these characteristics, it is not surprising that when the Center attempted to implement the GLPs, the process met with a certain degree of disdain. The scientists' general feeling was that they had done very well without such circumscribed rules and saw no redeeming value in their implementation. "Why is this necessary?" was a frequent question.

The following list summarizes some of the early attitudes of the investigators:

- GLPs would inhibit scientific experimentation due to the need to develop detailed protocols, Standard Operating Procedures (SOPs) and final reports. Simply put, the regulations would adversely affect their ability to publish in a timely fashion.
- GLPs were just another intrusion by management into an area previously reserved to the scientist. Reflected in this attitude was the feeling that it was illogical to expect someone unfamiliar with their work to inspect, understand and appreciate the intricacies associated with development of protocols, conducting the study and assembling a comprehensive report.
- There would be too much oversight, in in-life inspection phases, for example. The idea that someone would actually observe how closely someone was adhering to an SOP in conducting a technique was embarrassing at best and unnecessary at the least.
- The regulations would stifle creativity. This comment was made more frequently than any other. It was thought that individuals might see research avenues worthy of pursuit with respect to certain agents, but decide that because a study would be under GLPs, it would take an inordinate amount of time and effort. Instead, it would be to the investigator's advantage to conduct other studies of a non-GLP nature.

I believe it is fair to describe these feelings as being consistent with a high degree of apprehension.

Another factor that played a major role in the pace at which the GLPs were accepted during their initial implementation was the Agency's or Center's perception of where they fit in the scheme of things. How involved did management need to be? Could not the investigators do what was necessary without management's devoting an extraordinary amount of time to the process? Coupled with this quandary was the vague notion that perhaps the Agency was not or should not be subject to GLPs. Additionally, management and bench scientists shared the impression that the government laboratories were not the problem, that the GLP regulations were created to correct problems in the industrial sector. Consequently, the leadership necessary for providing direction and displaying an appropriate level of concern was less than that needed for a change of this magnitude.

We therefore had a situation in which the investigators felt threatened and were somewhat apprehensive and the Agency or Center was not certain of its role in the process. In part, these early attitudes were the basis for the less than satisfactory performance in our first inspection.

THE 1980 INSPECTION

The 1980 inspection detailed eighty-four deviations, a large number of which did not involve studies, but problems with the facilities. We were not psychologically prepared for the extensive and detailed inspection of the facilities and audit of studies. Numerous ideas were put forth as to why we thought such a meticulous inspection was conducted. Most prominent among them was that we were or should be the standard by which industry should be measured, and thus more attention had been focused on FDA studies and facilities. Whatever the reason for the level of detail associated with the inspection, the results caused us to begin asking questions about our approach to and management of GLP studies.

Some of the major deviations noted during the 1980 inspection were:
- Incomplete protocols; there were segments of some studies for which protocols had been misplaced or not written;
- Deficient and/or nonexistent SOPs;
- Nonfunctional Quality Assurance Unit (QAU); the staff necessary to provide a fully functional QAU was inadequate;
- Animal feed storage room insufficient;
- Unkept diet-mixing room;
- Animal rooms in poor condition; wall coverings that were loosely attached, light diffusers missing; occasional holes in walls of animal rooms and corridors;
- Calibration of all balances not accomplished;
- Poor documentation, use of pencil and correction fluid;
- Inadequate archives, storage and retrieval systems.

In terms of public relations, the result of the inspection and eighty-four deviations was that the trade journals and newspapers became very interested and reported the results in depth. The following are representative excerpts.

FDA Labs Fail to Maintain SOP's Required
Under GLP, Audit Charges

The Center for Food Safety and Applied Nutrition failed to maintain Standard Operating Procedures (SOPs) for many elements of the nonclinical studies conducted at the Food and Drug Administration's downtown FB-8 building, according to a Good Laboratory Practice inspection audit conducted in September jointly by scientists from the Baltimore District and Center for Veterinary Medicine.

GLP Deficiencies at Center for Food Safety and Applied Nutrition's Beltsville Facilities Noted

Good Laboratory Practice deficiencies at the Beltsville laboratory facilities of the Food and Drug Administration may be addressed as part of the Center's overall effort to institute an effective quality assurance program which covers the Beltsville facility as well as FB-8.

This was an embarrassing situation, to say the least. However difficult it was, the first response was to accept the criticism in as positive a manner as possible. This does not mean that we agreed with all comments made by the inspectors, but it was not an exceptionally difficult job to determine those points considered "most valid."

The following excerpt summarizes the post-inspection philosophy.

FDA Accepts GLP Criticisms

Management of the Center for Food Safety and Applied Nutrition's laboratories must accept a large share of the responsibility for failure to comply adequately with the GLP regulations as documented in the inspection report.

It is clear that the Center for Food Safety and Applied Nutrition's toxicology laboratories are poorly managed and research projects are hampered by inadequate administrative support, animal housing facilities, coordination, and an inadequate system of quality assurance.

CHANGES IN ATTITUDES AND ACTIONS

The Director and Deputy Director at the Center made it clear that there had to be changes in attitudes and actions to prevent a recurrence of the criticism. The first step was the cessation of all research at the Center. As projects were completed, new studies were not initiated, and studies were held in abeyance for a period of about nine months. During this period, SOPs for all phases of GLP studies were drafted, reviewed by supervisory personnel and redrafted. SOPs for the Quality Assurance Staff, Veterinary Medical Officer and every facet of the Center's research program which related to GLPs were completed. Curriculum vitae were updated for all personnel, animal rooms were repaired, and these activities were, of necessity, accomplished within the Center's budget.

There were no new hires to whom to assign the responsibility of planning and assisting the scientists in accomplishing these tasks. Individuals were detailed from other areas in the Center to work on the various tasks. The group that had the primary responsibility for coordinating the work was called the "Quality Assurance Task Force." In what was truly a team effort, volunteers worked evenings and weekends to complete various tasks. The entire Center adopted the attitude that we as a group would get the job done, and I do not believe I am overdramatizing this effort.

The objectives of the Quality Assurance Task Force were to:
1. Identify each deviation from the inspection;
2. Develop a corrective action plan;
3. Assure that SOPs for all areas of laboratory work were completed;
4. Develop and present a training program.

One example of the management plan used to correct the deficiencies is illustrated in Table 1. Each deviation was listed in the plan, along with the section of the act to which the deviation applied. The individual or individuals responsible for the corrective action were listed, together with the data by which the corrective action(s) should be completed. As noted in Table 1, a training course was to be conducted by the Center. Table 2 lists the topics covered in the course. Each individual associated with the GLP studies, from laboratory technicians to division directors, was mandated to attend the course. After the lectures, extensive discussions were held to explore certain issues in more depth.

TABLE 1
Example of Management Plan To Correct Deficiencies

Deviation	Regulation Section of Act	Corrective Action	Responsible Individual	Deadline
Management not assuring that deviations are corrected	58.31 (g)	1. Center should conduct a training program for all line management 2. CAU report deviations 3. Head of Division checks that de-deviation is corrected 4. Include adherence to quality control procedures in performance objectives for study director		

TABLE 2
Topics Covered in Training Course

I. Background and History of GLPs
II. Review and Interpretation of Regulations
III. Writing Standard Operating Procedures
IV. Quality Assurance Unit
V. Protocol Preparation (Form)
VI. Writing Final Reports (Forms)
VII. Contents of GLP Inspection by EDRO
  a. Entrance to Facility
  b. Facilities
  c. Data Audits
  d. Exit Interview

THE 1985 INSPECTION

The true test of any training exercise is whether performance is subsequently improved. Although management was now involved very heavily, and study directors and others had accomplished the corrective actions outlined in the management plan, the question remained as to whether these improvements would be reflected in a later inspection. In September 1985 the Center was again inspected. Six studies were reviewed and only eight deviations noted. (See Table

TABLE 3
Deviations From Last Inspection (September 1985)

1. Test article-carrier mixtures were not analyzed for test article concentration in the mutagenicity studies.

2. Some data for analysis of test article-diet mixtures on Study #BRQ-173-T were not used and the documentation does not indicate the reason for this.

3. The humidity level in animal room #5430 fluctuates widely (i.e., 23%-75%) outside of the 40%-55% acceptable range specified in ARB SOP #15.

4. Proper functioning of the light timers in room 5430 is not monitored and documented for conformance to protocol specification.

5. Protocols or SOPs for Studies BFQ-141-T and BFQ-201-T do not state the acceptable ranges for the concentrations of test article dosing solutions.

6. Records are not maintained to document daily monitoring of the refrigerators and freezers in room 4458 used to store test articles, feed samples, and dosing solutions from Study BFQ-201-T.

7. The feed for Study BFQ-201-T was used prior to 8/14/85, the date analysis for interfering contaminants was performed.

8. The QAU did not inspect a critical phase (the preparation and administration of the test article (DON)) of Study BFQ-201-T on 7/25/85.

III.) While this is not perfection, compared to the 1980 experience it certainly represents a success story.

The prevailing attitude is that GLPs are an accepted fact, to the point that investigators treat some non-GLP studies as studies of the GLP type, developing SOPs and the information usually reserved for GLP studies. Additionally, one of the major benefits of our having undergone an extensive reorganization of our approach and follow-up regarding GLPs has been a fully functioning QAU. It required some time for investigators to view it as an ally rather than an adversary. Once that occurred, the willingness to accept QAU suggestions and critiques increased.

CONCLUSION

Thus it appears that we have settled into the practice of accepting and working harmoniously with the GLP regulations. Of course, there are occasions when management has to intercede to ensure that compliance is maintained. We believe that management must play a strong role in leading the organization into areas of major change, and that scientists will adapt when shown that such change is to their benefit in terms of improvement of the quality of scientific studies.

INDUSTRIAL MANAGEMENT VIEW OF QUALITY ASSURANCE FOR FOOD AND DRUG ADMINISTRATION REGULATED PRODUCTS

Richard L. Steelman
McNeil Pharmaceutical
Spring House, PA

ABSTRACT

This paper will deal first with general principles which govern the attitudes, degree of emphasis and commitment which management brings to quality assurance, then with specific examples of the need for an ongoing process to improve quality, and finally with some examples of the process for implementation and maintenance of improved quality.

The following factors critical to assurance of high quality products for FDA review and approval will be discussed in detail:

1. A process that defines the quality of every activity leading to a final product and involves all of management and the work force to make it happen.
2. Personnel with the proper training, experience and ethics.
3. An organizational structure which permits and forces information to flow in every direction.
4. A willingness to share the company strategy, plan, goals and responsibility with all employees.
5. A budget which is adjusted to an appropriate number of projects.
6. Controls—in the form of regulations, guidelines, ethics, government, activist groups.
7. A belief that industry and FDA have the same end goal—safe and efficacious products.

1. Address correspondence to: Richard L. Steelman, Ph.D., McNeil Pharmaceutical, Welsh and McKean Roads, Spring House, PA 19477-0776.

2. Key words: management, quality, toxicology.

3. Abbreviations: EIR, Establishment Inspection Report; FDA, Food and Drug Administration; GLP, Good Laboratory Practices; IND, Investigational New Drug; NDA, New Drug Application; SOP, Standard Operating Procedure.

INTRODUCTION

After an overview by Dr. Frank Press, you have listened to Dr. Gene McConnell's presentation describing what quality means to the National Toxicology Program. In a more specific vein, you have heard Dr. Sid Green present the background leading to the implementation of Good Laboratory Practice regulations within the Food and Drug Administration (FDA). My assignment is to move away from these broad topics to focus on perspectives of the management of industrial research on products for submission to the FDA.

In preparation for this task, I have tried to broaden my personal views by talking with other managers from the pharmaceutical industry. Before attempting to pass on to you this global view, I have to disclose some biases and teachings which are unique to my present employment at one of the Johnson and Johnson (J&J) family of companies, McNeil Pharmaceutical.

All of the J & J Companies are governed by a unified and critically important policy statement called "Our Credo." Since its origin the Credo has been a constant reminder of the five major responsibilities we all have as employers and corporate representatives. Most documents start with key ideas and the Credo is no exception. It begins, "We believe that our first responsibility is to the doctors, nurses, hospitals, mothers and all others who use our products. Our products must always be of the highest quality." The Credo goes on to describe our responsibility to those who work with us, our responsibility to our management, to the communities in which we live, and to our stockholders. But all of these responsibilities depend on our achieving products of the highest quality.

Some might think that the credo concept is merely motherhood and apple pie. The October 1985 issue of the AMA publication *Management Review* describes some informal research carried out by Johnson and Johnson in collaboration with The Business Roundtable's Task Force on Corporate Responsibility and with the Ethics Resource Center in Washington, DC. A list was compiled of those major corporations which had "a codified set of principles stating the philosophy that serving the public was central to their being" and for which there was "solid evidence that these ideas had been promulgated and practiced for at least a generation of their organizations." The performance of these companies over the last three decades was then examined.

The findings were impressive. On an average these companies had an annual compound growth rate in profits of 11 percent, which works out to a 23-fold increase in profits over 30 years. This is compared to only a 2.5-fold increase in GNP during the same period and only a 5.3-fold increase for all Fortune 500 companies. Thus a corporate policy of high ethics, emphasis on quality and social responsibility clearly produces a good return on investment.

The second teaching that I want to discuss is an often quoted statement made by General Robert Wood Johnson. When speaking about management he said, "Management is cause, all else is effect." Think about that for a minute—it sounds like an exaggeration at first. Management is cause, all else is effect. You cannot find an exception to this powerful statement. It does not say managers are more important persons than others, but it does say that management sets all things in motion and produces all effects, both good and bad.

My personal biases, born over 35 years in this industry, can be summarized by saying that product quality is *the* most important corporate concept and management sets good quality in motion. Remember that *you* are management, not just the next level above you.

AN INDUSTRY-WIDE PERSPECTIVE

Moving to an industry-wide perspective, what is necessary to achieve quality products for FDA review and subsequent marketing?

First, we need an agreement about what constitutes a quality product. Philip B. Crosby, one of the leaders of the quality revolution which is sweeping through modern business practice, says that "quality has much in common with sex. Everyone is for it. (Under certain circumstances, of course.) Everyone feels they understand it. (Even though they would not want to explain it.) Everyone thinks execution is only a matter of following natural inclinations ... and, of course, most people feel that all problems in these areas are caused by other people."

That humorous analogy does not help us much. Mr. Crosby teaches that quality is conformance to requirements. Requirements have to be set or negotiated for every activity involved in the research, development, manufacture, marketing and sales of the potential product. This process of setting requirements and conforming to them in the context of toxicology studies is well known in terms of animals, food and water. Subsequent papers in this symposium will be presented by leaders in these fields. But the process must be carried to every level of personnel and every activity, no matter how minor. The quality, yes even the believability of the results of an Ames *Salmonella typhimurium* test for mutagenicity, must be checked against the requirements for performance for each of the five commonly used strains of bacteria employed in the test.

Let's examine next the concept of quality vs. the Good Laboratory Practices (GLP) regulations. The GLP regulations foster the concept and implementation of quality but they do not begin to guarantee quality. They foster the concept because they speak to proper training and experience of personnel, adequate resources for the assigned work load and assignment of study director to be responsible for each study. The primary thrust of the regulations describe in great detail how every activity must be documented and retained in permanent files.

Cage cleaning is a good example. The Standard Operating Procedure (SOP) for washing dog cages may say that the water temperature must reach 180° F for four minutes in order to destroy bacteria on the cages. A temperature recorder records the line water temperature for the entire period that the cage washer is in operation. If this recording is signed, dated and retained, it meets the SOP requirement that the water temperature reached 180° F. It becomes satisfactory documentation for GLP purposes. But water coming out of that line is sprayed around inside the cage washer and may cool 20° before hitting the cage. At this lower temperature, it does not kill bacteria and the cage is unsuitable for service.

In order to do a quality job, a "turn pill" may need to be fastened to the cage itself to record the proper temperature for bacterial kill. The color change of this indicator pill now becomes the requirement for quality and the SOP must be rewritten to document this new event. So it is not enough to document, you must document the right thing.

Here is another example of how the GLPs fail to ensure quality. For many years industry and the FDA have conducted and reviewed LD_{50} tests in rodents. The GLP procedures helped us document the strain, age, weight of the animals used, the conditions of testing such as temperature, humidity, housing (single vs. group), dose, volume, vehicle, etc. Only recently have Zbinden and Fluri-Roversi (1981) challenged the test itself and shown that it was improper, imprecise and led to a wasteful use of animal resources in a way that also caused unnecessary pain to animals.

Since industry and FDA have accepted that for most situations a modified version of the LD_{50} test can produce satisfactory results using fewer animals and causing less pain, the classical LD_{50} test is used only infrequently for very special experiments in most laboratories. In this example, documentation of an existing test did not produce quality results. The purpose of the test had to be reexamined and new specifications written to achieve new goals.

I don't want to create the feeling that the GLP's were not needed, because they were. They remain a valuable tool in the drive toward error-free experiments and suitable data audits. The problem is that they require so many resources to implement and they have received so much management attention (the dreaded EIR and Form 483) that attention has been diverted from some other real quality problems.

Here are some examples of quality toxicology concerns. Are two-year rodent carcinogenicity tests useful or misleading? Is an 18 month dog chronic toxicity study more useful in predicting human toxicity than a 12 month test? Is behavioral teratology a useful addition to safety testing of drugs? These are million dollar questions that are not getting management attention and relate to the quality of the toxicologists' products: the investigators' brochure and the preclinical portions of the IND and the NDA. If we return to the definition of quality as conformance to specifications, then the message for toxicologists is clear. We have to include in the specifications not just how to do the test, but what the results mean. What is an acceptable result? Have the tests been adequately validated, do they really predict human toxicity, have we spent the effort and money on post-marketing followup or epidemiology studies necessary to ensure good predictability? When was the last time you talked to the phase I and phase II clinicians on a project to find out how useful the animal data were to them and how they could be improved in the future?

As I talked with my colleagues from other companies, they frequently mentioned organization structure and proper budgeting processes as key determinants of quality. Since most research and development areas include a team approach to project development, the organizational structure must permit information to flow up, down and sideways equally well. In order for specifications to be negotiated between two or more parties, a clear set of specifications is necessary. This is just as important for the preparation of a vehicle by pharmaceutical development for use by the chronic toxicity group as it is for the final licensing agreement between two companies to co-develop a product. If the line operation does not permit easy flow of communications, then working groups, teams, or committees may facilitate the flow.

Budgeting is an important determinant of quality. There is never enough money to buy capital equipment and to staff at the desired levels for all of the opportunities available. It becomes imperative to match the dollars to the projects in a realistic manner. This is a tightrope walking exercise with too much money spent or not enough money spent knocking the walker off the rope into the abyss below. Managers at all levels have to be sensitive to morale, overtime levels and signs of fatigue such as illness, absence or increased turnover. Short periods of overload can be helped by temporary personnel, summer students, and overtime, but remember, these all carry both positive and negative implications to GLP compliance, accident rate and quality.

One of the important features of the GLP regulations is the insistence on a master schedule which shows all of the ongoing projects and the study directors assigned to each. This master schedule permits the local inspector or home office reviewer to estimate the adequacy of the study director staff for the volume of work to be controlled or directed at any given time period. This is, of course, only a rough indicator since the experience, training, maturity and energy of a study director all affect how many studies he or she can effectively manage.

I have been talking about factors critical to assurance of high quality products for FDA review and hopefully, approval. There are only three critical factors left:

1. A willingness to share the company strategy, plans, goals, and responsibility with all employees.
2. Controls, in the form of regulations, inspections, government, ethics and activist groups.
3. A belief that industry and FDA have the same end goal—safe and efficacious products.

The topic of sharing company plans, goals and responsibility with all employees came up recently in a conversation with a manager from a consumer products pharmaceutical company. He was describing a situation in which a project milestone had been missed. The project was the marketing of a sustained release dosage form of an existing tablet product. In tracking the cause of the delay it was determined that the analytical group, the pharmaceutical development group and the toxicology group were all working with slightly different formulations of the final product. These subtle changes, believed to be improvements by each group, had not been communicated at any forum where all three groups were represented. The concept of sharing plans had been violated. Every entry level management course teaches the importance of communicating the plan and getting the workers to buy into the plan. Why don't experienced managers always do this? There are many reasons or excuses. The most frequent and sometimes even valid reason is lack of time. "I meant to pass that on but a crisis came up," or "I had to go to another meeting." If you or your staff are using or hearing that type of excuse often instead of rarely, then some time needs to be spent on communications and sharing of responsibility.

Controls form a fundamental factor in a quality product. Toxicologists are among the most inspected people in the world. Specifications are set on the animals you use, their food, water, bedding, air, cage room, facility and so on. We have FDA, EPA, HPB, BGA, AAALAC, USDA, OSHA and the rest of the alphabet looking at our background, training, experience, facility and finally our product—the research report. In addition to institutional and governmental regulations and guidelines, we have controls in the form of codes of ethics and pressures from activist groups. And if you don't think activist groups exert control pressure, talk to toxicologists from the cosmetic industry!

The last critical factor for quality that I want to emphasize is the belief that industry and the FDA have the same end goal—safe and efficacious products. In a talk at the 1985 Project Management Institute annual meeting, Dr. Arthur Hull Hayes, former commissioner of the FDA, said that he believed that there was no difference in the characteristics of the FDA staff and the industry staff in the areas of integrity, ethics, objectives and goals.

Both groups want safe and efficacious products on the market in a time frame that permits proper evaluation. The FDA does not want to approve an unsafe product and the industry does not want to have to recall an unsafe product. Regarding quality there is a key difference between management willingness to take prudent business risks and willingness to take safety or medical risks. There are no prudent medical risks.

CONCLUSION

What I have said to this point can be summaried very easily:

>   Management is cause, all else is effect.
>   Quality is the most important corporate concept.
>   Management sets quality in motion.

As you listen and participate in the specific topics remaining in this symposium, I want you to think how management would react or influence the outcome of each topic—and then remember your leadership role, for you are management.

REFERENCE

ZBEINDEN, G. and FLURI-ROVERSI, M. (1981). Significance of the LD_{50} test for the toxicological evaluation of chemical substances. Arch. Toxicol. **47**:77–99.

INDUSTRIAL MANAGEMENT VIEW OF QUALITY ASSURANCE FOR ENVIRONMENTAL PROTECTION AGENCY REGULATED PRODUCTS

Robert A. Scala
Research and Environmental Health Division
Exxon Corporation
East Millstone, New Jersey

ABSTRACT

Quality assurance in toxicological studies is an important management function for both industry and EPA. For the most part, quality means "doing it right the first time." Management has many incentives for that to happen. Using an analogy with safety, the importance of quality, the responsibility for quality and the consequences of poor quality are outlined. Scientist-scientist interactions with EPA are also discussed in terms of their impact on quality. The role of industry and EPA management in setting goals and insisting on adherence to them is viewed as a way of minimizing adversarial relations between scientists and quality assurance staff.

A FABLE

Once you have sat through presentations from NTP, FDA and the pharmaceutical industry on quality assurance in toxicology, there really isn't much more you want to hear, even if the topic is defined in terms of EPA's needs and regulations. For novelty's sake, I thought of reciting aloud the full set of EPA quality assurance regulations. (Our QA Manager expects us all to have them memorized anyhow.) The result of that would probably be lunch at 11:10, not 12 noon as scheduled.

Instead, I decided I would tell a fable. From that story I will attempt to extract the role of management in the quality process and close with an analogy that, in our organization, we feel well describes the purpose and status of quality assurance.

"In an earlier, more peaceful time, the *animals* carried out the toxicity studies on new pesticides or industrial chemicals in an informal yet somehow orderly

1. Address correspondence to: Robert A. Scala, Ph.D., Research and Environmental Health Division, Exxon Corporation, P.O. Box 235, East Millstone, NJ 08873.
2. Key words: goal adherence, industrial management, quality assurance, toxicological studies.

27

fashion. Many studies were conducted in the same rather large house, often with more than one species present. The animals assigned themselves to their cages as they wished. They also assigned someone to snap the lights off each day for activity time and on again later for rest time. The *humans* were permitted to leave their offices each day and were trained to feed and care for the animals. Because humans were slow learners, many times the animals failed to receive the proper dose of agent, or failed to be provided with adequate feed and water or failed to have their quarters cleaned.

The leaders of the animals concluded that this way of doing the studies was wasteful, inefficient and could even produce misleading results. They were especially concerned at the number of humans who could not do simple mathematical computations correctly, operate simple weighing devices or even record numbers accurately. These leaders of the animals sought to bring order to the conduct of the studies by the humans, and they did so in the following way. Reasoning that it was their lives that were at risk in these experiments and yet these studies were needed for new products, the leaders reviewed the work of the humans; assessed the needs and shortcomings; put in place the necessary facilities, training, procedures and controls; appointed several of their number to oversee the humans and found in a short time that there was a vast improvement in the overall operation.

This project became known as 'Doing it right the first time.' Alas, however, not all animals in the house seemed to be interested in it. They found many excuses for not participating—'things were all right as they were,' 'who cared if there were occasional errors,' 'it's too expensive.' The humans, of course, knew nothing of this. They merely went about their daily tasks of feeding the animals, caring for the quarters, etc. Some were involved in the new project; the others associated with the nonparticipants, totally unaware of 'Doing it right the first time.' So with time there came to be two classes of animals in the house. Most were active participants in the project; a few weren't.

The difficulty came in the utilization of the data from these studies. In the earlier times, the principal users were other animals in gray houses in a humid city by a river. They knew, because they themselves had done such studies, who was committed to 'Doing it right the first time' and who wasn't. But with the passage of time and changes in circumstances, the animals in the gray houses changed and these, along with other animals, were not so likely to believe the humans had really learned. They began to talk about certain animals looking in on the humans to assure that they did their work properly. In time these 'checking animals' wrote guidelines and procedures and ultimately convinced their fellows in the gray houses in the city by the river that only 'checked' studies were acceptable. The rest is history. Today the animals are of three kinds. The first are those who were always 'Doing it right the first time.' These are somewhat unfriendly to the 'checking animals,' finding their role superfluous. The second group of animals became convinced of the value of 'Doing it right the first time' and saw the 'checking animals' as a way to help them achieve that goal. The third group is fortunately a diminishing type. They never did comprehend that there is no market for their studies, and are slowly disappearing from the house. The animals in the gray houses in the city by the river take full credit for this improvement in quality." But then, this is only a fable.

MANAGEMENT AND QUALITY

Classical textbooks on management (meaning those written in an age of alliteration and before our heightened awareness of sexist language) describe the role of managers in terms of men, money and machines. Management employs these resources in the most effective fashion to provide a needed product or service. Where does quality fit in? A shoddy product or service certainly stimulates no repeat business. The marketplace is a fine discriminator of quality. In the fable, the value of "Doing it right the first time" was evidence to the "doers," and there was in place the best of all quality systems. That consisted of a conviction from the bottom up and from the top down of the value and importance of quality.

In the ideal case, the concept of quality permeates an operation. Workers strive for it, management encourages and recognizes it, and the marketplace selects on that basis. Management needs no lectures on the value of "Doing it right the first time." Waste, loss, inefficiency, downtime, rejection, user dissatisfaction, worker disaffection, loss of customer loyalty, the contagious nature of sloppy practices in any endeavor, all flow from lack of quality. Management is aware of all this. The cutting edge of the issue for managment is in the verification of quality, especially by third parties. Who will define quality? How is it recognized? At what point have things progressed beyond "Doing it right the first time" and into the realm of inappropriate expectations? In the fable, the "checking animals" were valuable in seeing that the studies went along properly. If the "checking animals" lose sight of their support role and wish their function to be the final product, then the animals may no longer have a quality problem, but they will have substituted a problem of scientific credibility and research purpose.

Most managements view their responsibilities in the sense of team function, with leadership. Visualize a symphony orchestra. Each instrument makes its own contribution. The quality of the product is a function both of the quality of each performer and the ability of the conductor to blend and integrate so that the whole is harmonious.

So as not to do violence to the published program, I would like to make some specific observations about the interaction of industry scientists with their counterparts in EPA. This is a quality assurance item on the broadest scale and one in which management has a strong interest. At the outset, this interaction has a potential for conflict, but not of the sort which you would expect. We are long past the image of government scientists clanking about Washington in white armor defending a hapless public from sinister, fire-breathing industrial dragons. Today, in my view, our conflicts are largely those of thoughtful scientists seeing the same data with different eyes. Conflict resolution, on the part of management in industry and the EPA, consists in large part of establishing open lines of communication, insisting on documentation and/or verification of scientific positions, making possible the use of referees or other third-party participation, insisting that good science makes for sound regulation and realizing that bad science, especially bad toxicology, will haunt you for years. One of the best guarantees we have that EPA management will hold that position is the presence of Dr. John Moore as Assistant Administrator for Pesticides and Toxic Substances. He has consistently shown himself to be open to ideas, suggestions, new approaches, different interpretations, etc. *if you have the documentation.* Are we that open?

CONCLUSION

I'd like to close with a final analogy that is full of meaning for the petroleum and chemical industries. Management views quality in the conduct of toxicology studies the same way it views safety in the laboratory. (See Figure 1.)

It doesn't take much imagination to substitute the word *quality* for *safety* in Figure 1 to have an unmistakable profile of quality studies in toxicology. (See Figure 2.) Most of us believe this to our very core and have tried throughout our

---

FIGURE 1. Management's View of Safety.

1. Safety is the responsibility of each individual in the laboratory.

2. An unsafe act can not only hurt you but your fellow worker as well, so everyone must take precautions.

3. Unsafe behavior can result in loss of life, limb and jobs.

4. Safety is a state of mind, an attitude, a constant presence influencing each person's behavior.

5. Safety is not inherent but must be learned by repeated training and reinforcement.

6. There is no excuse or justification for doing a job in an unsafe fashion.

7. The evaluation of a manager's performance should include safety as one of the job elements.

FIGURE 2. Management's View of Quality.

1. Quality is the responsibility of each individual in the laboratory.

2. Poor quality can not only affect you but your fellow worker as well, so everyone must be involved.

3. Poor quality can result in loss of jobs.

4. Quality is a state of mind, an attitude, a constant presence influencing each person's behavior.

5. Quality is not inherent but must be learned by repeated training and reinforcement.

6. There is no excuse or justification for doing a job in a sloppy fashion.

7. The evaluation of a manager's performance should include quality as one of the job elements.

careers to put these attitudes and behaviors in place among our people. We were doing it not only before there were EPA QA guidelines but, for many people here in this room, before there was an EPA! For the most part, literal compliance with the guidelines is easy once the mind set is created in the individual. If we let the activity become adversarial or, even worse, if it becomes a contest between industry and EPA ("you'll never find out what we're doing," or "I'll find something if I dig hard enough"), that's the time when management on both sides must exercise another of its functions—discipline—and be sure that the goals and priorities of the workers are consistent with the goals and priorities of the organization. The kind of behavior just illustrated is not on the priority list of either industry or EPA.

PANEL-AUDIENCE DIALOGUE
QUALITY MANAGEMENT
PERSPECTIVES

Chairperson:
Robert A. Scala
Research and Environmental Health Division
Exxon Corporation
East Millstone, New Jersey

Panel:
Ernest E. McConnell, Richard J. Ronk, Richard L. Steelman

Bill King (Procter & Gamble): Dr. McConnell, you mention that there are five steps in assuring the quality of a study from beginning to end. The last of those steps was what you called a "global audit." I presume this is by the quality assurance organization, but my question is, what role do you see quality assurance playing in the other steps, or even in all five steps?

Ernest McConnell (NTP): I think that, obviously, quality assurance is concerned in every step along the way. In the National Toxicology Program, we have a great deal of effort that goes into making sure that the laboratories are well qualified to do our studies before we even put a study in there. So we start at that point by making sure that the physical nature of the laboratory is able to do the job and that the various discipline leaders in that contract laboratory are qualified. Then we have a peer review process which we use in the design of the study before it even goes into the laboratory.

Once the laboratory has been selected and the study is about to go in there, we have a team that goes to that laboratory to make sure that everyone in the lab, particularly the principal investigator, knows what we're after. In other words, we go through the protocol step-by-step; then, periodically during the study, we visit that laboratory and do a kind of audit, you might say, of the study in progress. In other words, we physically go into those animal rooms, see where the animals are, look at any early deaths that might have occurred, look at the weight gain, the feed consumption, etc. Then, when the study is completed, we have several steps that we go through in evaluating the data; and, then, finally this global audit, as I called it, is where we try to put the study back together to

33

see if you or anyone else would agree that we did a competent job in carrying out that particular study.

Kimberly Perry (Monsanto): I have a general question for any of the panelists. Two of you have made comments about including in the performance objectives for study directors, their adherence to QA procedures. I think this is important, but how can management ensure that study directors will not try to hide their mistakes, that they will openly talk about the problems with studies they have?

Sidney Green (FDA): The way it's handled within the center is that the quality assurance unit is responsible for inspecting all of the studies under Good Laboratory Practices and, once a study is inspected, let's say, a critical phase of the study, and there has been an observation, a deviation, that deviation is recorded, and the study director, his supervisor and the division director are made aware of that deviation. That's about as far as it goes if the deviation is corrected within five to ten days and, in most instances, they are very minor and can be corrected during this time period.

Now, if that deviation is not corrected within five to ten days, then it's bounced up to a higher level, and other individuals get involved. Obviously what occurs at the rating period is an evaluation of the study director and the other persons who have not followed through to take care of that deviation.

Robert Scala (Exxon): Let me add to that. What you're really talking about in my mind is "concealment," and any system of performance evaluation, in fact, any system of proper management, has to have checks and balances to assure that concealment doesn't occur. If you'll just look at the kind of audit trail that's followed for financial documents, you'll know that we have to be susceptible in our work to the same form of audit, which means multiple parties are involved, certain levels of authority are designated for certain types of things. Also, as a statement of policy and practice, openness demanded between the various levels of organization with a clear understanding that fair dealing is the only accepted way of business. Any organization that pays off on other than that is inviting a problem. It happens. We all know that, but I think it becomes part of the organizational culture. It starts the day the person joins the organization in whatever position, this idea of open and complete reporting—open and complete documentation of what you do—which documentation, then, is subject to review by others.

Richard Steelman (McNeil): I'd like to comment further that in a relatively small organization, when you evaluate study directors, you're really not looking at them any differently than evaluating any of the other scientific staff because the study director's job description is an integral part of the basic job description. So, we don't have any particular look at how a person performs his study director function versus his overall toxicology functions. We just look at the entire spectrum of their activities.

Bill Hollis (National Agricultural Chemicals Association): Sid Green, the importance of academic research, peer reviewed and published in reviewed journals, has an impact on the decision making process; and yet, we find that those institutions do not have, in any way, the level of quality assurance and GLP systems that I think the government has now instituted. You've had your very vivid experiences, and we ours. Is it possible that we might include in this triumvarate, this third leg, to the research community of the academic institutions to encourage them, now, to begin to think of establishing or accommodating, with the assistance of government and their own peers, a quality assurance program as well as observing some GLPs in their studies?

Green: To the extent academic institutions are involved in the types of studies that are conducted by toxicological laboratories, be they government or industry, than they ought to be aware of the fact that we certainly need to make sure that the data can be assured, obviously, to the extent possible. If they do not have a fully functioning quality assurance staff or a quality assurance unit which can conduct internal inspections, then it certainly behooves them to try and establish some internal means of auditing and assuring their data. I would think that the government would not mind assisting. Again, I would have to say, to the extent it could, whatever that means, in trying to bring that about. We are quite willing to share information, to share experiences, if it means that in the end we are all getting good quality toxicologic data.

Carl Schultz (Cosar Inc.): A comment on the earlier question that was asked regarding the study director. I think the key role of the study director is the implementation of the GLPs. One of the problems I have observed commonly in industry, government or academia, is that job description or the responsibility definition of the study director is unclear. Most of the time, study directors are defined as toxicologists or biologists. Their primary role is coordination of the study management. The role for coordination is often not understood and not taken as seriously as the person takes the toxicology end. That's the area I'd like to see if we can have a little more discussion on the specific responsibility that are SOPs for the study directors. Are they implemented?

Steelman: That's a critical question. It's one that we have debated a number of times and, as a result of those debates, have held meetings and gone back and changed the SOP for what we're requiring or how we're describing a study director. It generally does revolve around the question of not how you perform your function within the department, but how you perform it in the other areas where you're exerting this coordinating role that you described. How do you ensure that the pharmaceutical development section or department or division does all of the things that they are supposed to do? How do you ensure that your obligation to carefully archive all the material at the end of the study is fulfilled? That's the area where study directors have the most difficult problems. I don't know that we've reached an answer, but we've tried, basically, to hone the definitions of what we do mean when we say, "coordinate." We've described in detail that this doesn't mean that they are the principal responsible for that, but it means that they should contact the principal person responsible for that activity and ensure that it's been done to the satisfaction of that directly responsible person or the person responsible at the lowest level of responsibility, if you will.

McConnell: In our experience, we found that in those areas where we've had problems in specific studies, quite often, you could track it from the study director on down. There's absolutely no doubt about it. That person who's the study director exudes whatever it is that he or she exudes and that is reflected the whole way down. If the study director is a little on the sloppy side, and it's been my experience that, not all the staff, but that those who are so inclined, will also mimic that. But if the person is fastidious, is sharp, is on top of that study, then the people down the line also realize that that person is concerned and will try a little bit harder.

We've had studies where we've had some problems in which a study director did not know what room the animals were in when we confronted the person. When you find that kind of situation, you can be pretty sure that your study is going to have some problems.

Green: I think that was a problem early on in the FDA, but it actually was corrected, I think, just by constant emphasizing to study directors what their actual roles and responsibilities were. This was done by top management on down; so now, study directors are well aware of what their responsibilities are, and of course, if they are not aware when they are conducting a study, they are made aware at the rating time, the performance evaluation.

Andrew Tegeris (Tegeris Labs): It is really rather sad that there are no official courses, accredited courses, that would present QA personnel the opportunity to learn how to conduct QA studies. I don't know how you'd go about this. I have to think about who to assign to this very significant aspect of our work. We think that, perhaps people who have had study coordinator or principal investigator experience would be good candidates for this. I often thought that perhaps accountants would be good QA personnel. The point I'm coming to is this: The one official government program does exist.

EPA does have programs and courses which are repetitive, which are excellent, where they teach their personnel how to do QA audits. I asked some of my friends at the EPA whether I could send a candidate we had to take this course, and the answer was, "No, I could not." I think that this is something that should be addressed.

Green: I share your concern about training individuals who are conducting good laboratory practices studies. I probably would have answered in a similar fashion if you had posed that question to me—that, no, the training course conducted by the center does not allow for individuals from industry or outside the center or government to attend.

Dexter Goldman (EPA): If the question had been asked very recently, I was undoubtedly the person who said "No," because of simply a conflict in the amount of time and space we have and who is going to be paying for what. I think there are courses—I don't know what their quality is—in some places, such as New Jersey. As to whether you're going to learn anything or not, I don't know. I believe that there is, at one institution in the Washington area, a graduate level course within the medical facility that deals with how to be a study director and how to approach quality assurance, but there is no other organized thing that I know of.

Scala: It has been mentioned that perhaps accountants might be ideal for this role, but I think other than the fact that accountants bring a mentality of careful approach and very good accounting techniques to a problem, I'm not sure that they are ideally suited for this role.

McConnell: I question whether most universities would be able to pull this off because most of the people in the university, the toxicologists and so forth, they do not have the background that would be the type where you could understand what's required of government agencies, and so forth, regarding good data, or trackable data, if you will. So, I would say that if a course were to be put together, it would almost have to arise out of government. I'm not saying I know how to get that done, but I think you brought up a good issue, and something that we, individually or corporately, ought to think about.

Nona Karten (Microbiological Associates): The Society of Quality Assurance has just established an education committee of which I am a member. We will be designing some programs to meet the needs of professionals, and we hope, next year at the Society of Quality Assurance meeting, to have at least one day set aside for training sessions. If anyone has any ideas and recommendations on the subject, we would like to hear from you. Dr. Carrie Whitmire and Bob Cypher of Hazleton Bionetics, Alice Malloy of F.M.C. and I comprise the committee, and we would appreciate hearing from any of you.

Tully Speaker (Temple University): There is a need for a course. Like most universities, we simply cannot, on an economic basis, ordinarily think in terms of complying with GLPs in the punctilio of detail that is required. But because there is a need for a course, I will offer the facilities of Temple to serve as coordination center; if we can enlist government cooperation, certainly we can enlist industrial cooperation. I'd be happy to put together such a course and offer it in general.

Tegeris: It's a basic principle of marketing that you should give the market what the market wants. I think there is a definite need for establishing QA programs throughout the country. I think the proposition of having a society offer courses once a year is what is needed. First of all, not everybody in the country can participate in these. To expect the government to do this, even though I think and I agree it is really the government's responsibility to institute a program like this, I just don't think it's going to be done; at least, it's not going to be done in due time. I do think that officials in government could very easily notify universities around the country that, indeed, there is such a need, and then let them pick it up. That way official programs, well-developed programs, will be available throughout the country for everybody.

Laila Moustafa (World Health Organization): I'm very glad to see that this question was raised, but it is not only within this country that there is a need; it is an international issue, and I know this is not going to be the immediate remedy for the problem, but it is an avenue for information exchange and training programs by utilizing the World Health Organization, International Program for Chemical Safety, where we do have what we call manpower training courses offered in the different regions of the World Health Organization. These courses are usually organized by the region, and headquarters eventually help in developing these programs to meet the immediate need of that region. So, in the Mediterranian countries, the need would be different than, for example, in the American continent and the Asiatic continent. I would encourage you very much to make that contact.

Carrie Whitmire (NTP): In the course of getting our laboratories into GLP compliance and into a quality assurance mode, there was a great deal of training that had to take place. We offer this to any of our laboratories that come on to our Master Agreement. We have also taken this into consideration when we had contracts at universities. There are at least four universities which I have personally visited and helped them in setting up a quality assurance program.

Goldman: In the days I was with NTP, I got beaten enough times to ask two very simple questions at a laboratory because there are two undefinable management personnel—one is quality assurance and the other is the safety officer. The question that we always asked was, "Why was this person selected for that function?" You got some interesting answers. I would like to ask a question of Dr. Steelman and Dr. Scala, and that is, you have an in-house procedure for communication on quality control. I would like to ask, if you contract out or subcontract out any of your operations, how do you assure yourself that your in-house standards are met by your subcontractors?

Scala: I think the answer to that is that we don't have 100 percent assurance that we will have the same kind of control and understanding of the quality assurance process when we contract out. We do contract out, I would say, depending on the year, 5 to 10 percent of our work. That's done for various reasons. Sometimes it's done to enable us to have the contact with the outside world that we don't get when we do everything inside; other times it's done because we lack expertise in a specific type of experiment. But, whenever we contract out, whether it be in this country or abroad, we site visit not just with the study toxicology and internal study director staff, but with the quality assurance staff as well. We interview members of the quality assurance staff of the company that's going to do the work, and we talk to them about procedures, prior inspections that they have had, the results of those inspections, and their communication process—how they communicate with their management. So, in summary, we attempt to get as much of the same kind of information as we believe we have in-house about those facilities where we contract the work. I have to admit that it's not 100 percent.

Steelman: We, too, do very little outside contracting, and we also have a pretty good handle on the outside contractor's QA system. A long time ago we became convinced of the value of the unannounced visit. We had gone through the usual professional courtesies in years past, and then we realized that this gave people a chance to tidy things up. One learns a considerable amount on an unannounced visit. You don't have to parachute in at midnight, but just show up on a Tuesday morning at 9:00 when they didn't know you were coming. You'll learn a lot.

Rob Dewoskin (Research Triangle Institute): I'd like to ask the flipside of the question about education. Dr. Steelman mentioned that you can have conformance with the GLPs but not necessarily have a guarantee of quality. His quality means conformance with specifications, fitness for use, satisfaction of the consumers' need and so forth. These criteria, that may or may not parallel the GLPs, are very important in evaluating the quality of the study. How is it that quality assurance unit people become informed of these criteria, which, as I say, may or may not parallel the GLPs?

Steelman: I'm glad you asked that question. A Philadelphia politician told me that that actually means, "I wish you had died in your sleep last night." It's actually a dodge that's used to delay while you try to think up an answer. Even with that dodge, I can't think up the answer. Can anybody help me?

Dewoskin: May I suggest an answer? There's a lot of controversy as to the level of education the quality assurance unit people should have. It originally started with people who had no science training who were simply around and were, literally, accountants with check lists. Current views are that they should have scientific training. I think a good start would be as part of the study director's responsibilities, to have the study director write down the list of criteria, the things they feel are important, to go along with the other kinds of criteria and aspects of the study that come from the GLPs. The quality assurance people, are very well informed, already, but in determining what is critical to look at, it would be more useful if study directors could have that written down rather than having quality assurance people trying to guess what's important and what isn't; or inspectors, I might add.

Scala: I think the point you made about having at least some people in your quality assurance unit trained in the scientific discipline is a good one, although we have arguments from time-to-time that our particular people may be over-trained in those areas. That gets into the issue of the quality assurance people interpreting the science rather than the quality aspects.

McConnell: I think, also, that the issue is one which is almost institution-specific. If you examine the mix of studies done in any particular laboratory, the kind of business that the institution is in, I can think of two or three other possible criteria which would say that the kind of training you'd want for your QA person is, maybe, different. The kind of relationship you want between the QA group and the study director can also be different. So I would say it's hard to lay down a hard and fast rule, but would support your idea that there should be some kind of understanding within the organization as to what each party's role is. I think that's just common sense.

Jeb McCandless (Atlantic Richfield): I would be more interested in having a list made out as to what the study director does not want QA to look at. I think the audit would be much more interesting.

Robert Kapp (Exxon): I think we all concur that QA is an integral part of our business here. From a management perspective, I'm the ever-vigilant manager, and I wanted to ask a few questions. Is there some way that each of you could quantify the QA effort for us? For instance, how many QA staffers per study load? How many audits per study? What types of audits? These sorts of things. How much is enough? I guess what I'm looking for is, is there some kind of barometer of adequacy that you might be able to quantify for this group with respect to each of your shops? Is that a fair question, or an unfair question?

McConnell: We've done some sort of analysis. It's always hard to tie these kinds of numbers up very tightly. But originally, when GLPs become part of our studies, we were interested in what would this cost or what does this cost, at the time because we were already, we felt, pretty close to it. Then, we've added to that, as I said, our pathology reviews and our corporate-type audits, and we figure, including government personnel costs—these site visits and so forth, I've told you about—plus the cost that's sort of buried in one of these studies that the contractor charges us, between 15 and 25 percent of the cost of the study is in the quality assurance of that study, or is for the quality assurance.

Green: Someone indicated that he'd be more interested in what the study director would say that he does not want the QA to look at—that's quite a different approach from, I think, the way we usually look at quality assurance. The QAU, once it begins inspecting a study, is able to inspect any facet of that particular study regardless of whether the study director feels that they should or should not do so. Now, if there is a deviation and if the management in the center—branch chief, division director or what have you—feels that the deviation is not one that should be in the quality assurance area, but rather the scientific concern, then there's a discussion that is held. Of course, that's sort of ad hoc, and there's really no clear rule as to who wins or who loses there. It simply depends upon the issue, and how it is decided, but study directors really have no recourse. I think I'm correct again, in saying within the center, to whether they can or cannot allow the quality assurance unit to inspect any and all aspects of a study conducted in the center.

In regard to quantitating quality assurance activities, that's really not been done, at least within our organization as of now, and it may be due to the fact that we have inadequate staff, and they've not been impacted to the extent that they would indicate that, "Well, look, we're overburdened now; we can't do a good job, so you guys are going to have to provide additional folks for us to get the job done." But I certainly can see that happening in the future, particularly when we move to Beltsville and expand our operations. But here again, I really can't say anything with respect to quantitativeness. We'll just have to see how it goes, and depending upon where it goes, add individuals to the staff.

Steelman: Regarding those questions that the study director might not want asked, I agree with Sid Green. We don't have any areas where we don't want them to ask questions; we don't have any areas where we don't want them to inspect, even though that sometimes ties us up for a lot of hours. What we do have is areas where we don't want to see their comments on the QA report in the same context that we're getting their GLP comments. That's a little fuzzy; what I really mean is that we want to have them separate their comments about things like safety, about things like the science that's involved, about things that we don't believe are integral parts of the GLP process. We want those comments, but we want them separated in the report. They've been kind enough to do that for us after a few years of back and forth negotiations.

Regarding the quantification, again, very much the same answer. We have attempted to quantitate how many studies a study director can handle for the very same reasons. Each study director brings a different degree of experience and training and, particularly, energy to the job. I can recall one study director we had who had a very large number of studies. When the FDA inspector came in, he said, "I don't believe that any one person can manage properly and be study director of all these studies." And we said, "Well, let's let you meet her." He did, and he became convinced in a very short period of time that this person had the necessary background, training and energy to handle all of those studies, and she did that by answering every question he asked without reference to anyone else or any pieces of paper. So, I think it depends largely on the individuals in terms of how many data points they audit, how much of the data is enough—and that's a matter of experience—and the bottom line there is, how well have your inspections gone; what kinds of problems have been turned up by your audits; are they trivial or are they major, broad problems? I don't think that you can get a list from each firm as to how much is enough.

McCandless: My point was that I don't think it would be advantageous to have a study director make up a list of things to look at any more than it would be appropriate for them to make up a list of things not to look at.

Luke Brennecke (Pathology Associates, Inc.): Having done a large number of retrospective audits, I have seen what you can find, and what you can't find by looking at a study at the very end. Oftentimes, you wind up seeing those faults that were revealed throughout the study, but it's already too late to do anything about. So, the people on both sides are dissatisfied—those at the laboratory for having had their hands slapped, and those at the regulatory agency for seeing that a study was done incorrectly from the start. Based on that, at the risk of having a lot of contract laboratories groan, I think it's important to emphasize that studies, regulatory visits and audits should be done early and often during the course of a study. When you get to the end of a study many things that have been done wrong can no longer be remedied. If you get the planning done correctly from the beginning and check up on that during the course of the study, many of the problems can be alleviated.

Tegeris: Addressing the matter of the cost of doing studies, I am sure that our sponsors, both in the pharmaceutical and chemical industries, do spend somewhere between 15 and 25 percent of the cost of the study to audit it. Considering the fact that the costs for performing the studies, particularly the long-term studies, are getting to be rather prohibitively expensive, there is quite a bit of duplication in this effort. The sponsor spends a lot of in-house money to QA the studies, and then pays the contract laboratory a certain amount of money to QA studies. I would propose that if the contractor were to make their QA files open to the sponsor, if a joint approach were to be followed here, whereby the contract laboratory basically does the type of QA that the sponsor and/or the government wants, I think this would be a worthwhile effort, and this would certainly cut down on the cost of the studies.

J. C. Bhandari (Dynamac and NTP): I'd like to comment on the question regarding the quantification of the QAU responsibilities. I'm talking from experience on the industry side and now, providing the quality assurance support for NTP, and I believe the NTP does have a lot of good information, particularly a guideline SOP that defines what and how much, in a very systematic way, should be looked at and should be done. I'm thinking about some of the information with the industry, in general, or having some sort of a forum where that can be shared. I'm not suggesting that the NTP has the most ideal answer, but based on my experience, it is much more systematic, and it does make a lot more sense, and I do know that in the industry it is not as comprehensive as that.

McConnell: The only thing that I can say is that anything we have is subject to freedom of information and requests and anything else. We'll provide anyone with anything they request as long as we have the wherewithal to get it done. Basically, whatever we have is yours, you've paid for it.

Dan Todd (CDC): Having watched the medical missionaries in epidemiology evolve into an agency, which has as one of its centers professional development and training, I think what we're seeing here is, in its early infancy, the need, and hopefully, all of our support, with the government's support, to help NTP become that kind of a program where they can offer the kinds of assistance that we have requested in terms of oversight and quality assurance. I don't know that Dr. McConnell would regale that idea, but I think, based upon the work they have done, that the proficiency, the efficiency and the expertise that this kind of charge needs must be made and needs to be accepted. In its infancy, of course, it will take awhile.

Scala: Let me second what you've said. We've sensed it in our own organization over time, as we started with a very informal type QA activity, in fact, in anticipation of the government's position on this. Then, we watched it evolve into a formal activity working with outsiders and with our own staff, trying to learn how to audit. I think what you say is absolutely right—we're in a maturing area., and I think these kinds of exchanges, meetings such as this, the formation of a professional society, are all marks along the track of maturation, and I think we can all learn very much from each other here.

Chapter II
MANAGEMENT OF QUALITY

MANAGEMENT OF QUALITY

Donald H. Hughes
Ivorydale Technical Center
Procter and Gamble Company
Cincinnati, Ohio

CHAIRPERSON'S REMARKS

This session covers the management of quality. The objective is to present and discuss quality assurance programs that are used both by industry and government by examples and appropriate comparisons. What we are after is to not only see where we have been but also to find out what Good Laboratory Practices are and then go beyond that in the future to where we need to go and how we plan to get there. How do we assure ourselves that we have a good quality study? How do you know when the study is good? What type of informtion needs to be available to determine that a study is adequate for decision making? That really is the bottom line. Decision making has to rely on solid data. The information given to the manager who is making the decisions is absolutely vital for an appropriate, correct decision.

AN INDUSTRIAL APPROACH TO QUALITY TOXICOLOGY STUDIES

Jerry M. Smith
Rohm and Haas Co.
Philadelphia, Pennsylvania

ABSTRACT

Industry must not only sponsor and conduct toxicology studies of the highest quality, it must also sponsor and conduct full, complete toxicological evaluation programs of the highest quality. Because of the large investments required, both in resources and time, quality must be built into each step of a program. This requires a complete integration of toxicology efforts with those of non-toxicology research, manufacturing, marketing, sales and regulatory agencies. Without complete integration, a valid, high quality toxicology study may be conducted, but be inappropriate for evaluating and assessing the hazard or risk that may be associated with the uses of a chemical, product or process.

Overall quality begins with a highly qualified toxicologist (toxicology program director) who has responsibility for obtaining from appropriate sources information on use or proposed use, potential exposure and known toxicological properties of the material and structurally related materials. With these data the toxicologist develops a toxicology program. Following the development of a program, the toxicology program director, working with specific study directors, experts and statisticians, designs specific protocols. Following the design of specific protocols, the quality assurance unit reviews the protocols, verifies the qualifications of scientists, technicians, the laboratory conducting the studies and procedures to be followed.

During the course of the study, the quality assurance unit, the toxicology program director and appropriate experts monitor critical stages of critical studies. Upon completion of a study, the study director, with appropriate assistance from experts, reviews the data and prepares a draft report with appropriate evaluation of the study. With confirmation from the quality assur-

1. Address correspondence to: Jerry M. Smith, Ph.D., D.A.B.T., Rohm and Haas Co., Independence Mall West, Philadelphia, PA 19105.

2. Key words: good laboratory practices, good toxicology practices, hazard identification, risk assessment, risk management.

3. Abbreviations: GLP, Good Laboratory Practices; GTP, Good Toxicology Practices; SOPs, Standard Operating Procedures.

ance unit that the data reported in the draft report represent the raw data and that procedures were appropriately followed, the study director and the monitoring toxicologist review the assumptions and conclusions of the report for consistency with data generated by the study and with other available data.

The final report is approved by a senior non-participating toxicologist such as the laboratory director. As segments of the program are completed, the toxicology program director reviews data from appropriate studies, makes his evaluations and assessment of hazards and risk. The final assessment is reviewed by the Director of the Laboratory and other experts, as appropriate.

INTRODUCTION

Good regulations for the control of the toxic hazards of chemicals, whether for drugs, pesticides, household products or industrial chemicals, depend on quality toxicology programs which in turn depend on quality toxicology studies. The recognition of the need for quality toxicology studies led to the development of Good Laboratory Practices (GLPs) which are now generally practiced throughout the world by the toxicology community. The purposes of GLPs and audits are to assure the quality and integrity of test data; to assure that an independent reviewer can reconstruct the study and reach valid conclusions about the study; and to assure that the process will contribute to and improve the protection of health and environment. There is little question that GLPs and audits have contributed to an improvement in the overall quality of toxicological and preclinical testing. However, after almost a decade of GLP guidelines and audits, it is obvious that they do not assure the good practice of toxicology and safety evaluation. Good Toxicology Practice (GTP) includes not only quality studies and identification of hazard, but also evaluations of all toxicology data permitting the safe use of beneficial products. That is, GLP and audits of toxicology and preclinical studies assure the quality of studies, but GTPs assure the quality of hazard and risk assessments necessary for continued use of existing products and the introduction of beneficial new products. No one is more aware of this than the corporate or industrial toxicologist who has overall responsibility for providing not only hazard identification information but also assessments of hazards and risk for risk management decisions.

To assure ourselves that we were practicing good toxicology and that our system of toxicology program directors and quality assurance auditors was providing the best assurance against failed and flawed programs and studies, we evaluated our total toxicology effort. We examined both our productivity and quality, and in the process identified and examined our points of vulnerability and control.

PRODUCTS OF TOXICOLOGY

Toxicology evaluations and reports of individual studies as well as comprehensive evaluations and reports of toxicology programs are the products of toxicology. Individual toxicology findings, determinations and observations are products of toxicity units and other testing units. As with any product, quality is dependent upon specific need for the product; design of the product; quality and consistency of raw material and components; assembly of the product; and performance of the product. Therefore, the products of toxicology begin with study and program requests; includes experimental and program design, findings, determinations and observations; and concludes with report preparation, health hazard risk assessment and use of the assessments for health hazard risk management. Obviously, GLP is only a component of the products of toxicology or GTP.

UNACCEPTABLE PRODUCTS OF TOXICOLOGY

Normally to control quality, standards of performance are set and performance measured against the standards. GLPs, data audits and inspections identify variances, reject invalid studies and reports and cause studies to be repeated. While this process results in improved quality of toxicology reports, it is not cost effective and does not necessarily improve the quality of future products. To improve quality in a cost effective manner, it is necessary to identify, analyze and correct the causes of poor quality and prevent them from recurring. We identified four types of problems that lead to poor or unacceptable reports or toxicology products: Flawed Studies/Reports, Fraudulent Studies/Reports, Inappropriate Studies/Reports and Non-relevant Studies/Reports.

Flawed Studies/Reports. A flawed study or report is one that is incorrect or of such poor quality that it cannot be used. It results from poor or inconsistent use of raw material, execution of procedures, recordings of findings or preparation of reports. These are the errors most commonly found by quality assurance units, outside inspections and data audits. Strict adherence to GLP normally minimizes the issuance of flawed studies or reports and corrective steps can minimize the recurrence of the errors under similar testing circumstances.

Fraudulent Studies/Reports. A fraudulent study or report is one that has been deliberately falsified. Fortunately, fraudulent studies or reports occur rarely, but when produced, they can have catastrophic consequences. If the falsifications are premeditated, routine GLP, inspections and audits may not detect the deceit. However, if fraud is attempted by altering properly collected experimental data, inspections and audits are usually successful in detecting the deceit.

Inappropriate Studies/Reports. An inappropriate study or study report is one in which even though the study may have been experimentally valid or applicable to a different issue, the study design or results are inapplicable to the issue under investigation. In addition, an inappropriate comprehensive or summary report may be one that correctly quotes referenced sources but does not comprehensively report information derived from experiments or primary sources. This most frequently occurs when authors of the summary or comprehensive report are not knowledgeable about the toxicity of the material under investigation and rely on secondary and tertiary reference sources. This is one of the more grievous errors made today in efforts to evaluate potential health risks. GLPs, inspections and audits do not address these problems; they can be addressed only by open peer reviews.

Non-Relevant Studies/Reports. Non-relevant or irrelevant studies and reports are very similar to inappropriate studies and reports. Nevertheless, I believe that a separate category is beneficial. Normally, these are inappropriately designed studies that lead to non-relevant study results and reports. As is the case with inappropriate studies and reports, it is in the misuse of the results in comprehensive or summary reports that the quality of toxicology programs is compromised. As with inappropriate studies and reports, GLPs, inspections and audits do not address these problems; they can be addressed only by open peer reviews.

POINTS OF VULNERABILITY

Given that the products of toxicology are reports, and that the potential problems are ones of flawed, fraudulent, inappropriate, or non-relevant reports, and if the goal is to achieve and maintain the highest quality and productivity, an examination of points of vulnerability and controls is in order. The resources and activities required to conduct studies and prepare reports comprise the points of vulnerability.

Inspections and data audits are designed to check points of vulnerability within an organization and to ensure that only studies of acceptable quality are used for regulatory purposes. Internal examinations of points of vulnerability provide useful information to the management of toxicology laboratories. These examinations cannot only assure that the laboratory will successfully pass a GLP inspection and that results will be acceptable for regulatory purposes, but also provide important information to enhance both the quality and productivity of the toxicology laboratory.

Staff. The most important key to a quality, productive toxicology effort is the staff. It is obvious that the staff must be sufficient in number, of the highest quality and have the expertise to address toxicology and regulatory issues. An industrial toxicology effort must first have adequate experienced staff to manage toxicology programs while maintaining full integration with non-toxicology research, manufacturing, marketing, sales and regulatory agencies. These toxicology program directors are necessary whether or not a corporation has a toxicology laboratory. They should be experienced in toxicology programs and have an extensive understanding of toxicology testing. If a corporation has an in-house toxicology effort, the staff must also include study directors and investigators with extensive working knowledge in the areas of testing. Also, the frequency of testing should be sufficient to maintain proficiency. Outside consulting experts should be used to augment internal expertise as necessary. A cadre of experienced, highly qualified toxicologists is essential for maintaining GTPs.

Standard Operating Procedures. Standard operating procedures (SOPs) are both a benefit and a hazard to good toxicology practices. When SOPs are kept current and used, they enhance the conduct of the study. When appropriate, they enhance both the conduct of the investigation and evaluation of the results. However, if SOPs are allowed to become obsolete, and used noncritically or are substituted for more appropriate procedures, erroneous or nonrelevant results may be generated.

Special Procedures. Special procedures are often necessary to obtain the best results and require tailoring to the specific circumstances. However, if used without a full understanding of the usefulness and limitations of the special procedure, inappropriate, erroneous or nonrelevant results may be generated.

Experimental/Program Design. There are many standard protocol designs and regulatory requirements that have been published or are otherwise available to the industrial toxicologist; too frequently they are followed noncritically. Information from previous studies on the material under investigation or a structurally related substance often suggests that a modified or different investigative approach would provide better information for evaluation of potential health risk. This information must be used for GTP.

Materials and Methods. Even though SOPs and study design specify the materials and methods to be used in the conduct of a study, outside suppliers and support services may not be fully informed of the standards or criteria necessary to fulfill the requirements of the study.

Observations. Observations of effects of materials upon the test subject have been, are and will continue to be one of the most valuable sets of information obtained from toxicology studies and constitute the essence of discovering the unexpected. Effects or signs of effects observed in the toxicological laboratory are the integration of many lesser effects occurring within the test subject. Therefore, the preciseness of the description of the observation can profoundly influence the interpretation of the effects during the evaluation phase of the study or program. Poorly trained observers or inadequate observations remain one of the more vulnerable points for GLPs. GTPs require frequent observation by highly trained, experienced professionals. It should be noted that many so-called carcinogenicity studies have poor observations of toxicity.

Evaluations/Assessments. Evaluation and assessment of the results of toxicology studies and programs are the most difficult and least precise steps in hazard evaluation and characterization, yet the regulator and the public demand great precision from the process. Unfortunately, most regulators, the less experienced toxicologists and non-toxicologists rely primarily upon yes/no data and on calculated risk numbers. This is the area in which inappropriate and nonrelevant studies and reports are most frequently used. As stated previously, the most frequent and growing misuse of valid studies, i.e., experimentally reproducible studies, is in the process of extrapolating from hazard identification to risk management decisions. In this process, appropriateness, relevance, hazard assessment and hazard characterization are completely ignored. The results of such evaluations of health hazard and risk management are of poor quality, erroneous, wasteful of resources and counterproductive. GLP can check study conclusions against recorded observations, but GLP does not assure GTP.

51

Archives. Poor management of archives, ranging from loss of original data to the inability to retrieve information in a timely and orderly manner, does more than cause doubts about archive competence. It adversely affects quality and production because of the inability to adequately review historical data on structurally similar materials or to examine the types of material that have produced similar effects. This impedes both experimental and program design and decreases the quality of evaluations and assessments.

POINTS OF CONTROL

With an understanding of what the product is, what the potential problems are and what the points of vulnerability are, points of control become obvious as one examines the flow of work from the initial toxicological request to the issue and distribution of final study and comprehensive reports. The flow of work may differ from laboratory to laboratory, but in general includes request for work; administration preparation; experimental preparation; experimental execution; report preparation; report review and signature; and report issue and distribution.

Request. The program director and study director sit at an important control point, particularly with reference to the object of the study and program. By understanding the object of the study and program they can improve the quality and productivity of toxicology by minimizing the initiation of inappropriate studies and programs.

Administrative Preparations. Administrative preparation not only includes the scheduling of personnel and toxicity units, but also includes proper review of literature and design of studies and programs. Again the program director, along with the study director, performs the crucial task of assuring that the study design address the objectives not only of the study but also of the program.

Experimental Preparation. In preparing for the experiment, the selection of the "raw material" to be used, from selection of the animals and their diets, to the selection of methods to be used in measurement of responses, is critical. SOPs and the quality of the technician performing the measurements and observations can make the difference between a quality experiment and an invalid one.

Experimental Execution. All of the preparatory work will be wasted if the technicians and professionals conducting the study do not make appropriate and accurate observations and record these observations according to the study protocol. Furthermore, those conducting the study must go the extra step to record unusual happenings that were not anticipated, but are critical to understanding the toxicity of the text material.

Report Preparation. The report must be carefully written to accurately reflect the response of the test system to the conditions of exposure to the test material. The report must condense the data so that they can be easily and correctly interpreted by outside experts, yet tabulate them in such a manner that a reviewer can follow the flow of the experiment through each step. The report

TABLE 1
An Industrial Approach to Quality Toxicology Studies

	Request	Admin Prep	Exper Prep	Exper	Report Prep	Review	Issue
Standard Oper. Proc.	v	+	+	+	+	+	vv
Staff		+	+	+	+	v	v
Experiment Design	v	+	+	+	+		
Materials & Methods		+	v	+	+	+	
Observations			+	v		+	
Evaluation			v	v	v		
Archive			+		+	v	

+ – slightly vulnerable.
v – vulnerable.
vv – toxicology department lacks control.

must completely describe the materials and methods so that the study may be repeated, if necessary.

Report Review and Signature. The report of a study must be reviewed not only by the study director but also by the program director and a nonparticipating senior scientist for correctness of data interpretation. The appropriateness and relevance of the experimental design and results must be carefully reviewed against the conclusions of the report. Where appropriate, results from other studies and evaluations should be used to enhance the interpretation of the results.

Report Issue and Distribution. The report and evaluation must be distributed to the appropriate individuals responsible for making a health hazard risk assessment. The issuance of the report(s) must contain all information needed for an outside reviewer to make a full evaluation of the health hazard potential.

VULNERABILITY/CONTROL ANALYSIS

We prepared a Vulnerability verus Control matrix table and rated vulnerability as none, slight, vulnerable and very vulnerable and recommend that anyone interested in assessing weakness and strengths of his good laboratory and toxicology practices do the same (Table 1; see also Table 2). We found our procedures to be most vulnerable at the extremes of the process of toxicity testing and evaluations; that is, at the request or initiation phase of a program and the use/misuse of the information generated.

TABLE 2
Vulnerability/Control Analysis

Step	Vulnerability	Control
Request	Individuals might directly contract for tox studies by-passing Tox. Dept.	Accounting; budgeting; director/ mgr. awareness
Experimental Preparation	Invalid test sample	Retention sample; blind (coded) samples
	Incorrect chemical analysis	Use-dilution analysis; validated reagents
Animals	Inappropriate/improper test animals; pedigree records;	Commercial breeders; certified health records; randomization procedures
	Improper feed	Certified diets
Experiment	Mis-dosing	SOP; some computer prompting visual aids; analysis of diets; sample accountability
	Observations	SOP; supervision; training; multi-person responsibility; audit
	Equipment failure	Standards and calibration
Report Prepartion	Recorded data vs. reported data	Audit
	Misrepresentation of the data	Review process
Review	Change/modify interpretation	Agency review; TLAB; peer pressure
Issue	Substitution of reports; modification of reports; failure-to-report; non-full disclosure	Senior manager review

A request to do a test, study or an evaluation without a clear and fully understood objective by the requestor and the study and program directors is wholly inadequate. Both the program and study directors must understand the objective and purpose for the request in order to properly design the experiment(s) and program and evaluate the results obtained. The industrial toxicologist is most vulnerable when asked to evaluate a toxicity test for which he has no prior knowledge of the use of material under study nor the overall objective or purpose of the study.

During the administrative preparation, the design of the experiment is most vulnerable to inappropriateness. Standard protocols, which are commonly used, make possible a reproducible study, but not necessarily an appropriate study. Furthermore, study and program directors must be cognizant of outside pressure which can adversely influence the program and study designs.

Finally, the toxicology program director and study director must be alert to the potential distribution of the reports and evaluations and prepare the reports to minimize misinterpretation of the data and evaluations.

CONCLUSIONS

In conclusion, GLP, inspections and data audits usually do an adequate job of assuring quality and validity, i.e., reproducible studies. However, GLP does not assure GTP, which is dependent on a highly qualified staff and on peer review.

THE NATIONAL TOXICOLOGY
PROGRAM APPROACH TO QUALITY

Carrie E. Whitmire
National Institute of Environmental Health Sciences
Research Triangle Park, North Carolina

ABSTRACT

The National Toxicology Program's management approaches to assuring the quality of toxicology studies are multi-faceted. Management of National Toxicology Program (NTP) study quality begins early, with multi-level peer review of project concept and project proposal, and continues throughout the study to the completion of the research articles and technical reports. Peer reviews are performed by NIEHS internal committees, NTP Executive Committee, Ad Hoc Committees and Board of Scientific Counselors, as well as by the scientific community at large through publications in the open literature.

Major management tools for assuring the quality of NTP toxicology studies are the Statement of Work and approval of contract laboratories under the Master Agreement (MA). Toxicology study awards to MA approved laboratories are competitive, based on the review and evaluation of proposals developed for the conduct of individual studies.

Chemical Managers (CMs) are the primary scientists responsible for chemicals selected for study by the NTP. Their involvement begins with protocol design, a step that is peer reviewed by the NIEHS/NTP Toxicology Design Committee. The CM then acts as the focal point for information, tracking, evaluation, writing and presenting for peer review the study's technical report and other publications.

Through procurement and oversight, the NTP manages the animal breeding program and monitors the quality and health of animals used. Chemical quality

1. Address correspondence to: Dr. Carrie E. Whitmire, N.I.E.H.S., P.O. Box 12233, Research Triangle Park, NC 27709.

2. Key words: conduct, data, management, quality, toxicology.

3. BSC, Board of Scientific Counselors; CBDS, Carcinogenesis Bioassay Data System; CEC, Chemical Evaluation Committee; CM, Chemical Manager; GLP, Good Laboratory Practices; MA, Master Agreement; NCI, National Cancer Institute; NIEHS, National Institute of Environmental Health Sciences; NTP, National Toxicology Program; PO, Project Officer; QA, Quality Assurance; QAU, Quality Assurance Unit; RFP, Request for Proposal; SOP, Standard Operating Procedure; TDC, Toxicology Design Committee; TDMS, Toxicology Data Management System; TRTP, Toxicology Research and Testing Program.

is managed through procurement, analysis and stability determinations prior to shipment to laboratory facilities. Environmental and personnel safety requirements are defined before a competitive award is made.

At each laboratory, the NTP monitoring process is performed by a project officer and a team of discipline leaders. Quality assurance data auditing, both in-life and retrospective, is carried out in a highly structured manner. Prior to peer review and publication, study data are audited and the technical reports validated and reviewed by NTP staff. This management of study quality gives better assurance that the collected data support the published results.

INTRODUCTION

During the first section of this conference, management perspectives of quality in toxicological studies were discussed and the meaning of quality to the NTP was defined. The results of toxicology studies performed and sponsored by industrial groups and by the world's governments have significance for everyone. The results of these studies influence health and quality of life, not only for this generation but probably for generations to come. Today it is not only important to preserve a clean environment and the health of the world's population, but also to work to ensure that the quality of life will continue to improve for each new generation. These are but some of the reasons why the quality of toxicology studies must be scrutinized to assure that it is the best possible. Too much is at risk to set quality standards below what is reasonably possible to achieve.

As the size of toxicology programs increases, the number of safeguards to quality must be increased. Realizing that the cost of assuring such quality is not insignificant, management should incorporate the mechanisms for control of quality into toxicological studies. In the course of planning, the cost of repeating long-term toxicology and carcinogenicity studies, both in terms of money and the effects on quality of life, must not be discounted. The NTP represents one of the largest programs studying the toxicology of materials of public interest. The purpose of this paper is to present methods used by the NTP to assure management, the public and the scientific and regulatory communities of a quality product.

The NTP, a coordinated effort of several government agencies, represents a substantial effort to provide the nation with information on the possible health hazards of chemical exposure. In such a large program, it is essential that considerable review of our activities take place. Thus it is vital that quality controls be built into our work. The period between the initiation of planning for a toxicology and carcinogenicity study and publication of a technical report averages five to seven years. This brings about a pyramid, consisting of studies in the planning stage, studies in progress, all of the studies in some stage of report preparation and, finally, data which must be preserved for all studies carried out since the inception of the National Cancer Institute Bioassay Program in the 1960s. Because of these factors, the management of the National Toxicology Program applied special measures to assure quality.

PEER REVIEW

Peer review is one aspect of providing an assurance of quality to the NTP. The scope of studies performed by the NTP is broad and complex, necessitating an integrated, stepwise system of review (Figure 1). Each step improves the program's quality. There are two major external review committees and a number of external and internal review committees that act in an integrated fashion. Some of these will be discussed in the following paragraphs to demonstrate the review process that takes place.

The NTP Executive Committee is composed of heads of research and regulatory government agencies (Figure 2). It provides primary oversight, a forum for discussion of science policy issues and timely information exchange among the various agencies. This committee acts as the major advisory group for selecting and setting priorities for specific chemicals to be studied. One of its important tasks is to review and approve the NTP Annual Plan, which details plans for the coming years and results from the previous year.

The NTP Chemical Evaluation Committee (CEC) is a subcommittee composed of members of the agencies making up the Executive Committee. It reviews the chemicals nominated for study by academia, government, industry, labor and the public and develops a list of chemicals proposed for study. After additional input from the public and the NTP, the Board of Scientific Counselors (BSC) reviews the list in order to establish information related to priority and need. The Executive Committee reviews the recommendations of the CEC and BSC, determines if a chemical should be studied, deleted or deferred, and refers the selections to the NTP Steering Committee.

The NTP Steering Committee is made up of representatives of the NTP, consisting of the National Institute of Environmental Health Sciences (NIEHS), the National Institute for Occupational Safety and Health and the National Center for Toxicology Research. The committee was formed in 1980 to strengthen coordination and promote interagency working relationships within the NTP. The Committee plans agendas for upcoming NTP meetings, reviews ongoing programs and projects and proposes new programs, and makes agency allocations for chemicals approved for toxicologic characterization by the Executive Committee.

The NTP Board of Scientific Counselors is composed of eight non-governmental scientists appointed by the Assistant Secretary of Health, Department of Health and Human Services. The Board provides scientific oversight in identifying needs, determining the program's scientific adequacy, and evaluating the merit of various aspects of the program.

The NTP Board of Scientific Counselors' Technical Reports Review Subcommittee is composed of members of the Board and Ad Hoc Experts representing different backgrounds and views. These individuals are responsible for examining draft Technical Reports for toxicology and carcinogenesis studies, a process which takes place in public sessions, with comments and questions requested from the individuals or groups attending these open meetings. Relevant and appropriate comments concerning the reviews and summary com-

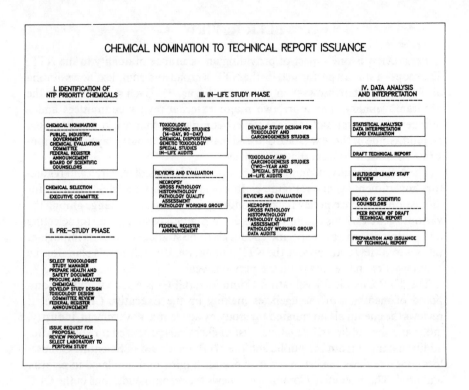

CHEMICAL NOMINATION TO TECHNICAL REPORT ISSUANCE

I. IDENTIFICATION OF NTP PRIORITY CHEMICALS

CHEMICAL NOMINATION
PUBLIC, INDUSTRY, GOVERNMENT
CHEMICAL EVALUATION COMMITTEE
FEDERAL REGISTER ANNOUNCEMENT
BOARD OF SCIENTIFIC COUNSELORS

CHEMICAL SELECTION
EXECUTIVE COMMITTEE

II. PRE—STUDY PHASE

SELECT TOXICOLOGIST
STUDY MANAGER
PREPARE HEALTH AND SAFETY DOCUMENT
PROCURE AND ANALYZE CHEMICAL
DEVELOP STUDY DESIGN
TOXICOLOGY DESIGN COMMITTEE REVIEW
FEDERAL REGISTER ANNOUNCEMENT

ISSUE REQUEST FOR PROPOSAL
REVIEW PROPOSALS
SELECT LABORATORY TO PERFORM STUDY

III. IN—LIFE STUDY PHASE

TOXICOLOGY
PRECHRONIC STUDIES (14—DAY, 90—DAY)
CHEMICAL DISPOSITION
GENETIC TOXICOLOGY
SPECIAL STUDIES
IN—LIFE AUDITS

REVIEWS AND EVALUATION
NECROPSY
GROSS PATHOLOGY
HISTOPATHOLOGY
PATHOLOGY QUALITY ASSESSMENT
PATHOLOGY WORKING GROUP

FEDERAL REGISTER ANNOUNCEMENT

DEVELOP STUDY DESIGN FOR TOXICOLOGY AND CARCINOGENESIS STUDIES

TOXICOLOGY AND CARCINOGENESIS STUDIES (TWO—YEAR AND SPECIAL STUDIES)
IN—LIFE AUDITS

REVIEWS AND EVALUATION
NECROPSY
GROSS PATHOLOGY
HISTOPATHOLOGY
PATHOLOGY QUALITY ASSESSMENT
PATHOLOGY WORKING GROUP
DATA AUDITS

IV. DATA ANALYSIS AND INTERPRETATION

STATISTICAL ANALYSES
DATA INTERPRETATION AND EVALUATION

DRAFT TECHNICAL REPORT

MULTIDISCIPLINARY STAFF REVIEW

BOARD OF SCIENTIFIC COUNSELORS
PEER REVIEW OF DRAFT TECHNICAL REPORT

PREPARATION AND ISSUANCE OF TECHNICAL REPORT

FIGURE 1. Review process for NTP toxicology studies, starting with chemical nomination through issuance of the Technical Report.

ments are incorporated into the final published Technical Report.

Ad Hoc Panels are established by the NTP BSC, as needed, to provide specialized expertise for special projects, such as Chemical Carcinogenesis Testing and Evaluation.

The Toxicology Research and Testing Program (TRTP) Management Committee consists of key staff and Branch Chiefs of the Toxicology Research and Testing Program of NIEHS. This committee represents an internal review and decision making group which is active in the NIEHS portion of the NTP. It was established to ensure coordination and communication among the NIH segment of the NTP and is responsible for planning, review and implementation of NIEHS NTP activities.

The Toxicology Design Committee (TDC) is composed of NIEHS scientists representing a broad range of expertise in toxicology and carcinogenesis research. Members include experts in carcinogenesis, chemistry, biochemical toxicology, pharmacokinetics, reproductive toxicology, genetic toxicology, pathology and statistics who act as an oversight and advisory committee for the Chemical Manager.

The CM prepares a briefing package and presents this material to the TDC peer review committee, generally in two phases. New chemicals for study are presented for the prechronic studies, at which time the background scientific data are reviewed and the proposed study design presented. The second phase occurs after completion of the prechronic studies and includes a discussion of the findings and the proposed study design for the chronic or 2-year studies.

The TDC committee recommends to the CM any modifications, deletions or additions the members believe will produce a study that better meets scientific needs. This review is conceived from the scientific point of view and does not consider the economics of carrying out the study. Once the protocol has been completed by the CM it receives additional review for scientific approval and NTP management approval of both the scientific content and the cost of the study.

Ad Hoc Peer Review Panels are composed of both government and non-government members with expertise in the area to be reviewed. NTP establishes the panels to review proposals submitted from establishments for carrying out research and other activities to be performed in studying NTP chemicals. Based on the merit of these proposals, the contracts office proceeds to award contracts to carry out the tasks as prescribed in the federal procurement regulations.

Various other committees play special roles in overseeing the quality of the NTP plan and accomplishments, providing examples of management involvement in assuring quality.

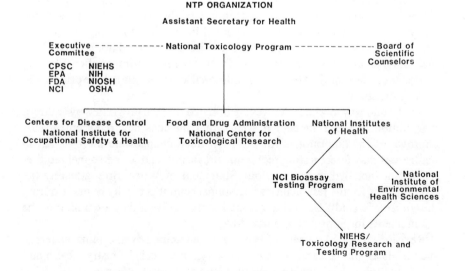

FIGURE 2. Organization of the National Toxicology Program.

NTP MASTER AGREEMENT STATEMENT OF WORK

The MA Statement of Work is considered one of the cornerstones for assuring quality in NTP toxicology studies. "Guidelines for Carcinogen Bioassays in Small Rodents" was first published by the National Cancer Institute (NCI) in 1976 (Sontag, 1976), and represented the first concerted effort to standardize studies carried out by the NCI Bioassay Program. Further efforts were made to standardize bioassays by the use of a single prime contractor. With the establishment of NTP in 1978 and the phaseout of the prime contractor activities in 1982-83, the NTP issued its first general Statement of Work for the conduct of acute, 14-day repeated dose, 90-day subchronic and 2-year chronic studies in laboratory animals in March 1981. This Statement of Work was revised in March 1982, October 1982 and January 1984 (all unpublished). The Statement of Work is currently undergoing review for additional updates to reflect current state of the art in toxicology/carcinogenicity studies in laboratory rodents.

Change in the testing program has been continuous and, when appropriate, is handled by modifications of the contracts. Such changes can involve the individual studies or the Statement of Work as a whole. New editions of the Statement of Work result from the state of the art of toxicology and the needs of NTP. The state of the art is based on new scientific findings and the need to improve study quality in response to changing requirements of the regulatory agencies to improve the quality of life.

The Statement of Work can be changed in two ways. First, changes occur gradually and are incorporated into the study requirements by modifications to the contracts and the Statement of Work. NTP has numerous tests in progress at any one time, and changes initiated into an ongoing study can only be made if they affect some aspect of the study remaining to be completed. For example, the period from initiation to completion of a study requires 24 months. If the study was in the twentieth month, it would be possible to change the tissues which should be examined at terminal sacrifice, but it would not be possible to incorporate additional animals needed for a 65-week interim sacrifice. Existing contracts can be modified to include additional animals only if done prior to the start of the study.

The second way in which changes are initiated into the program is by issuing a new edition of the Statement of Work that includes new requirements for approval of the laboratories for the MA. Such changes are more global in nature and may affect testing requirements, facility and/or personnel requirements not included in the previous Statement of Work. Strengthening the requirements for the test facility or personnel cannot generally be made during the course of a study. Such changes are less disruptive if they are built into the requirements for approval of a new MA.

Revisions in the Statement of Work are contributed by discipline leaders in such fields as animal care, clinical chemistry, analytical chemistry, health and safety, pathology and quality assurance, and by project officers.

Today, it is a general requirement that the contractor be capable of performing dosed feed, gavage, dermal and dosed water routes of administration and/or inhalation route of administration. All contractors must be capable of performing routine hematology, urinalysis and clinical chemistry studies in-house or by subcontract. Another change which has gradually occurred in the program is to seek out those facilities which have capabilities in various special studies which are included in studies from time to time, such as sperm morphology and vaginal cytology, immunological or behavioral studies. Special studies in neurobehavioral toxicology is the only special type of study for which capabilities are optional. Such additions to the testing program, either on an individual chemical basis or across the board, offer opportunities to evaluate the significance of such procedures in detecting specific types of toxicity. Other less routine special studies that contract bioassay laboratories are unable to carry out are performed in parallel either at NIEHS or through contracts established especially for studies of these types. Examples include nonroutine reproductive, immunotoxicology or metabolism and pharmacokinetic studies.

The Statement of Work is a valuable tool, not only in selecting testing laboratories but also as a reference or guide for laboratories interested in conducting state of the art toxicology studies. Each time a Request for Proposal (RFP) is advertised for a new MA competition, numerous requests are made for copies of the RFP (and Statement of Work); these requests far exceed the number of laboratories responding for MA awards. The list of requests demonstrates that many people other than testing facilities are interested in the standards which the NTP has established for its testing program.

The Statement of Work also serves as a guide for monitoring, inspecting and auditing the work carried out at the test facility. It is the bible of standards which the facility uses in writing their Standard Operating Procedures (SOPs) and is the standard by which NTP staff monitor and evaluate the correctness of the SOPs and what is practiced at the laboratory. A member of the QA/GLP monitors determines that a copy of the Statement of Work is available to the Quality Assurance Unit and to other parts of the program, such as chemistry and pathology.

SELECTION OF NTP CONTRACT LABORATORIES

The selection of laboratories qualified to perform toxicology/carcinogenicity studies is one of the most significant phases of contracting. In order to select a qualified laboratory, it is necessary to define the requirements of the study, how it is to be accomplished and the evaluation criteria for selecting the laboratory. In the NTP, the Statement of Work not only defines what is to be done, but also how it is to be done. The selection criteria flow from this.

Within the federal government, procurement procedures are well defined. The MA mechanism consists of issuing a RFP with the Statement of Work for what is to be done. Each proposal is evaluated strictly on its response to the Statement of Work against pre-established evaluation factors. This evaluation is done by a peer review committee selected primarily from outside government, based on individual's knowledge and experience in toxicology testing. The committee is selected to assure that expertise is available to evaluate capabilities in animal care, analytical chemistry, clinical chemistry, toxicology, pathology, and health and safety as related to toxicology/carcinogenicity studies. It is not the intent of this paper to discuss federal procurement regulations, but to demonstrate that the NTP procedures for the selection of test facilities are impartial and assure that quality facilities are available for carrying out NTP studies.

Once this evaluation has been completed based on the initial responses of the offering laboratories, site visits are made by a qualified group of experts in the various disciplines to evaluate the facility of each offerer whose proposal was found to be in the competitive range. ("Facility" is used here to mean the building, equipment, experience, personnel and management to carry out the proposed work.) This site visit is a second assurance that quality laboratories are available to carry out the NTP studies.

Based on the recommendations of the site visit team, best and final questions and other evaluations by the contracting officer, the MA Awards are made. These awards do not consist of any contracts to carry out work, but rather indicate that a given laboratory is qualified to bid on NTP studies. The complexity of the studies varies greatly from RFP to RFP. Specific awards are based on the laboratory's ability to carry out a particular study and are influenced by specific routes of administration, i.e., inhalation, gavage, dose feed, dosed water, and the capability to perform special studies such as neurobehavioral toxicology. On the basis of these established qualifications, competitive awards are made based on responses to RFPs for specific bid packages of chemicals to be tested. This is a third test of the facility's ability to carry out particular studies and takes into consideration their understanding of the specific problems related to those studies.

In order for this system to work in a program as large as the NTP, there must be an adequate number of laboratories approved under the MA to meet NTP toxicology testing needs. Study monitoring is more efficient and cost effective when a number of studies are carried out at one facility, another advantage of using the MA contracting mechanism.

The life of a MA allowing the laboratory to bid on new packages is five years, subject to biannual review to determine if the facility is still qualified. After this five-year period, the laboratory must respond to a new MA announcement and again be approved for continuation on the program. MA orders issued under an earlier MA continue through completion for administrative purposes, whether or not a new MA award is made. Receipt of one MA award is no guarantee that it will continue or that a new one will be awarded if the quality of work deteriorates. If facility or personnel changes occur during the life of the MA, such changes are subject to approval by NTP so that continued quality can be ensured.

In summary, the MA provides a ready source of approved laboratories to bid on the packages of chemicals requiring toxicology studies. Bidding on test packages allows further evaluation of each responding laboratory's capacity to carry out specific studies. NTP is looking for the best laboratory to do the best job for each study at a reasonable price.

NATIONAL TOXICOLOGY PROGRAM
MONITORING SYSTEM

During this conference, various aspects of the NTP monitoring system for assuring quality will be discussed. An overview of this system as an aspect of assurance by management of NTP testing program quality will now be given. Several types of monitoring established by NTP management take place at the MA toxicology laboratories. Such collaborative monitoring acts as a check and balance to bring about the best possible studies.

1. Project Officer. Under federal regulations, the Project Officer (PO) is the government agent responsible for monitoring and evaluating all technical aspects of the work performed under the contract. At NTP, the PO is assisted in this task by a team of discipline leaders.

2. Discipline Monitoring. Due to the complexity of toxicology studies, NTP has found that greater expertise can be brought to the program when disciplines are divided into animal care, analytical chemistry, clinical chemistry, toxicology, pathology, health and safety and computer data collection.

A. Health and Safety. During the chemical study design phase, it is essential that chemical-specific health and safety information be incorporated to ensure adequate protection of laboratory personnel and the environment. This information may influence the procedures utilized and possibly limit the highest dose used.

During pre-award site visits for the selection of laboratories under the MA, facility design and health and safety practices are reviewed to assure protection of personnel and the environment. During chemical studies, laboratories are monitored through the monthly reporting requirements detailing modifications to the laboratory's health and safety program, medical and biological monitoring, health and safety training, ventilation monitoring, chemical monitoring results, personnel injury/incident reports, chemical spills and releases, waste disposal, training and updates on health and safety attention items noted during previous reports or site visits.

Site visits, program reviews and monthly reporting reviews continue through the course of each study and are directly tailored to the specific needs of each chemical study. Such chemical health and safety monitoring can improve the quality of the study by recognizing, evaluating and controlling possible sites of contamination and resultant inadvertent exposure to the test material. The Statement of Work discusses many aspects of the Chemical Health and Safety Program for NTP testing laboratories.

B. Analytical Chemistry Monitoring for NTP toxicology studies is initiated before the study is contracted to the laboratory. The study's quality depends on the quality and accuracy with which the chemical is selected and defined. The form of the chemical to which the public is exposed must be considered, as must the stability and solubility of that form when the route of exposure to animals is defined. Mixtures must be considered if the workforce or the public is to be exposed in that manner. Whenever possible, the source of the chemical needs to be the most likely source of potential public exposure. This becomes particularly important when naturally occurring materials are studied, since significant differences in chemical composition may occur based on the source selected. Examples of this are asbestos and talc.

The material to be studied is procured by an analytical chemistry support contract laboratory. As part of quality control, the analytical laboratory determines the identity, purity, stability under various storage conditions, solubility, procedures for homogenous mixing of dose formulations and the best procedures for analyzing the bulk material and the chemical/vehicle mixture. For inhalation studies, the laboratory, in consultation with analytical chemistry discipline personnel, undertakes an extensive study to determine the best way to produce an atmosphere containing the chemical. The nature of the atmosphere depends upon the physical/chemical nature of the chemical (particulate, gas or aerosol).

Upon receipt of the bulk chemical at the laboratory, the chemical's identity and purity are also defined. Subsequently, the substance is checked at four-month intervals to ensure that it maintains its integrity while on study.

Analytical procedures are defined for sensitivity based on the dose levels to be used in exposing animals. This process may be difficult when animal toxicity data are not available. Occasionally more sensitive analysis procedures are required for the chronic study based on toxicity found in the prechronic studies. As a check on the accuracy of dose preparation, the animal facility routinely analyzes dose mixtures. In addition, NTP has established a referee analysis program whereby a dose mixture sample is analyzed by both the laboratory and an independent analytical chemistry laboratory. These referee analyses are initiated with the first preparation for the subchronic study and others are carried out at least five times during the chronic study.

C. *Animal care* is an important part of assuring quality in toxicology studies. A study is only as good as the test system; therefore, NTP provides high quality, healthy rodents of uniform genetic background through contract breeding facilities. These facilities are provided with breeding stock from NIH to be used in rederiving their breeder stock in isolators. All rederived rats and mice are associated with known microorganisms to obtain uniformity between animal sources. Each production colonly is monitored for parasites and serum titers for a variety of rodent viruses. The genetic quality of these animals is monitored on a routine basis to ensure genetic uniformity. Retired breeders are also examined grossly and selected tissues reviewed microscopically to determine the overall state of health.

Hematology, urinalysis and clinical chemistry proficiency testing are required of all new MA Agreement laboratories.

D. *Data Collection* creates records which remain a mark of quality long after the study has been completed. Well-organized, complete records provide a means of data tracking of the study as defined by the protocol and substantiate the conclusions expressed in the final report.

A team of computer scientists works with NTP to assure proper functioning of the on-line Toxicology Data Management System (TDMS) as well as the Carcinogenesis Bioassay Data System (CBDS) used since the start of the program to analyze the studies not collected on TDMS. The on-line TDMS system is monitored at the laboratory regularly to assure that problems are found and resolved early in the study.

E. Quality Assurance / Good Laboratory Practices (QA / GLP) monitoring is carried out routinely by the laboratory as well as by NTP and GLP contract monitors and auditors. The program has required GLP compliance since October 1981 and the contractor's performance is monitored regularly by the PO and all discipline leaders as well as by NTP quality assurance personnel. In-life audits are performed at the laboratory and retrospective audits take place at the archives prior to publication of the technical reports. The number of in-life audits is to be expanded as a part of the monitoring service in an effort to find problems early and assure that corrective actions are begun. QA monitoring is carried out to ensure that the laboratory QA unit is a functioning unit consisting of well-qualified individuals. The interaction of management with the QA unit is considered an essential part of the system for assuring quality of toxicology studies. The fact remains that unless both the sponsor and the laboratory management are involved, quality will suffer. Quality must start at the top. "The speed of the leader determines the rate of the pack."

3. Chemical Managers (CMs) Monitoring. The CMs play an important role in the quality of toxicology studies at NTP. Each chemical selected for study is assigned to a member of the NTP staff based on expertise, interest and workload. The CM is responsible for knowing and understanding the relevant scientific literature, consulting the appropriate industry and other experts in the field of toxicology, and discussing the chemical with the agency or individual nominating that chemical. CMs are also responsible for contacting government regulatory agencies interested in the chemical for their input concerning the regulatory needs which the NTP study design must meet. CMs prepare and present a draft experimental design to the Toxicology Design Committee, which is composed of NTP scientists with various areas of expertise. This review ensures that the experiment is designed to measure relevant endpoints.

Based on findings in the literature and discussions with other scientists working with the chemical, the CM may recommend that the chemical not be studied. This recommendation may be based on the discovery that adequate studies are already in progress to answer the questions related to toxicity and carcinogenicity or that such information already exists. The recommendation may also be made for the chronic study based on findings of the prechronic studies carried out by NTP.

The CM's duties include all phases of the study, from the design through the actual review and publication of the results. CMs interact with the PO and all discipline leaders to assure the quality of the study. They are the contact points for industry, public and government agencies for study design and progress through the review and publication of the results. They attend scientific meetings and report on study findings. Thanks to the CM's responsibility for a chemical, the quality of all aspects of the study is always being monitored and necessary status information is available to NTP management when problems occur requiring decisions regarding the study findings. This access allows the

67

early alerting of interested regulatory agencies, industry, the person and/or party nominating the chemical and the public when the findings have been confirmed by the integrated review of the various disciplines involved in decision making related to toxic and/or carcinogenic findings.

ARCHIVING OF DATA AND MATERIALS

Preservation of data and materials generated by the NTP is not related to the quality of the toxicology studies. Nevertheless, it is an integral part of the program to make available quality data for review by the public sector and regulatory agencies. The usefulness of the data depends on the quality of preserved data files and the means of storage and access by interested parties. NTP has attempted to meet these needs.

Data from all toxicology and carcinogenicity studies are preserved at the archives located in Research Triangle Park, North Carolina. Since testing was initiated by NCI in 1961 and continued by NTP in 1981, the amount of material stored at the archives is massive. The archives consist of data on 287 reported studies, and on 89 studies for which the technical reports are in some stage of preparation for publication. Files arrive at the archives almost daily and must be inventoried and entered into the filing system. It is estimated that today these files contain the data for 375 prechronic and chronic studies as well as 43 prechronic studies for chemicals which were not carried to the chronic stage and 44 for which chronic studies are now in progress. It is further estimated that there are approximately 1000 file drawers of paper files, 4400 boxes of bags of wet tissues (averaging 70 bags/box), 3000 boxes of paraffin blocks of tissues (averaging 375 blocks/box) and 4.2 million slides.

The archives is not a stagnant storage area. Retrospective audits by NTP support contractors are carried out there on a continuing basis. In addition to the NTP audits, audits by the regulatory agencies and industrial auditors are also conducted. The archives is the site of review of wet tissues, blocks, slides and paper data.

Considerable thought has gone into storing this material to provide safety and accessibility. Individual rooms have been allocated to slides, blocks, wet tissues and paper data files. Extensive filing and inventory systems have been defined for these materials. The Food and Drug Administration GLP regulations have stipulated that filing systems will provide ready access to these materials by test article, date of study, test system and nature of study. By computerizing the inventory, the location of individual studies at the archives is easily determined.

During the past two years another safeguard to data preservation has been initiated. All paper files are being microfiched and the original and a copy of these fiche are being prepared for storage at the archives. These files provide a means of preserving the paper files indefinitely and reducing the continuing requirements for additional space. The NTP's intent is to preserve the original files for at least three years after Technical Report publication or so long as there is expressed interest. After this period the microfiche copies are to be preserved and the original paper files destroyed. The question of how long to retain the wet tissues is now being considered. However, none will be destroyed until the interest of NTP, regulatory agencies and the public sector has been reviewed for each chemical. This process of selection is intended to provide a means of retaining a manageable amount of paper files and wet tissue files while still preserving microfiche copies of all paper files and slides for all studies.

The quality of the data preserved at the archives is only as good as the original files. With the initiation of retrospective audits prior to publication, missing data are requested from the laboratories and the files are being made as complete as possible. Initiation of data collection by computer has also improved the process of preserving data and obtaining more complete data files. The major concern with computerization is preserving the program to recall these data and the instrumentation required to receive them. Based on these problems, it will be essential to preserve hard copies of the material collected by computers on microfiche for ease of access over the years. This approach eliminates the need to maintain a library of discs along with a museum of hardware and software on which to run them. Every attempt is being made to preserve the paper files by microfiching and to preserve the slides as long as possible, as it is recognized that the value of this material makes it irreplaceable.

ACKNOWLEDGEMENTS

The author wishes to thank the following for their help in assembling the materials for this paper: Dr. D. W. Bristol, Dr. D. Canter, Dr. R. Chhabra, Dr. J. E. Huff, Dr. C. W. Jameson, Dr. E. E. McConnell, Mr. A. T. Prokopelz, Dr. G. N. Rao, Dr. M. L. Vernon and Dr. E. Weisburger.

REFERENCES

DOUGLAS, J. F., HAMM, T. E., JAMESON, C. W., MAHAR, H., STINSON, S. and WHITMIRE, C. E. (1981). Monitoring guidelines for the conduct of carcinogen bioassays, U.S. Department of Health and Human Services, Public Health Service, National Institutes of Health, NIH Pub. No. 81-1774, June 1981, National Toxicology Program, Technical Report Series No. 218. Available from National Technical Information Service, U.S. Department of Commerce, 5285 Port Royal Road, Springfield, VA 22161.

GREISHABER, C. K. and WHITMIRE, C. E. (1984). Effects of Good Laboratory Practices on chemistry requirements for toxicity testing. In: Chemistry for Toxicity Testing. (C. W. Jameson and D. B. Walters, eds.), pp. 221–225, Butterworth Publishers, Boston, MA.

JAMESON, C. W. (1984). Analytical chemistry requirements for toxicity testing of environmental chemicals. In: Chemistry for Toxicity Testing. (C. W. Jameson and D. B. Walters, eds.), pp. 3–14, Butterworth Publishers, Boston, MA.

SONTAG, J. M., PAGE, N. P. and SAFFIOTTI, U. (1976). Guidelines for carcinogen bioassays in small rodents. National Cancer Institute, Carcinogenesis, Technical Report Series No. 1, Feb. 1976, U.S. Department of Health, Education and Welfare, Public Health Service, National Institutes of Health, #NCI-CG-TR1, DHEW Pub. No. (NIH)76-801. Available from Superintendent of Documents, U.S. Government Printing Office, Washington, DC 20402, Stock No. 017-042-00118-8.

INDUSTRIAL MANAGEMENT APPROACH TO SCIENTIFIC RESEARCH QUALITY

Judith K. Baldwin
Research and Environmental Health Division
Exxon Corporation
East Millstone, New Jersey

B. Kristin Hoover
Toxicology and Product Safety
ARCO Chemical Company
A Division of Atlantic Richfield Company
Newtown Square, Pennsylvania

ABSTRACT

Aspects of managing quality research programs from definition through planning, evaluation and quantification of goals to be achieved are discussed within the context of business concerns and economics.

INTRODUCTION

The petrochemical industry conducts toxicological research in response to management goals and regulatory requirements (U.S. Congress, 1976). Management recognizes as good business the assessment and communication of toxicity information associated with its processes and products. Corporate policy statements on this issue generally state the need to protect employees and consumers by meeting or exceeding, if necessary, all regulations regarding the manufacture, distribution and use of potentially toxic materials. These policies have led to large corporate multitiered testing programs. Even the most basic toxicology programs, whether conducted in-house or in an independent laboratory, require expenditures above testing costs for program management, interpretation and dissemination of the information derived. The quantity of information derived relates to expenditure. Quality, an equally important attribute, may not be as obvious. This paper will provide a management perspective on some of the key elements involved in data quality.

1. Address correspondence to: Dr. Judith K. Baldwin, Research and Environmental Health Division, Exxon Corporation, P.O. Box 235, East Millstone, New Jersey 08873.

2. Key words: evaluation, management, quality processes, standardization, uniformity.

3. Abbreviations: EPA, U.S. Environmental Protection Agency; GLP, Good Laboratory Practice.

DEFINING QUALITY IN AN INDUSTRIAL CONTEXT

Quality is often considered a nebulous concept without means of assessment or quantification. Unfortunately, this results in quality becoming a statement without a program for achievement. Quality is a process. That process requires the management of all aspects of operations that affect the final product. Management sets the objectives and policies which determine the quality standard of the work or product needed. Achieving a standard of quality within cost constraints is part of the process. Quality in research or manufacturing is achieved by maximizing the return on investment, i.e., deriving the most out of each dollar spent through improved operations and minimizing costs by reduction of waste of time, money and resources. Quality is increased as costs are reduced by identifying and preventing problems throughout the process.

The management principle of the greatest quality for the least cost is directly applicable to industrial research efforts. The creation of the quality assurance unit under Good Laboratory Practice (GLP) regulations (Food and Drug Administration, 1978; Environmental Protection Agency, 1983; Organization for Economic Cooperation and Development, 1982) was a recognition of toxicology as a manageable business with standards. The regulations emphasize the quality of conduct and documentation rather than the report content. The standards of documentation set by these regulations reflect the guidelines controlling other industries in which the public acceptance of information and services needs to be clearly demonstrated, such as banking (Goldman, 1985). In business terms, management expects the quality assurance process in toxicology testing to be proactive and cost effective by error prevention, performance assessment and compliance documentation.

IMPLEMENTING QUALITY IN INDUSTRIAL RESEARCH

Industrial management concerned with high quality standards and corporate toxics policy has set into place quality assurance units. Compliance with GLP regulations is often cited as a minimum standard for all studies. The strong emphasis on documentation and tracking inherent in GLP regulations was recognized as a useful starting point for all study records. Likewise, the function of the industrial quality assurance unit begins, but usually does not end, with the GLP regulations. These regulations specify that the quality assurance unit consists of qualified individuals reporting to the highest levels of management. Quality assurance professionals are responsible for tracking the entire program through the master schedule and observing and evaluating both process and product.

All of the elements of production are recognized by the GLP regulations. These include facilities, equipment, maintenance, training, record keeping, storage, standardization of operations and completeness and conformance of the product—the study report (Food and Drug Administration, 1978; Environmental Protection Agency, 1983; Organization for Economic Cooperation and Development, 1982).

Toxicological testing is too costly in terms of capital and resources to allow for production of substandard reports or flawed studies. Unfortunately, unless there is evidence of absolute fraud, information from poorly conducted studies is seldom disregarded. The Environmental Protection Agency (EPA) considers studies not conducted in compliance with GLPs to be unreliable for purposes of demonstration of no risk, while reserving the discretionary right to acknowledge noncompliant studies (that is, subminimal standard studies) for purposes of showing adverse effects (Environmental Protection Agency, 1983). The low rejection rate for large studies is based on the prohibitive costs of repeating studies or the undesirable consequences of poor data. Management plans for proper conduct rather than face the prospects of early termination, production of expensive but unreliable data or, worse yet, showing adverse effects that may or may not be attributable to the material under test.

Industrial management cannot afford quality assurance functions that evaluate only product. Identifying poor studies at the report stage is too late to minimize losses by termination of the study. It is poor study conduct, not the use of quality assurance, that generates most added toxicology costs. Much like fixing "lemons," identification of erroneous data points in a report does nothing but cause tables to be rewritten. Poor documentation confounds interpretation. Toxicologists are forced into positions of having to make conclusions based on poor data in much the same way that pathologists may be expected to read around autolysis or disease. It is a more effective use of resources to assure research quality by providing process quality under cost effective conditions leading to an acceptable product and reliable, useful data.

Quality is not quantified by the number of report errors identified and corrected. Quantification comes instead in the reduction of errors by operational improvements. Quality improvements are seen in toxicology by planning for quality, providing process quality, and preventive action.

Because of the unique position of industrial quality assurance units in the organizational structure, they are expected to provide for quality in each step. It is at each step that quality must be quantified in terms of reductions.

PLANNING FOR QUALITY

During the planning phases, protocols and contracts are reviewed for compliance, clarity of objectives and details sufficient to meet objectives. Questions are asked such as, does an "n" of 50 significantly improve statistical power over an "n" of 40? Is single caging worth the expenditure to enhance individual observations and reduce losses from cannibalism? Has the method of determining test material concentrations been clearly identified? Will the method chosen produce sufficiently accurate and precise values to determine actual exposure? Will there be enough variation in target concentrations to allow for a less precise analytical method? Have the acceptable control performance values been determined so that test results can be clearly validated or invalidated during the course of the study? Have identifiable milestones of performance over the course of the study been determined and documented so that studies with little chance of producing valid results may be terminated at 6, 12 or even 24 months? It is hard for scientists to realize that management has the responsibility for preventing losses even if it means stopping a $100,000 study after $98,000 has been spent. The concept of taking a one-time loss rather than spending another $10,000 fixing a flawed study is one which is difficult for scientists who have committed so much personal effort.

Another aspect of quality planning includes an assessment of chances for success. Can the laboratory conduct 100 enzyme determinations in an eight-hour period without introducing zeitgeists (sampling errors introduced by diurnal variations) or instrument-related bias? Have data recording systems been clearly defined? Are record forms or computer systems tested in place before the study starts? Does every person in the study team understand how to record data such as the number of decimal places, time of day, accurate units, and proper use of paginated titled forms? Actual confirmation of the soundness of data recording systems avoids the use of data recorded on paper towels.

The protocol review and study planning phase examine key study operations to make certain that they proceed as scheduled. It is at this time that quality assurance selects and schedules the phases to be inspected as part of their quality assurance plan. Some programs conducted within a single facility are repetitive and conducted frequently enough to permit a randomized selection of study elements for review. The randomized selections provide for a total operations overview over a period of time. Long-term studies or single, contracted studies are not properly assessed by that method; rather, a majority of phases are assessed at regularly scheduled intervals. Regardless of the inspection schedule, the protocol, standard operating procedures and GLPs are the standards by which study conduct will be evaluated at the time points necessary to maintain and protect quality.

INSPECTING FOR QUALITY

The most basic principle of quality inspection is conformance to standards of all phases of conduct so that all aspects of data, including observations, fit within acceptable tolerances. If the key determinant of toxicity is evaluation of dermal carcinogenic potential, then observations must be made on all animals at regularly scheduled, documented intervals throughout the course of the study. Obviously this is a repeated inspectional procedure. It has been our experience that a quarterly verification usually identifies errors in data recording or changes in observation procedure that are likely to lead to a loss of precision.

In dermal carcinogenicity studies, a quarterly verification of animal identity, mortality and tumor incidence by 100% verification (British Standards Institution, 1979) of data against the animals provides important information. For example, are the positive controls exhibiting tumors at the same rate normally expected, or is the rate elevated indicating infection or the need for improved husbandry practices? Early mortality resulting from those conditions precludes tumor development in the test groups. Is the level of moribund sacrifice different for tumor-bearing animals versus those without tumors, thus introducing statistical bias? Do animals die shortly after the first documentation of tumor development, indicating that observational frequency may be declining? Are there any other conditions which may affect study outcome, such as unequal exposure to fluorescent lighting, irritation sufficient to influence tumor yield, or evidence of environmental stress factors which may affect the immunological profile of the test model? This information is necessary in order to make determinations on study termination. The consequences of continuing a study without confidence that it meets standards range from the cost in marketing losses that a false positive result would cause to liabilities arising from false negative results.

Quarterly inspections of process and data quality also shorten the time to issuance of a final report. This is because only the data generated in the period since the last quarterly inspection need be checked for accuracy. All previously generated data will have already been verified. Therefore, seven-eighths of the in-life data are ready for incorporation into the report immediately upon study termination.

Having accurate data at the end of the in-life portion of the study provides a base for assessing quality in the next portion of the study—pathology. The incidence of in-life tumors and the number examined by the pathologist indicate the care taken in histopathological preparation. The in-life tumor number is usually lower than the number found by histopathological evaluation. This provides the first check that all lesions observed in-life have been accounted for. The quality of histopathological evaluation is judged by a performance standard related to the study endpoints. This is determined by statistical comparison for degree of detail and consistency of reported incidences of three selected findings in multiple negative control groups. These negative control groups can either be nested within the program or across programs conducted within a reasonable time period.

If inconsistencies are found, the cost of slide reevaluation is justified. Following review of a second or possibly third opinion, an appropriate evaluation is made. A pathologist found to be inconsistent with regard to degree of detail or diagnosis may then be required to pass a pathology service validation assessment before further participation. Since the data elements leading to the pathologist's report have been evaluated for quality, the report review becomes a simple check that all data were clearly, completely and consistently reported.

ACHIEVING UNIFORMITY OF QUALITY

Other types of chronic studies have different key endpoints, such as test material exposure determinations and completeness of tissue harvest. These endpoints require frequent inspections and well-planned quality assessment. Regardless of study type and specific endpoints, well-conducted assessment programs provide a unified overview of the many facets that simultaneously contribute to the quality level of the study. The findings of each phase or operational inspection are considered for their effect on the quality of the whole study. For example, were a number of small, seemingly insignificant errors found in dose calculations, preparation and administration, reflecting a larger problem in poor training or lack of attention to detail? This is more alarming than a single misdosing occurring in a lifetime study. Small repeated errors lead to a higher overall error rate than does a single mishap.

Assessments are made by each inspector against recognizable standards or according to previously agreed-upon specifications so that uniformity is achieved. Inspections are made on a continuum. When consistency of operation is important to conduct quality, a number of short, repetitive inspections are made by one or two inspectors. If different staff members conduct separate inspections, each inspection report is reviewed against the previous records and discussed. The number and degree of errors detected and subsequent corrections are assessed for unnecessary repetitions. Thus the different aspects of study conduct or disciplines employed are reviewed at the point of their impact upon the study and in relation to study quality by either a single evaluator or an identified unit working in concert.

PREVENTING PROBLEMS

The real test of the ability to manage for quality comes as problems or potential problems are identified. Error estimation is not enough. Management also expects appropriate solutions to problems and adjustments necessary to prevent potential error sources. Therefore, quality evaluation reports must identify errors thoroughly and present possible strategies for solution to prevent future repetitions. Serious problems must be communicated to management in a timely and useful fashion. Management needs precise evaluations to act appropriately and quickly. Although audit reports contain all findings, communication occurs on other levels to expedite corrective actions. Less severe process errors and potential problems are communicated at the staff level for immediate, on-the-spot correction. Serious problems are referred immediately to the study director for resolution. If resolution is not achievable or implemented soon enough to prevent further deterioration of quality, management must make decisions to terminate or refocus resources or commit further funding to achieve the goal of producing desirable data.

In the past, the timeliness and interaction between the evaluator and the evaluated was the subject of much debate. Once practice standards were adopted and management performance goals were set, each has seen a commonality of purpose.

QUANTIFYING COSTS

How much does all of this evaluation cost? Just as management defines the depth and scope of the test program by budgetary allowance, management is also interested in evaluation costs. These are not quality costs. It has been stated that quality is free because it is conformance to a standard of performance set by management (Crosby, 1979). It is nonconformance to standards that costs. Of course, evaluation of conformance, a function of doing business, has some associated costs. Just as how many tests are needed and how many tissues shall be examined and how many different statistical analyses are worthwhile are appropriate questions, so is how much evaluation. Inspection of 100% of the data points may make management uneasy. This is easily cured by a reduction to 10%, which has been traditionally acceptable. A more useful tool for evaluation is statistically based auditing (British Standards Institution, 1979; Hoover and Baldwin, 1984; Hoover and Baldwin, 1985), which predicts data accuracy within confidence ranges using a sample of considerably less than 10% for data arrays larger than 2,000 points.

The principle of 10% inspection has some pitfalls. Management is responsible for liabilities associated with nonconformance. Mutagenicity assays, which are relatively inexpensive short-term tests, often have little emphasis placed on the evaluation of their conduct. Unacceptable data or reports merely signal the need for repeating a study. Unfortunately, a single so-called "cheap study" with false results, whose errors would have been easily found upon evaluation, may not be evaluated under the "look at the every tenth study" inspection process. This could ultimately prove exceedingly costly in terms of unnecessary actions, missed reporting and even penalties; any saving would be unreal in the extreme.

CONCLUSION

Basically, the management of quality in toxicology is no different nor more costly than management of quality in any other endeavor. Management defines the standards, sets the goals, puts the resources at the disposal of the production units, and evaluates process, operations and products. The benefit of these evaluations and corrective measures, when necessary, is seen when study data are saved rather than fixed. While costs are associated with quality assurance, its appropriate use results in studies being conducted properly and reported accurately the first time, providing assurance to the user that the information is valuable and useful in determining hazards that may be appropriately used in risk assessment. Indeed, it must be viewed as a necessary part of the cost of doing business and not as something separate and optional when conducting laboratory studies.

REFERENCES

BRITISH STANDARDS INSTITUTION. (1979). Guide to the Use of British Standard 6001, Sampling Procedures and Tables of Inspection by Attributes.
CROSBY, PHILLIP B. (1979). Quality Is Free. McGraw Hill, New York.
ENVIRONMENTAL PROTECTION AGENCY. (1983). Toxic Substances Control; Good Laboratory Practice Standards. Final Rule. Fed. Reg. 48(230):53922–53944, November 19.
FOOD AND DRUG ADMINISTRATION. (1978). Nonclinical Laboratory Studies:

Good Laboratory Practice Regulations. Fed. Reg. 43(247):59985–60025, December 22.

GOLDMAN, DEXTER S. (1985). The EPA's Quality Assurance Program for Pesticides and Toxic Substances and its application to Laboratories in OECD countries. Presented at the 14th International Meeting on Good Laboratory Practice, Cambridge, England, April 1-3.

HOOVER, B. K. and BALDWIN, J. K. (1984). Meeting the quality assurance challenges of the 1980s: team auditing by toxicologists and QA professionals. J. Am. Coll. Toxicol. 3:129–139.

HOOVER, B. K. and BALDWIN, J. K. (1985). Hard data for hard decisions. Presented at the 189th National Meeting, American Chemical Society, April 28-May 3.

ORGANIZATION FOR ECONOMIC COOPERATION AND DEVELOPMENT. (1982). Good Laboratory Practice in the Testing of Chemicals. Final Report of the Group of Experts on Good Laboratory Practice. Paris.

U.S. CONGRESS. (1976). Toxic Substances Control Act. Public Law 94-469, October 11.

NATIONAL TOXICOLOGY PROGRAM APPROACH TO MONITORING STUDY PERFORMANCE

Douglas W. Bristol
Toxicology Research and Testing Program
National Institute of Environmental Health Sciences
Research Triangle Park, North Carolina

ABSTRACT

The two management systems developed by the NTP to monitor study performance are a reflection of the size of the program (188 studies underway at 18 laboratories as of October 1, 1985), the interdisciplinary nature of toxicology research, and the provisions of government contracts. The first system involves a project management team approach which is led by the NTP Project Officer. The primary monitoring performed by the Project Officer is supported and amplified by the rest of the project management team, i.e., Chemical Managers (NTP study directors assigned for each chemical), Discipline Leaders, and Contract Officials. A separate quality assurance system provides input to the project management team and to NTP management through the conduct of GLP-compliance inspections and audits of studies in progress as well as retrospective data and report audits. Oversight and direction for the monitoring effort is provided by the NIEHS Toxicology and Research Testing Program management officials. The organization of NIEHS as well as the activities and interactions of the various members of the NTP project management and quality assurance teams are presented and discussed as they relate to the monitoring of study performance.

1. Address correspondence to: Dr. Douglas W. Bristol, Toxicology Research and Testing Program, N.I.E.H.S., P. O. Box 12233, Research Triangle Park, NC 27709.

2. Key words: management system, oversight, project management, quality assurance, study performance.

3. Abbreviations: CTEB, Carcinogenesis and Toxicology Evaluation Branch; ETU, Environmental Toxicology Unit; GAO, Government Accounting Office; GLP, Good Laboratory Practice; MA, Master Agreement; MAO, Master Agreement Order; NCTR, National Center for Toxicological Research; NIEHS, National Institute of Environmental Health Sciences; NIOSH, National Institute of Occupational Safety and Health; NTP, National Toxicology Program; OAM, Office of Administrative Management; Path QAS, Pathology Quality Assessment; PI, Principal Investigator; PO, Project Officer; PWG, Pathology Working Group; QA, Quality Assurance; RFP, Request for Proposals; SOPs, Standard Operating Procedures; TDMS, Toxicology Data Management System; TRTP, Toxicology Research and Testing Program.

INTRODUCTION

The National Toxicology Program (NTP) conducts scientific studies on chemicals of public health and regulatory concern in order to provide definitive documentation regarding their potential toxic effects. The specific types of studies performed on each chemical are designed to best answer the particular toxicologic interests identified and tailored to meet the special needs of regulatory and non-regulatory scientists. Collectively, the studies performed run the full gamut of modern-day toxicology. Thus, the NTP draws upon considerable scientific resources to perform the studies needed to accomplish its mission.

Performance standards have been developed over the years for conducting the most common and well-defined types of toxicity and carcinogenicity studies. These standards are documented in the NTP General Statement of Work for the Conduct of Acute, 14-Day Repeated-Dose, 90-Day Subchronic, and 2-Year Chronic Studies in Laboratory Animals (revised July 1984). This document is used in the process which identifies laboratories that are both interested in and capable of performing these "core" NTP studies under a Master Agreement (MA) with the National Institute of Environmental Health Sciences (NIEHS). This paper describes the organization of the NIEHS and the approach it uses to monitor studies performed at MA laboratories under the provisions of the NTP Statement of Work.

As of October 1, 1985, studies involving a total of 188 NTP chemicals were in various stages of conduct at 18 different MA laboratories. Because of the enormity and complexity of this program, the NTP uses two systems to monitor and evaluate the studies being performed; they are called the project management and quality assurance (QA) systems. The project management system focuses on all aspects of the MA laboratories' operations. It represents a team approach spearheaded by Project Officers, coordinated by program managers, and supported by Chemical Managers, Discipline Leaders, a Contracting Officer, and Contract Specialists. The QA system consists of Good Laboratory Practice (GLP) compliance inspections and data audits at laboratories, plus retrospective data and NTP Technical Report audits. The two systems interact and are coordinated so that they provide feedback to assure the quality of the work performed from both the scientific and the data integrity points of view.

ADMINISTRATION OF NTP

Most toxicologic evaluations of NTP chemicals are performed either in-house or under contract by NIEHS; however, some chemicals are evaluated by the National Institute of Occupational Safety and Health (NIOSH) or by the National Center for Toxicological Research (NCTR) when special interest and expertise are contributed by staff scientists at those institutions. At the NIEHS, the Toxicology Research and Testing Program (TRTP) administers the studies conducted on NTP chemicals from the time when individual chemicals are selected for evaluation to the publication of a NTP Technical Report.

The organization of the TRTP is shown in Figure 1. The QA Unit reports to the Director of TRTP. The Contracts Office provides support to TRTP through a team of Contract Specialists led by a Contracting Officer in the NIEHS Office of Administrative Management (OAM). Each of the four Branches shown in Figure 1 has distinct programmatic responsibilities and differs in the degree to which its resources are utilized for basic research, methods development and validation research, studies of NTP chemical effects, and direct support of NTP studies conducted at MA laboratories. The activities of the four TRTP Branches are coordinated by the TRTP Director and a TRTP Management Committee.

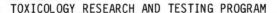

TOXICOLOGY RESEARCH AND TESTING PROGRAM

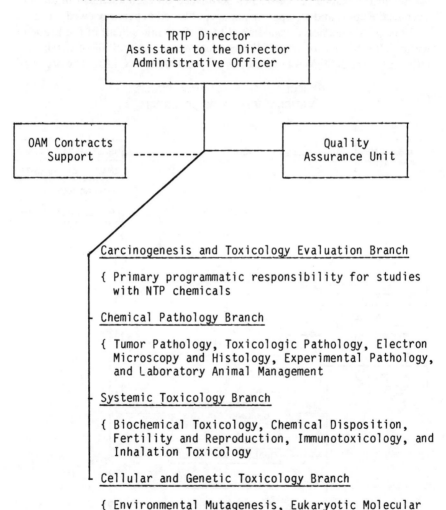

FIGURE 1. Organization of the Toxicology Research and Testing Program (TRTP).

The manner in which the TRTP Branches interact to accomplish the toxicological characterization of NTP chemicals is outlined schematically in Figure 2. The "core" toxicology and carcinogenicity studies performed under the NTP General Statement of Work by MA laboratories are represented by the central column, which includes prechronic (normally 14-day and 13-week) and chronic (2-year) studies. The Carcinogenesis and Toxicology Evaluation Branch (CTEB) has the primary administrative responsibility for these studies. Special or specific studies performed either in-house or under special contracts are represented by the left and right columns and are primarily the responsibility of other Branches in the TRTP. The goal of the overall evaluation process is to document the results of the studies performed on each chemical in an NTP Technical Report and as separate papers published in peer-reviewed journals.

While NTP chemicals are assigned to staff scientists in all of the Branches within TRTP, most of the NTP Chemical Managers and all of the Project Officers for the NTP MA laboratories are located in the CTEB. The organiza-

TOXICOLOGICAL EVALUATION PROCESS
NATIONAL TOXICOLOGY PROGRAM

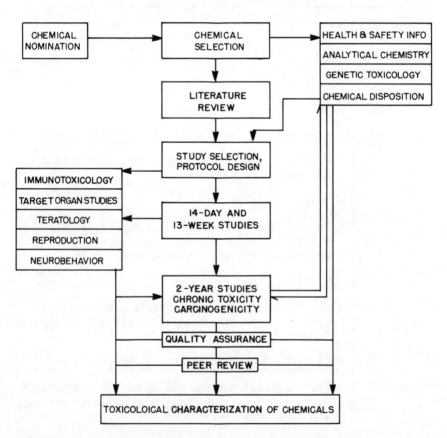

FIGURE 2. Schematic for studies performed with NTP chemicals.

tion of CTEB is shown in Figure 3. The functional structure of the Branch enables this group of about 25 full-time senior staff to coordinate the simultaneous study of over 300 NTP chemicals, 188 of them at MA laboratories plus those for which studies are being designed or reported. Managers for Study Design, Study Performance, and Study Reporting facilitate and coordinate the efforts of Chemical Managers, Project Officers, and Discipline Leaders throughout NTP in their respective areas of responsibility and inform the CTEB Chief of progress, changes made or needed, and problems encountered. In particular, the Manager of Study Performance ensures that standards are

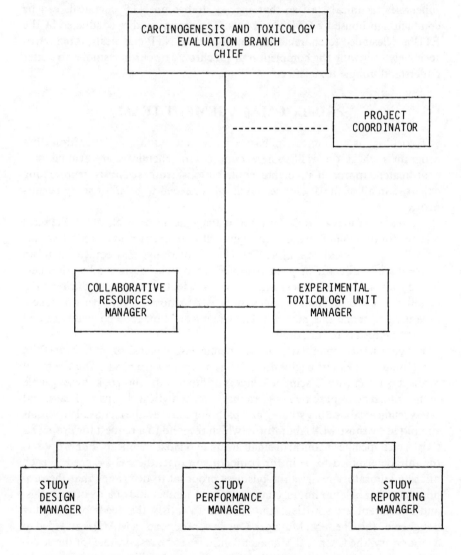

FIGURE 3. Functional organization chart for Carcinogenesis and Toxicology Evaluation Branch.

applied to studies conducted by NTP MA laboratories in a uniform and consistent manner. The Manager for Collaborative Resources oversees several functions, including: chemical procurement; all aspects of analytical chemistry and chemical health and safety protocol development; Discipline Leader activity in the areas of Chemistry and Health and Safety; and liaison between the TRTP and the Contracts Management Office through a Collaborative Services Section for the updating of the NTP General Statement of Work, award of MAs, and award of MAOs for the actual testing of chemicals. The Manager of the Experimental Toxicology Unit (ETU) maintains research facilities and supervises technical staff so that special studies on NTP chemicals can be conducted in-house by CTEB scientists. The special studies conducted by the ETU are designed to characterize the toxicity of NTP chemicals, often retrospectively following the completion of prechronic or chronic studies to better understand unique toxic effects.

PROJECT MANAGEMENT TEAM

Toxicology is an interdisciplinary science that requires collaboration. In a program such as the NTP where hundreds of chemicals are evaluated, a coordinated approach involving contributions from scientists representing expertise in all of the disciplines involved is needed to monitor study performance.

Chemical Manager Role. Project management for each NTP chemical selected for toxicologic evaluation begins with the assignment of a Staff Scientist called a Chemical Manager. The Chemical Manager is equivalent to an internal study director or principal investigator who designs all studies performed on a given chemical and provides scientific oversight during their conduct. The project management system used to monitor study performance is organized to make this possible. The Chemical Manager also evaluates and reports the results of the studies.

The coordinated interaction of the Chemical Manager, Project Officer (PO), and Discipline Leaders begins during the contract award phase. The Chemical Manager, along with Discipline Leaders or other staff who are knowledgeable in the critical areas of toxicology, animal care, analytical chemistry, health and safety, clinical laboratory studies, and pathology, review the technical proposals submitted by those MA laboratories which respond to a request for proposals (RFP) on a specific chemical or small group of related chemicals. For proposals that are determined to be in the competitive range, the PO assigned to each offering laboratory reviews the business proposal to determine that the proposed number of labor hours, labor-hour mix, number and quality of materials, and equipment are sufficient and suitable to satisfy the needs of the study designed by the Chemical Manager. Once a contract (i.e., a MAO) is awarded to a laboratory, the Chemical Manager continues to be responsible for the scientific aspects of the study, but the primary responsibility for managing the technical, contractual aspects of study performance shifts from the Chemical Manager to the PO.

Project Office Role. In each contract awarded to a MA laboratory, the responsibilities and limitations of a PO's authority are clearly stated. An example taken from the special provisions section of a recently awarded contract follows:

The Project Officer is responsible for: (1) monitoring the Contractor's technical progress, including the surveillance and assessment of performance and recommending to the Contracting Officer changes in requirements; (2) interpreting Scope of Work; (3) performing technical evaluation as required; (4) performing technical inspections and acceptances required by this Master Agreement Order; and (5) assisting the Contractor in the resolution of technical problems encountered during performance. *The Contracting Officer is responsible for directing or negotiating any changes in terms, conditions, or amounts cited in the Master Agreement Order.*

For guidance from the Project Officer to the Contractor to be valid, it must: (1) be consistent with the description of work set forth in this Master Agreement Order; (2) not constitute new assignment of work or change to the expressed terms, conditions, or specifications incorporated into this Master Agreement Order; (3) not constitute a basis for an extension to the period of performance or Master Agreement Order delivery schedule; (4) not constitute a basis for any increase in the Master Agreement Order fee and/or cost.

In the course of carrying out these broadly-stated responsibilities which emanate from Government acquisition regulations, the NTP project management system requires that the PO does not act alone, but rather serves as the NTP's focal point for interaction with the MA laboratory. The PO evaluates information about the status of NTP studies performed at a contract laboratory continuously. When studies proceed ideally, i.e., without incident and on schedule, the extent of interaction by the PO with both contractor and NTP staff is limited to routine inspections, evaluations of progress, and review of reports. However, when unexpected results or technical problems are encountered during the conduct of a study, the PO is obliged to inform the Chemical Manager, Discipline Leaders, the CTEB Manager of Study Performance, and the Contract Specialist so that a proper response and course of action are developed. The PO must look in particular to the Chemical Manager for oversight guidance so that the goals of the original study design are not thwarted. The Chemical Manager will assess the impact with the PO, the Manager for Study Design, Study Performance, or Study Reporting, Discipline Leaders, and other NIEHS experts, as needed. Once a proper course of action has been determined, the PO works with the Contract Specialist and with the MA laboratory to implement the decisions made as quickly as needed. Thus, the PO serves as an interface between NTP project management staff and MA laboratory personnel.

The NTP's project management system approach to monitoring study performance encourages and requires that Chemical Managers and other NTP staff have direct contact with MA laboratory staff; however, changes to a particular study cannot be made unless they are processed through the responsible PO. The PO assigned to monitor the MAOs awarded to a laboratory and the Principal Investigator (PI) for each NTP contract at that laboratory must work with their respective contract offices to accomplish the proper administration of the contract requirements. This approach helps to avoid the problem of having too many individuals making important decisions in isolation.

Contracting Officer Role. The Contracting Officer is the government representative responsible for directing or negotiating any changes in the terms, conditions, or amounts cited in each MAO awarded to a contract laboratory. The Contracting Officer is assisted in carrying out this responsibility by Contract Specialists who are assigned to administer the contracts at one or more MA laboratories.

Both the PO and the MA laboratory are required to keep the Contract Specialist informed of technical progress and problems so that, if changes to a study are needed, they can be made using proper administrative procedures. In effect, this requirement provides administrative oversight as well as formal documentation of steps taken by NTP staff to monitor the technical aspects and progress of studies.

Discipline Leader Role. Discipline Leaders are experts in each of the various scientific areas which contribute to the conduct of NTP studies. The NTP identifies scientific experts among the TRTP senior staff to shoulder scientific oversight responsibility for the following discipline areas: Animal Care, Biostatistics, Chemistry, Computer Data Management, Health and Safety, Anatomical Pathology, Clinical Pathology, Quality Assurance, and Toxicology.

From the point of view of monitoring study performance, Discipline Leaders have two key responsibilities. First, they establish and maintain standards for the organization and conduct of studies as described in the NTP General Statement of Work. Second, they actively assist all POs and Chemical Managers in monitoring study performance through a variety of activities. These include participation in Annual Program Reviews and special site visits conducted at MA laboratories, review of monthly progress and special reports, assessment of histopathology quality, review of qualifications associated with proposed changes in key personnel staff at MA laboratories, and consultation as needed to evaluate performance or resolve technical issues of study conduct. The contributions of Discipline Leaders, combined with those of Chemical Managers and POs, ensure that NTP studies are conducted in accordance with state-of-the-art practices that meet the scientific needs for each NTP chemical under study.

Manager of Study Performance, CTEB Role. Because NTP studies are conducted at about 18 MA laboratories representing different levels of effort, approximately 12 POs with responsibility for from 1 to 3 laboratories are needed to monitor study performance. While the authority for all technical monitoring of a given MA laboratory is vested in the assigned PO, the responsibility for oversight of monitoring activities at all MA laboratories is given to the CTEB Manager of Study Performance. This individual coordinates, facilitates, and oversees activities of the project management team, especially those of POs. Responsibilities for this position include:

1. Chair a Monthly Project Officer Meeting where MA laboratory progress is reviewed and technical or contractual issues which impact on monitoring are discussed and resolved. While POs, the Contracting Officer, and a representative from Collaborative Services attend this meeting regularly, Discipline Leaders and other NTP staff attend on an *ad hoc* basis to discuss specific issues.
2. Participate in TRTP Quarterly Toxicology Studies Status Meetings where reports are presented covering progress of all activities associated with testing NTP chemicals from selection through reporting.
3. Organize and conduct PO/PI meetings as needed.
4. Develop or clarify policy and procedures within NIEHS that influence monitoring of study performance.
5. Maintain a PO handbook and schedule for Annual Program Reviews; provide training and support to newly assigned POs.
6. Review requests for contract modifications to ensure that they are necessary and within scope.
7. Represent NTP management as part of the project management team during conduct of Annual Program Reviews at MA laboratories.
8. Review PO Site Visit and Annual Program Review reports.
9. Assure completion of critical action items and assist POs in the resolution of unusual or particularly complex problems.
10. Inform the CTEB Chief about the overall status of study performance and monitoring at all MA laboratories.

By performing the above activities the Manager of Study Performance has frequent contact with NTP project management team members, NIEHS management, and MA laboratories. This provides an oversight perspective that cannot be obtained by other members of the project management team. The overall responsibility of this position is to utilize the contact and perspective gained to ensure that NTP studies are monitored effectively, uniformly, and consistently at all MA laboratories.

PROJECT MANAGEMENT ACTIVITIES

Studies of NTP chemicals at MA laboratories proceed in three basic stages: (1) prestudy organization, (2) an in-life phase, and (3) a post-life, histopathologic evaluation phase. A MAO may be awarded for the conduct of prechronic studies only (about 20 months for completion), for chronic studies only (about 3 years for completion), or for both prechronic and chronic studies (about 5 to 6 years for completion). Thus, the NTP project management system must monitor not only numerous studies, but also studies that are at different stages of conduct. Accordingly, while the Chemical Manager and PO are responsible for monitoring individual studies closely, the focus of Discipline Leaders and the PO is on all aspects of a MA laboratory's performance. This section outlines and highlights how the NTP project management system approaches the monitoring of study performance.

Prestudy Activities. The PO assigned to a MA laboratory is familiar with both the organization of the laboratory and the requirements for testing of a NTP chemical so that once a MAO is awarded, prestudy activities can begin. The Technical Proposal of the successful offeror is incorporated into the Statement of Work of the MAO. While it includes a general outline for the studies to be performed, the first order of business for the PO and PI (or Study Director at the MA laboratory) is to develop a detailed schedule of activities for the required studies. To accomplish this step, the NTP uses a computerized tracking system called the NTP Chemical Status Report for Laboratories, one of many reports available on a management system called CHEMTRACK. The Chemical Status Report organizes tracking information, by chemical, for each separate MA laboratory. A summary of this system is shown in Figure 4.

Fields 1 through 3 contain information that is incorporated selectively into other reports produced by CHEMTRACK, such as the NTP Management Status Report. Field 4 is specially designed for use by the PI, PO, and other NTP staff; this field is often used to prompt upcoming activities, to track special or nonroutine activities not included in Field 3 of the report, or to provide specific information about delays and problems. The PO is required to update all information in this report monthly. This is accomplished by way of mail and telephone conversations between the PO and the PI for each MA laboratory. It provides an effective mechanism for tracking the current progress of each study in considerable detail. It also serves as an effective vehicle for the PO and PI to discuss specific problems encountered; over a period of time, patterns show up which help the PO and PI to identify system problems affecting more than one study so that they can be addressed and resolved.

A subset of Field 3, which shows all of the events scheduled for conduct of a subchronic (90-day) study, is presented in Figure 5. Original dates, once entered into on the computer tracking system, are not changed unless a study needs to be restarted. Current dates are converted from estimated (E) to actual (A) as they are accomplished.

Close review of Figure 5 reveals that the chemical was received three days ahead of schedule and less than two weeks after the contract was formally awarded. By or at the time the contract was awarded, the NTP supplied the MA laboratory with analytical methods for analysis of the "bulk" chemical as well as for analysis of the concentration of the chemical in vehicle (c/v) mixture. In this case, the initial analyses to confirm both the identity and the purity of the

NTP CHEMICAL STATUS REPORT FOR LABORATORIES

Field 1. Information about study design, Chemical Manager, MA Laboratory, code numbers
Field 2. Comments section covering each phase, e.g., special studies, responsible pathologist
Field 3. Original and current dates (estimated or actual), by species, for each study event from contract award through contract closeout
Field 4. Special comments section for prompts or timely information

FIGURE 4. Organization of the NTP Chemical Status Report for Laboratories.

DATES SCHEDULED FOR A SUBCHRONIC STUDY

	RATS: FISCHER 344 (FC)		MICE: B6C3F1 (FCRF)	
	Original	Current	Original	Current
Contract Award:	02/01/85	02/15/85A	02/01/85	02/15/85A
Chemical Recd at Lab:	03/01/85	02/27/85A	03/01/85	02/27/85A
1st Bulk Anl Compl:	03/29/85	03/25/85A	03/29/85	03/25/85A
C/V Method Validated:	04/05/85	04/10/85A	04/05/85	04/10/85A
Subch Doses Rec'd PO:	NA	NA	NA	NA
Lab Protocol Apprvd:	04/16/85	04/26/85A	04/30/85	05/03/85A
Animals Ordered NTP:	04/18/85	04/18/85A	05/02/85	05/02/85A
Subch Start Date:	04/30/85	04/30/85A	05/14/85	05/14/85A
Subch Report Sent PO:	01/28/86	11/21/85E	02/11/86	12/05/85E
Subch Path Mat'l->QAS:	01/28/86	11/21/85E	02/11/86	12/05/85E
QAS Completed->PWG:		04/00/86E		04/00/86E
PWG Meeting Date:		05/00/86E		05/00/86E
SC PWG RPT, SL->LAB:				
Subch PWG Approval:		05/00/86E		05/00/86E

FIGURE 5. Subset of Field 3 from the chemical status report for laboratories; contract awarded for subchronic (90-day) and chronic studies.

chemical were performed without complication. The method for analysis of the c/v dosage mixtures was also validated (including review of the results by the NTP Discipline Leader for Chemistry) approximately on schedule.

While the chemistry work was being performed, the PO and PI were keeping each other informed so that the animal order could be confirmed and the Good Laboratory Practice (GLP) study protocol could be developed. For NTP studies, a separate GLP study protocol is written for each species by the MA laboratory and sent to the PO. The PO is responsible for sponsor approval, but, before signing, submits the protocol to the Chemical Manager for the study as well as to any other NTP staff who can provide significant input for formal review. For the study in rats shown in Figure 5, the PO sent the original protocol back to the PI for revision and resubmission prior to approval. This review step is very important because the GLP protocol provides a roadmap for the conduct of the study to be performed. It includes review of the Standard Operating Procedures (SOPs) that are incorporated into the protocol by reference. The PO will often invest additional time for review of the first protocol submitted when studies of a chemical are to be performed using staggered start dates for two species of rodents, because changes made will also apply to the preparation of the second protocol. The small delays encountered in approval of the GLP study protocols shown in Figure 5 did not interfere with either the receipt of animals as arranged by the PO and the Discipline Leader for Animal Care, or with the study start. The rest of the dates entered for events in Figure 5 relate to the in-life and histopathology phases of the studies. From the original dates projected and the current dates estimated at the last update, it seems that the current, estimated dates for pathology quality assessment (Path QAS) and peer review by a Pathology Working Group (PWG) could be rescheduled so that these subchronic studies can be completed ahead of schedule.

The Chemical Status Report not only provides the PO and the PI with an effective tool for organizing and tracking the technical aspects of studies performed on each NTP chemical, but it also enables the different members of the NTP project management team to coordinate interdependent activities and to utilize internal resources and time effectively. The data entered into the CHEMTRACK computer system for each chemical at each laboratory provide another report that gives an overview of activities for an entire MA laboratory. This report, called the Calendar of Deliverables for Laboratories or Deliv-cal, provides a chronological listing of important, future events and deliverables associated with the conduct of studies performed on all NTP chemicals under contracts awarded to each MA laboratory. It includes entries for originally projected dates, currently projected dates, chemical name, species, Chemical Manager name, and the name for each event or deliverable being tracked. Deliv-cal enables the PO to assess the status of current and future activities associated with all studies at a single MA laboratory. Discussion of this information with the PI provides a mechanism to spot potential problems in advance, to plan the start of newly awarded studies, or to reschedule events and deliverables as needed. The combined information available from the Chemical Status Report and Deliv-cal provides the NTP project management team with detailed information on the status of individual studies as well as a profile of all studies being performed at each MA laboratory.

One important prestudy-phase activity that is not tracked by computer is the site visit performed by NTP staff prior to the start of the first study associated with a NTP chemical. The PO arranges for the Chemical Manager who designed the studies to visit the MA laboratory either when the GLP study protocols are being written or at the time that animals are first exposed to the chemical. This visit enables the Chemical Manager to discuss the goals and special aspects of each study directly with the personnel responsible for its conduct. The Chemical Manager and PO can inspect the animals and facilities, review study-specific procedures, or provide information regarding special techniques or observations to be made, if necessary. The PO can also arrange to have a NTP expert participate in the study start site visit as needed; recently, the expert on dermal studies has made several such visits to provide instructions and assure that skin-painting techniques are uniform across all MA laboratories and in accord with revised guidelines given in the July 1984 Statement of Work. There are many benefits gained from prestudy site visits, and this practice will be continued.

In-life Activities. The in-life phase of a NTP study begins when the first animals are exposed to the chemical being evaluated. From this point to completion of the study, the NTP project management team uses several different tools for monitoring and evaluating performance. The PO, being primarily responsible for these functions, has frequent contact with the PI and other MA laboratory staff. One cardinal rule that applies to the interaction between the PO and the PI is that verbal communications must be frank and frequent so that surprises never appear in a monthly progress report or in any other report submitted by the MA laboratory. The Chemical Status Report provides a template for detailed assessment of study progress on a monthly basis. The update is scheduled to precede submission of the Monthly Progress Report from the MA laboratory so that the information is current and detailed.

The Monthly Progress Report is organized by sections and multiple copies are submitted so that it can be reviewed not only by the PO, but also by each Discipline Leader. This timely report is not subjected to QA review. It contains ten sections, each of which provides information regarding the current status of progress in one of the following discipline areas: Bioassay Status Summary, Animal Care, Chemistry, Toxicology, Health and Safety, Administration, Pathology, Biostatistics, Quality Assurance, and Chemical Status Report. Other sections to track special activities can be added by the PO and PI, if needed. Further details regarding the format and requirements for each section of the Monthly Progress Report are given in the NTP General Statement of Work.

The NTP Discipline Leaders and Chemical Managers review their respective sections of the Monthly Progress Report and provide written comments back to the PO. The PO then serves as a focal point for sorting out information and communicating with the PI or other MA laboratory staff. On those occasions when it is best for a Discipline Leader or Chemical Manager to communicate directly with their MA laboratory counterparts, conference calls are arranged by the PO, or if the PO is not involved directly, a memorandum to document the business conducted is written by the caller and distributed to the PO and other NTP staff. The appropriate use of internal memoranda is an important mechanism for keeping project management team members informed about technical issues, and to help document progress.

The NTP management team members can also review data for each chronic study at any time by using the NIEHS computerized Toxicology Data Management System (TDMS). The MA laboratory accumulates data for animal weights, food or water consumption, clinical observations, animal removal information, and histopathologic evaluations (microscopic) directly using computer terminals and discs. Data, after review by study personnel, are transmitted to a mainframe computer for storage and entered into a reports system called the Experimental Status System for review by authorized personnel. The advantages to monitoring offered by this system include the more timely and independent evaluation of study data whenever needed by a Chemical Manager and a better opportunity for detailed technical monitoring by the PO, e.g., to determine if procedures are performed at the MA laboratory according to the schedule laid out in the GLP study protocol, or to review original body weight data.

The NTP project management team also reviews a variety of other reports submitted periodically or in connection with the completion of specific studies. Periodic reports include: Annual Narrative, Water Analysis, Animal Survival (weekly, gavage studies only), and Dosage Mix and Analysis Schedule Reports.

Reports unique to each study include: Special Study Report (e.g., clinical pathology, or sentinel animal serology reports), Interim Sacrifice Report, Final Study Report, or reports that are required as unique deliverables by the MAO awarded for studies of a particular chemical. For some special studies, samples are collected from animals being exposed at the MA laboratory and shipped to a second NTP contractor where they are analyzed. In such cases, the second laboratory submits a report to the MA laboratory and to NTP staff for review. Examples include sperm morphology and vaginal cytology evaluation, evaluation of rat urine samples for mutagenicity, and micronuclei examination. The primary responsibility for monitoring work performed by the second contract laboratory is vested in the PO within TRTP who administers that contract. Monitoring assistance from the NTP project management staff is provided when requested by the PO.

The most active monitoring of study performance is achieved through the conduct of quarterly site visits and annual program reviews at MA laboratories. Details regarding the planning, conduct, and follow-up for an annual program review are provided in a PO Handbook that has been developed by CTEB staff. An earlier checklist for site visits and program reviews has been provided by Douglas et al. (1981).

The annual program review at each MA laboratory is planned and coordinated by the PO, and performed by a NTP project management team. It provides a comprehensive, on-site assessment of the status of NTP studies and all aspects of a MA laboratory's operations. During the two to three day review, Discipline Leaders, a Contract Specialist, the Manager of Study Performance, and other NTP staff, as needed, inspect the study animals, laboratory facilities, equipment, record keeping procedures, training files, compliance with GLP regulations, and safety practices. The NTP project management team members visit with their MA laboratory counterparts about technical aspects of laboratory procedures, operations, equipment, staffing, and management. They review protocols, SOPs, and study records to see that all technical aspects are in compliance with the MAO awarded for each different study as well as with the NTP General Statement of Work. These reviews are thorough and result in a wide variety of action items and recommendations which apply not only to the MA laboratory, but also to NTP staff as appropriate. It is the responsibility of the PO to follow all action items through to their completion and resolution during the upcoming year.

The PO and the PI prepare an annual program review briefing package which is distributed to NTP participants four weeks before the review. In addition to organizational information about the MA laboratory and the conduct of the annual program review, the briefing package contains: (1) information on the status and schedule of studies for each chemical, (2) method(s) used for animal identification, (3) the previous Annual Program Review Report and response from the MA laboratory, (4) site visit reports by the PO or other NTP staff since the last annual program review, (5) sections from the most recent Monthly Progress Report, and (6) information that deals with recent items of concern or interest. Separate copies of the most recent In-life QA Site Visit Report are also distributed to each NTP program review participant. About one to two weeks before the review, the PO conducts a pre-annual program review meeting attended by NTP staff (such as Chemical Managers) who can provide significant input into the meeting. The purpose of this meeting is to assess the currently perceived status of the MA laboratory and to identify any special needs that NTP participants have so that issues, problems, and progress can be evaluated during the annual program review. Following the meeting, the PO prepares a final agenda, by discipline area, and makes arrangements with the PI so that each NTP participant can meet with appropriate MA laboratory staff and cover important subject areas during the time-limited annual program review.

The annual program review usually starts with personnel introductions and a briefing. During the major portion of the review, the NTP participants inspect and discuss laboratory operations pertaining to NTP studies with the laboratory staff. During this phase of the review, the PO is responsible for facilitating and coordinating the activities of the NTP participants. Near the end of the review, the NTP participants meet in executive session. The PO coordinates the discussion of findings that are presented by each individual participant. The executive session is especially important in the assessment of problems or situations which have an impact on more than one discipline area and in the definition of action items and recommendations. The annual program review ends with a formal debriefing of the laboratory staff where findings, action items, and recommendations are enumerated by discipline area. The PO summarizes key findings, cites urgent action items, indicates where responsibility for the needed actions lies, and gives a timeframe for their completion.

The Annual Program Review report parallels the debriefing session. It is a complete statement of findings, action items, and recommendations for follow-up by the PO. It consists of a set of memoranda from each of the NTP review participants. The PO writes a cover memorandum which summarizes the action items in a manner that enables the MA laboratory to respond to each item and the NTP review participants to review each response in a straightforward manner. The PO sends the report to the CTEB Chief, through the Manager of Study Performance, for approval and then to the PI at the MA laboratory.

Quarterly site visits are less comprehensive than annual program reviews but are no less detailed. They are conducted by the PO, who may be assisted by project management team members when expertise is needed to deal with special problems or concerns. The main objectives of a quarterly site visit are to track the completion of action items, to assess the overall status of ongoing studies or laboratory operations, and to plan newly awarded studies. These visits are usually announced and last two to three days. They provide an opportunity to document the completion of action items or to indicate what further action is required to clear them. The quarterly PO site visits also involve inspections of animals, facilities, and procedures, as well as reviews of data, SOPs, schedules, and reports in preparation. The Site Visit Report is handled in the same way as an Annual Program Review Report.

Histopathology Phase Activities. This phase of a study begins with the scheduled necropsy of animals and ends with the submission of a Final Report by the MA laboratory. Details for the conduct of the various steps involved in histopathologic evaluation are provided in the Statement of Work. Histopathologic procedures are monitored and evaluated on-site by the PO and NTP pathologists during site visits and annual program reviews. During the past year, a policy was implemented in which the necropsy for each chronic study is attended by a representative from the NTP. NTP decided that the proper conduct of necropsies is so critical to the quality of each study that these special trips to MA laboratories are warranted.

As the histopathologic evaluations are completed for a study, materials (pathology narrative, computer tables of results, necropsy record forms, slides, blocks, and wet tissues) are submitted to the NTP Archives. The quality of these pathology materials is reviewed in a series of Path QAS steps. This process culminates in a PWG peer review of the histopathologic evaluations. This entire review process has been described by Boorman et al. (1985).

During the histopathology phase, pathology materials and study reports are received by NTP staff and support contractors. The PO, in effect, delegates responsibility for the evaluation and acceptance of these contractual deliverables to other members of the project management team. The PO remains responsible for assessing the technical progress of studies and the workload status at the MA laboratory. If deliverables are not acceptable and are returned to the MA laboratory, the PO must establish priorities and new schedules for their resubmission. It is very important that delays be projected using the Chemical Status Report and internal memoranda so that the interdependent schedules of the NTP project management system can be adjusted. While the PO performs tracking and coordinating activities, it is also important to keep the Contract Specialist informed so that proper contract administrative actions can be taken if serious problems are encountered during the completion of studies.

When post-PWG action is complete, the PO arranges for the remaining study records (paper records, microfiche copies, and computer disks), the remaining chemical, and any other materials to be sent to the various NTP Archives for proper storage or disposal. These items are inspected for acceptance. If they need to be returned to the MA laboratory for any reason, the PO coordinates activities for their final resubmission. When all technical and contractual work has been completed the contract is closed out by the PO and the Contracting Officer.

QUALITY ASSURANCE SYSTEM ACTIVITIES

The NTP QA system consists of a QA Unit which interacts with TRTP management and NTP project management system staff as described above. The major activities of the QA Unit are presented in this section.

The QA system is supported by two types of resource contracts which provide teams for: (1) QA Monitoring site visits to MA laboratories and (2) retrospective audits of data and reports at the NTP Archives. The NTP QA Unit presently consists of two senior staff who monitor and evaluate the work performed by its support contractors. It will be expanded during the coming year to include auditors with expertise in QA procedures for the review of toxicology, pathology, and chemistry data and reports. At the present time, these functions are being performed by NTP project management team members. When the TRTP QA unit is fully staffed it will conduct MA laboratory inspections and retrospective audits in addition to those performed now by support contractors only. This will provide the QA Unit with more detailed, first-hand knowledge that comes from performing these activities.

QA Monitoring at MA Laboratories. At the present time, the QA Unit staff participate in annual program reviews as the Discipline Leader for Quality Assurance. The focus of this activity is to assess the extent to which each MA laboratory is organized for and operating in compliance with GLP regulations. More detailed monitoring of MA laboratories is performed by QA contractor teams. These involve both GLP compliance inspections and detailed QA audits of study data. Support contractor QA data audits are targeted for studies that are likely to provide the best cross-section of a MA laboratory's operations at that point in time. They are scheduled so that the audit report will be available a few weeks prior to the annual program review conducted at each MA laboratory. Additional audits are scheduled as deemed necessary. The QA site visits provide feedback to the NTP project management staff regarding the current status of studies, laboratory organization, and compliance with GLP regulations. They give direction and emphasis to the technical monitoring performed by the PO and other members of the project management staff.

Retrospective Audits. Retrospective audits are performed by support contractor teams. The Audit Reports are reviewed and approved by NTP staff. This retrospective audit activity began in June 1983 and applied to all studies whose Technical Reports had not yet been published in final form. It also includes retrospective audits of studies performed on 32 chemicals for which NTP Technical Reports had already been peer reviewed, printed, and distributed, and which were identified by the NTP Executive Committee's Subcommittee on Data Audits as having potential impact on an agency's policy.

GAO REVIEW OF NTP'S OVERSIGHT OF CHEMICAL TESTING

From January 1984 to June 1985, the U.S. Government Accounting Office (GAO) assessed the adequacy of the NTP's oversight of its contract research activities. Prior to March 1982, most of those activities had been managed by a prime contractor. NTP files for 16 MA laboratories covering the period from July 1982 through June 1984 were reviewed; POs and other staff scientists were interviewed. The GAO performed a more detailed review of five laboratories that appeared to have some indication of problems to determine how corrective actions were taken. The more detailed review included discussions with contract laboratory staff as well as attendance at one Annual Program Review conducted by an NTP project management team. The GAO also reviewed NTP quality assurance reports for in-life and retrospective audits to assure that they were being performed and visited with four quality assurance support contractors to discuss and document how they carried out their responsibilities.

Full details of the review conducted by the GAO are contained in the report to the Chairman of the Subcommittee on Oversight and Investigations, Committee on Energy and Commerce, House of Representatives (1985). With respect to project management oversight of chemical testing by contractor laboratories, pages 17 and 18 of the GAO report included the following observations:

> NTP assumed full responsibility for project monitoring, reorganized its staff, initiated regular internal meetings to disucss and resolve common project management concerns, and began to establish new operating procedures for research oversight. All these changes help to ensure that problems occurring at contract laboratories are identified and resolved. Moreover, our review of NTP monitoring deocumentation in the 2-year period following NTP assumption of management responsibility for the oversight of testing contractors showed that NTP is following its established oversight policies and procedures in monitoring testing laboratories and is taking action to correct noted problems.

On page 24 of the report, the GAO observed that an increased emphasis on quality assurance activities has improved test reliability as follows:

> NTP's contracted live animal audits have provided additional assurance about the accuracy and reliability of tests while they are being conducted. It also has provided NTP with a more thorough means of identifying possible problems and, where such problems are identified, has enabled NTP to discontinue tests before additional work is performed. Similarly NTP's post-life data audits have resulted in NTP's identifying problems with completed tests and has provided a new means to anticipate and respond to possible concerns about tests' reliability and validity before issuing formal reports.

While it is clear from the GAO report that the NTP has organized itself effectively and is doing a thorough and professional job of monitoring studies performed by contract laboratories, it is also clear that a challenge to continue and to even improve upon its present efforts exists.

ACKNOWLEDGEMENTS

The author wishes to thank Dr. J. E. Huff for critical review and helpful suggestions made during the preparation of this paper as well as Ms. D. Galanides and Ms. L. F. Brammell for typing of the manuscript.

REFERENCES

BOORMAN, G. A., MONTGOMERY, C. A., JR., EUSTIS, S. L., WOLFE, M. J., McCONNELL, E. E. AND HARDISTY, J. F. (1985). Quality Assurance in Pathology for Rodent Carcinogenicity Studies. In: Handbook of Carcinogen Testing, H. A. Milman and E. K. Weisburger, ed. Noyes Publications, Park Ridge, NJ, pp. 345–357.

DOUGLAS, J. F., HAMM, T. E., JAMESON, C. W., MAHAR, H., STINSON, S. AND WHITMIRE, C. E. (1981). Monitoring Guidelines for the Conduct of Carcinogen Bioassays, U.S. Department of Health and Human Services, Public Health Service, National Institutes of Health, NIH Publication No. 81-1774, June 1981, National Toxicology Program, Technical Report Series No. 218. Available from National Technical Information Service, U.S. Dept. of Commerce, 5285 Port Royal Road, Springfield, VA 22161.

U.S. GENERAL ACCOUNTING OFFICE. (1985). Report: GAO/HRD-85-86. National Toxicology Program: Efforts to Improve Oversight of Contractors Testing Chemicals. June 28, 1985, Document Handling and Information Services Facility, P.O. Box 6015, Gaithersberg, MD 20877.

THE VALUE OF IN-LIFE AND RETROSPECTIVE DATA AUDITS

James E. Huff
National Institute of Environmental Health Sciences
National Toxicology Program
Research Triangle Park, North Carolina

ABSTRACT

Data audits are integral to the high standards of quality assurance. Good Laboratory Practice (GLP) regulations establish management responsibility for the proper conduct of nonclinical studies, whereas comprehensive data audits and active monitoring of ongoing experiments are the means of ensuring the integrity and quality of the study. Because of the impact of study results on public health issues relating to chemical toxicity and carcinogenicity, the data base upon which interpretive conclusions and decisions are based must be reconstructible.

To strengthen this view, the National Toxicology Program (NTP) uses a concentrated program of examining in full detail the experimental data—correspondence, records, reported findings, tissues/blocks/slides—from long-term toxicology and carcinogenesis studies conducted in laboratory rodents. Initial efforts emphasized retrospective evaluation of recently completed studies. Concomitantly, the Program decided not to issue formal conclusions or Technical Reports from any studies until a data audit was completed. Priorities were established to obviate delays in interpreting, evaluating, and announcing to the public these important data and conclusions. The decided priority guidelines for doing these data audits are: 1) studies on chemicals scheduled for public peer review where pathology data have been evaluated and Technical Reports are being drafted, 2) studies on chemicals for which Technical Reports were already written and approved by the NTP Board of Scientific Counselors Peer Review Panel but not yet printed, 3) studies on chemicals already printed and distributed as Technical Reports.

1. Address correspondence to: James E. Huff, Ph.D., N.I.E.H.S., N.T.P., P. O. Box 12233, Research Triangle Park, NC 27709.
2. Key words: carcinogenicity studies, in-life audits, retrospective audits, toxicology studies.
3. Abbreviations: GLP, Good Laboratory Practice; NTP, National Toxicology Program.

Audit procedures deal mainly with these eight aspects: 1) administrative information, 2) pretest animal data, 3) chemistry information, 4) dose preparation and administration, 5) environmental conditions (temperature, relative humidity, lighting, air changes), 6) in-life observations, 7) pathology, and 8) Technical Report. Of 110 completed and ongoing retrospective data audits, only one study has been judged inadequate for reporting. So far 11 laboratories have had one or more studies examined. Further, 25 ongoing studies have now received in-life data audits.

The scope of the effort is large and complex. To give some notion as to the involved magnitude, the Program has about 350 active ongoing studies, and for each chemical being investigated in two-year studies the experimental protocol involves exposing two species (usually rats and mice), both sexes in groups of 50-70 animals each, at 2 to 4 dose levels and controls. The resultant data divide into three major discipline areas: chemistry, toxicology, pathology.

The paramount logistical, technical, and scientific questions about the toxicology and carcinogenesis studies center on: 1) how much of the experimental data needs to be examined (audited) before the data can be deemed valid to support the conclusions and 2) how many/what type of discovered discrepancies need be found to potentially compromise a toxicology study? Answers to these remain subjective, and should flexibly reflect the nature of any problems observed and experience gained.

INTRODUCTION

Imagine all the people
living life in peace.

John Winston Lennon

From an historical perspective one benefic yet bleak episode that stunned our program was the disconcerting discovery that one of the 25 or so laboratories conducting several of our toxicology studies was not doing what many would consider patently obvious and necessary for good toxicology. Particularly disturbing was the awareness and eventual realization that our multiple, costly, and time-lengthening corrective actions were not successful. Immediately thereafter in early summer 1983, we instituted an encompassing activity of doing after-the-fact detailed reconstructions of completed experiments. We decided that the depth of these beginning data audits was essential and necessary. With the help of many staff, the overall scientific community, other federal agencies, industry, as well as stimulus from the Congress and the Government Accounting Office, we believe that the Program has gained considerably from this intense effort.

This paper concentrates on the status of what we have done and are doing with respect to in-life and retrospective data audits; gives some notion of the magnitude and direction of our past, present, and future efforts in this important area; and illustrates some decision making using information learned from retrospective data audits on our long-term toxicology and carcinogenesis studies.

BACKGROUND

audit: A methodical examination and review of
      a situation or condition [or toxicology experiments]
      concluding with a detailed report of findings.

After directing more efforts to making sure that the data results and reconstruction of experiments were adequate, guidelines were formulated for setting priorities in scheduling audits. The first priority was given to studies on chemicals scheduled for peer review in public meetings where pathology data have been evaluated and technical reports of the data were being drafted. The second priority comprised studies on chemicals for which technical reports had already been written and taken through the public peer review process, but had not yet been printed or distributed formally. The decision was made to attach lower priority for auditing these studies, since the data and conclusions were already known, and any significant public health issues would have been handled. The third priority was for studies on chemicals whose technical reports had been printed and distributed or made available to the scientific community that the NTP Executive Committee thought should be audited. In large part these priorities were established to keep new results of our recently completed studies flowing to the public.

A comprehensive audit includes a multitude of items designed to cover all important aspects of NTP studies. For instance, a typical experimental design for two-year toxicology and carcinogenesis studies includes both sexes of two rodent species, 60 animals/species/sex/group, 2 to 4 exposure groups in addition to controls, and a variety of specific endpoint studies.

In planning and doing actual audits on our studies, we assume no notions that the experiments were or were not indeed conducted properly. We initially separated the available files for examination into the general areas of chemistry, toxicology, and pathology. Any problems discovered or discrepancies observed from this disciplinary data sampling led to more in-depth investigations.

Accordingly, audit procedures deal mainly with eight aspects: 1) administrative information; 2) pretest animal data; 3) chemistry information; 4) dose preparation and administration; 5) environmental conditions (temperature, relative humidity, lighting, air changes); 6) in-life observations; 7) pathology; 8) Technical Report. Of the 110 ongoing and completed data audits on chemicals from several laboratories, only one study has been judged inadequate for reporting. So far 11 laboratories have had one or more studies examined.

In-life study audits have been accomplished at 12 laboratories, a number of other studies have been scheduled, and audit teams have visited and examined the chemistry support laboratories as well as the chemical repository. To conduct a single toxicology study in your own laboratory allows close supervision and complete daily control. Yet conducting many experiments at many locations adds other logistic, administrative, and scientific dimensions.

Because all records are open to public view, others are not only invited to evaluate our audit findings but will often do an independent audit of our archival data. This is good and this is proper. We learn much from this sharing and interactive process.

AUDIT FINDINGS

To give some idea regarding any problems or discrepancies that have been found and documented, four distinct and anonymous situations are described to illustrate the range of observations and to demonstrate the composite decision making. All findings are important; yet, in my opinion, the most critical is animal identification and the essentiality of being able to trace the recorded diagnosis from the technical report to the computer tables, to the PWG, to the pathology quality assessment, to the lesion on the slide, to the tissue block, to the organ/tissue in the bag, back to the animal. All labels and recorded information at each of these stages must correspond. If this cannot be done, then one has to make more difficult decisions. During site visits or audits of ongoing experiments, we emphasize these factors and expect to discover and correct early on any potential problems that could lead to confounding factors. This will be done on all ongoing studies; currently, however, retrospective audits on studies most often designed and monitored in-life by others are being examined with priority by our audit teams. Most ongoing and planned studies reflect recent designs and are monitored by program staff; in-life audits are accomplished during program site visits and by independent third-party teams. Thus, results will be better assured, and while retrospective audits of varying magnitude will always be done, fewer, if any unique discrepancies will be newly discovered.

These experimental data often form the initial phase of the risk assessment/risk management process. Because epidemiological data are often absent, public health decisions must be based largely on animal data, and this means that the recorded observations and resultant conclusions need remain above reproach. Yet, all those involved in doing toxicology research know there is no such thing as a perfect study, especially one that extends for two years. After all, data from studies in animals are used to advance science as well as to predict effects in humans.

To share some recent examples of audit findings and interpretations will permit some insight into the decision-making process and program views, however valid or imperfect these may be considered at some future time. Decisions are made now; and the silent undercurrent omnipresent is the important recognition that these unique experiments cannot be dismissed without considerable cause. Those carrying onagers have ample opportunity for disagreement, yet our data, records, and decisions are open to public witness. We must avoid the attitude that any flaw, no matter how trivial, will automatically make a study valueless, and hence could force repeating the experiments for minor discrepancies of an administrative origin, rather than for scientific flaws. After all, good science coupled with common sense and honesty equal quality assurance.

For one chemical we could find no records of chemistry—absolutely none. Does this invalidate the study? In many cases we would say "Yes." However, for studies involving this particular chemical, the carcinogenic response was positive without doubt. There were no animal identification problems, and two other studies in the literature supported the findings with the same target organ. Because bulk chemical samples are always retained, reanalyses were possible; thus a sample of the bulk chemical used to perform the studies was analyzed and the reanalysis confirmed the identity of the chemical studied. Using this information and that obtained from the records and audit, we decided to report these results.

In another instance, the key issue was animal identification. The data indicated a positive response. In about 20 percent of the animals, identification from wet tissues inside the bag did not correspond to the bag label. We attempted to reconstruct the experiment using the retrospective audit technique. When data from misidentified animals were censored, the positive response indeed remained, but the statistical evidence shifted from one sex to the other. The decision was made not to report these findings, but to design and initiate a new study.

In a third example, an equivocal carcinogenic response was observed, but the identification of some animals from their wet tissues did not match their bag label. These were equally distributed among the male and female animals, as well as among dose groups. After censoring data for those few animals having questionable identity, the results were not changed. We decided to report these data.

In the fourth example, multiple studies were done at the same laboratory. There were marginal identification discrepancies and uniformly poor record keeping. This, alone, may or may not have influenced reporting the data, but, more importantly, it was coupled with poor survival due to cumulative chemical toxicity. We decided that the studies should be considered inadequate, but to report the data since the findings were consistent for this class of chemicals.

Of course, others may have a different opinion or would have made a different decision. This is certainly possible and does not and should not allow cause to impugn either decision. There are differences of opinion and of data interpretations, of course. The NTP encourages an open process, perhaps being atypical in this regard, by making painfully known all the good and all the bad together for evaluation by the scientific community. We make the archives available so that others may search further.

In summary, data audits are integral to the high standards of quality assurance. Good Laboratory Practice regulations established management responsibility for the proper conduct of nonclinical studies, whereas comprehensive data audits and active monitoring of ongoing experiments are a means of insuring the integrity and quality of a study. Because of the impact of study results on public health issues relating to chemical toxicity and carcinogenicity, the data base upon which interpretive conclusions are made must be validated. Although retrospective and in-life data audits do not guarantee perfect studies, these audits provide more confidence that the results and conclusions reflect the collective data. Further, data audits provide witness that the laboratory conducts experiments in a credible and scientific way.

Recognizing steady advancements together with documented progress and universal endorsement in quality assurance, good laboratory practices, and data audits, we must all resist the easy temptation of becoming unduly comfortable with our gained efforts. We must continue to reach for excellence, and to never dull the sound of those clarion words Robert Frost gave us in his memorable "Stopping by Woods on a Snowy Evening": "But I have promises to keep,/and miles to go before I sleep,/and miles to go before I sleep."

ACKNOWLEDGEMENTS

I appreciate the steadfast help from Dr. D. Bristol and Ms. Loretta Brammell in completing this manuscript.

PANEL-AUDIENCE DIALOGUE
MANAGEMENT OF QUALITY

Chairperson:
Donald Hughes
Procter and Gamble Company
Ivorydale Technical Center
Cincinnati, Ohio

Panel:
Judith K. Baldwin, Douglas W. Bristol, James Huff,
Jerry M. Smith, Carrie E. Whitmire

Donald Hughes (P&G): I have one brief announcement. The National Toxicology Program puts together the NTP annual plan. It covers all the chemicals that are in the toxicology program, their status, who the chemical managers are, what studies are being conducted beyond the carcinogenesis bioassay, whether they are teratology, reproductive or short-term tests. Those copies are available. If you're on the mailing list, you'll receive them. If you're not on the mailing list, please contact Larry Hart, NTP.

Pat Royal (Stauffer Chemical Company): SOPs specify that the study director is to be the center, focal person of all studies conducted under GLPs and, yet, as I understand the program at NTP, the contract lab assigns a study director who works in coordination with the chemical manager at NTP. Who then is responsible for writing the final report? If there are conflicts between the study director at the contract laboratory and the chemical manager at NTP, how are these resolved? Likewise, in regard to this, do both the chemical manager and the study director from the contract laboratory sign the final report? And, at peer review, are the QA audits and inspection reports available for the people at NTP to review?

Doug Bristol (NTP): The principal investigator at the laboratory functions as indicated in the GLP regulations. The final report is written by the laboratory, signed off, after review by the quality assurance unit, by the principal investigator, as well as the other key personnel/staff. The report itself involves materials and methods, results, and discussions, but the histopathology results are discussed in the pathology narrative, which is subjected to the pathology working group (PWG), which is the peer review step for pathology. With regard to the in-life observations, I don't think we ordinarily run into controversies there. If we do, it's a matter of reviewing the data and straightening them out. With regard to the microscopic pathology evaluations, those are taken care of through the PWG process, and there is a mechanism for dealing with discrepancies following PWG review.

Carrie Whitmire (NTP): The final report, as required by GLP compliance, is the laboratory report; however, the technical report is the NTP report and will include more than just the in-life or just the animal studies. It may include special studies and other things that are done on the chemical, which will give a broader view than what is given. It will include both species and be a comprehensive report for that chemical; so, the technical report is not considered the final report as in GLP requirements from the laboratory. There is no sign-off by both parties as far as the final report under GLP compliance. That is purely and simply the laboratory's responsibility.

Bristol: The question also asked about the retrospective data audit reports. After the reports are reviewed by various disciplines and approved, the chemical manager is responsible for writing an interpretation of the audit findings in the technical report, the summary of audit findings, so, that's where the responsibility is handled.

James Albert (Dynamac Corporation): Three terms were used today relative to fraud, concealment and cover-up by study directors. Now, speaking for the study directors I've known in the past, I've found them very ethical. Are you finding things now that you would consider fraud, cover-up and concealment, or are you referring to, instead, what has been in the past? Lord knows we don't want to go back to anything like that, M.E.R. 29s and such.

Hughes: We're looking at things that had happened in the past. If we're dealing with fraud and concealment and cover-up, those are legal considerations, and that's not the purview of this session or this panel or this symposium; rather, we're dealing with the scientific issues. Obviously, there's a history that we can't overlook, but we are trying to go into the future and learn from the lessons and mistakes of the past.

Whitmire: I think we might have confused the audience even though we gave the correct answer. We receive a lab report; it is the responsibility of the laboratory; that's the final report. We receive a QA report that was done by an independent organization and this is summarized by the chemical manager and placed into the technical report. Is it available to the public? The answer is "yes." Copies of the audit report are available on request. This is complicated further by what we call the NTP evaluation of the data. We call that a technical report and these are peer reviewed in open session. These are the opinions and best judgment of our staff, collectively; sometimes they differ from the judgment and best interpretation of the laboratory.

J. C. Bhandari (Dynamac): You emphasized that GLP does not necessarily assure GTP, and I agree with that. Would you propose how we can accomplish both GLP and GTP? Would you make a proposal that the QAU consist of the expertise that has the adequate appreciation for GTP? Could you expound on that, please?

Smith (Rohm and Haas): I think we need to keep Good Laboratory Practices and evaluations of individual studies along the same courses they're on. Good

Toxicological Practices, as I think I mentioned, require open peer review; and I think that's the only way that you will be able to have and maintain Good Toxicological Practices. I know of no system, other than open peer review, that will accomplish that.

Bhandari: There's a problem with that. Particularly in your industry, there is a lot of data that you might not want to expose. Do you mean the peer review within the company, or within the staff unassociated with data study? Some companies may not be that big. I could only see it from a QAU point of view where, in fact, your quality assurance unit would have such expertise as to appreciate toxicology. So, how would you do the peer review, say, within a pharmaceutical industry or chemical industry?

Smith: Well, the peer review can be very complicated. It depends upon how deep you want to go into it. As a general rule, for all chemicals, whether pharmaceuticals, pesticides or otherwise, the data are prepared and submitted to a regulatory agency. They do undergo the review of the regulatory agency. The health safety data, in general, are available to the public. The data can undergo peer review through evaluation of the data in the files, and, finally, if something becomes an issue, there are processes you can go through, open peer reviews, such as the Scientific Advisory Panel under FIFRA or the data can be accepted and go through and be examined as part of the peer review of an NTP study. So, there are mechanisms of peer review. I encourage industry, including our own, to publish their data more frequently, to get them out for peer review; and there is a very, very strong movement in this direction. There are some parts of toxicological evaluations that are proprietary, but these are very minimal, and I think they are being handled very well, in general.

Andrew Tegeris (Tegeris Labs.): I was impressed by the archives of NTP; however, I did not see any attempts or effort toward preventing a major catastrophe, such as by fire. Recently, we have been getting a lot of inquiries as to what type of fire proofing we have in our archives. Along the same lines, how does one address this? How do you protect against loss from fire or against loss from any other major natural catastrophe? Should we have two archives, physically separated, or what?

James Huff (NTP): May I ask Dr. Hardisty, who is the leader of the NTP archives, to answer that question.

Jerry Hardisty (Experimental Pathology Laboratories): At the NTP archives, we have four separate rooms, one which has the slides, one which has the paraffin blocks, one with data and one with wet tissues. Each of those four rooms is separated by two-hour fire walls. Each of the four rooms has a dual fire abatement system—sprinklers and halon fire abatement systems. They all have monitors in them, which are monitored 24 hours a day by the security service, which will contact me and the fire department at exactly the same time if anything should happen. That's the protection that we've tried to establish for the program, for their materials.

Whitmire: We have been doing a great deal of microfiching, as I mentioned earlier, and there is another copy of the microfiche at NIEHS.

Tegeris: How long did you say you keep wet tissues—three years or five years?

Whitmire: We haven't totally decided, but I would think more than three years after the technical report is published. So, that gives you quite a considerable time there, and only then, after they have been reviewed on an individual chemical basis as to interest and need. This is taken up with our people, and then it will probably be published in the Federal Register before anything is destroyed.

Steve Harris (Consultant): I hope that we have more of these meetings in the future; I think they are important for all toxicologists and quality assurance specialists.

We've heard throughout the day words such as "cost effectiveness," "communication," "morale," "building blocks of management"—all good words, but I heard a new one today which I want to elaborate on more: GTPs, "Good Toxicology Practices." How do we improve good toxicology practices? I think one area which we didn't get a chance to elaborate on was training, even though it was brought up throughout the day. We have the Society of Toxicology, the ACT, the SQA, that within their by-laws generally recognize any of their members as expert in a given discipline, expert as a toxicologist. What about being an expert in practical toxicology? Do we, as toxicologists, really know what's going on in the laboratory? Do we know how to work with our staff? Our technical staffs are a reflection upon management. Study directors, directors of toxicology, managers of toxicology, have to tell the technical staff why something is or is not being done in a particular way. You can't tell them, "It doesn't make a difference; you're not a Ph.D. or M.D. or D.V.M.; don't ask questions, just get the job done because we've got to get the report out."

Those of us with advanced degrees have learned academic toxicology, but can we apply it in the workplace to improve good toxicology practices, in addition to improving our quality assurance practices? Directors of toxicology, managers of toxicology, consultants, have to be able to work with staff. We've got to be able to go into an animal room and show our staff how to retro-orbital bleed. We've got to be able to do C-sections. We've got to be able to come in on weekends and work and weigh litters. I've seen enough in laboratories, in the last year and a half around this country, to suggest that if you're going to improve the quality of conduct of studies, GLPs and GTPs, you've all got to be intimately involved with your staff. They are the backbone of your program from whatever level, especially animal husbandry, because you're going to fail if your animal husbandry program doesn't get off the ground right.

Whitmire: May I comment on that a moment? I appreciate your bringing that up because it's very important, but there are three things—there's teaching, there's supervision and there's teamwork. Unless you get all three, you don't have anything. You've got to work together as a team. In auditing, if a toxicologist finds something that might be related to the in-life treatment, the toxicologist has got to know. I have said this many times, and I'm probably getting a reputation for it, but unless you are a detective, you're not a good scientist, and you cannot do auditing or inspection; you've got to sense that something is wrong, and then follow up to find out why. You've got a peak in weight, or a dip—what caused it? temperature? humidity? lack of food? a water problem? What caused it? These are things that make the difference; solving it immediately, as soon as possible; not trying to solve it five years after the study and explain why we've got dips and peaks in various individual and collective animal data.

Judith Baldwin (Exxon): I'd also like to respond to Steve Harris' comment. It's a pretty odd comment that brings the discussion from the panel back to the audience. But I think it is very worthwhile because we're all considering training problems, or training programs, right now. We all see the need to improve training programs and QA, and probably those we have in basic laboratory practices and techniques. What you've said is very important. The emphasis need not only be on the formalization of those programs, but by leadership, by doing, by showing the hands-on technique; not just simply films, filmstrips, self-guided assessment. We need to pass on what we know, and that includes discussion about the importance of the work, as well as how actually to do it. Why do we ask people to do observations in a certain way? How do we, as toxicologists, use that to make interpretations? What's important to us? If we tell people what's important, they'll get the message to us because the people in the laboratory are our eyes, ears and hands.

Robert Kapp (Exxon): I'm deeply impressed by the efforts you made and everything I've heard here this afternoon. Let me ask you a question about figures. How many persons do you have on your staff? What's your budget? Finally, if you allow, what's the ratio between the costs spent for toxicology testing and monitoring?

Bristol: I think many of these figures are available in the National Toxicology Program annual plan; certainly, budget and breakdown.

Huff: Of course, any answer would not adequately address your question. Our program has about 140 scientists; that is, from the Masters through the D.V.M., Ph.D. and so forth. Roughly 90-some percent of our work is not done in our institute. We have an annual budget through the NIHS, NIEHS, NCTR and NIOSH, roughly of $60 million. I remind you that each long-term study, nowadays, to do a full characterization of toxicology costs about $1 million, and to put that in perspective with the retrospective audits, we find that audits on a two-species, two-sex, two-year experiment cost us about $30,000 each. These are the bare numbers and I refer you to the annual plan to get a breakdown in more detail.

Gerard Herro (G. D. Searle): This question is directed to Doug Bristol. You discussed the review of data capture by computers from contract facilities. Does this review ascertain whether the hardware and software are validated? And, if so, what do you consider adequate validation?

Bristol: I think the best answer to that question involves a little description of how we capture the data. Terminals are on the in-life data; terminals are in the animal room and data are captured on-line. The disk is taken back to the office. Local reports are printed out and reviewed by laboratory staff to see that they are complete, and so on, before the data are transmitted to the main frame computer, so that it is human review of all the data that constitutes the primary validation effort. The system itself was developed by NCTR, National Center for Toxicological Research, and the validation that they have done is a matter of record at NCTR; but, a few weeks back at the Society of Quality Assurance Meeting, there was a great deal of discussion on this very topic, and it's a problem that industry and government are facing, I think, at this very time. We relied, primarily, on the human review of the data on a day-to-day basis.

Sharon Keener (Consultant): The results of the NTP studies eventually enter the scientific data bases, and there's been a lot of concern recently about data quality indicators and perpetuation of error in interpretation of study results as it relates to risk assessment. I was wondering what, if anything, has the NTP planned to do if they find that during a retrospective audit of their studies, that the study results may indicate that they are seriously flawed? Would they print a retraction or try and alleviate that?

Huff: Yes.

Baldwin: There's a number of us who are concerned about quality of the reports and the data that are out there in the literature because we all use the data bases to make certain assessments. I think it's an idea whose time has come.

Sid Siegel (The National Library of Medicine): Data quality indicators and data documentation completeness are an approach to identify how reports can be better used. We're now proposing experiments on material that's *a fait accompli*, to identify what we have to do with the swamp that's out there now. There are about 330 studies on our generic design chart. We consider the first 200 to be the responsibility of the National Cancer Institute, and we feel more responsible for the latter 130, and, as priorities for data audits, we are emphasizing those studies coming off now, but we have 32 studies that have been identified by our executive committee that are those already printed, and some of these do include NCI studies. I know Dexter Goldman from EPA has also requested us to look at some older studies; and he has done some as well. So, they're not untouchable. We're having enough trouble with the 130 to go back further.

K. K. Tripathi (Dynamac Corporation and NTP): One area that has not been emphasized enough is the chemistry, analytical chemistry. I thought I had better point it out. NTP has very, very elaborate procedures, and they have, in their SOP, initial analysis of the chemical for purity, identity, stability, homogeneity and all of those things. The bulk chemical analysis—chemical use log, animal room samples, then, you have the method of validation—all of these things, water, feed, some of these things are very, very important.

Hughes: Thank you, and chemistry is, also, very expensive.

Donald Hooker (Procter & Gamble): NTP uses the outside experts from industry and academia to do peer review and act on advisory boards. When it comes to scientific quality, are there any plans in the near term to have outside experts in quality assurance take a look at the quality assurance program that you designed and the results of that program?

Bristol: I wouldn't count it out, but, at this particular point in time, the focus of our program is what was presented on the inspections and audits performed at our laboratories on the studies that are being conducted, so that we can have the feedback there, and, also, on the catching up with regard to the retrospective audits. I think part of my new position will involve planning down the line, and, in that area, I think there's probably a need for seeking out other thoughts and ideas as an aid to that planning.

Whitmire: I'd like to say one thing there. We do have some expert assistance on this. We have audited materials that have been audited either just before they come in or after they have come in, before the reports are in, and the findings are not unlike on what I have seen of them, so far. So, I think we have a "Catch 22" there, or an expert panel that does serve and that is "you," the public.

Bristol: There are two other places where we do get input from experts, and those are among the quality assurance support contractors who support the activities that we have ongoing now. They represent some very fine expertise, and the way that they perform the job is not strictly rote; in other words, there is much interaction, suggestion, responses and so on. So, we get input there, and all NTP technical reports are peer reviewed, and that, also, represents a step where we get inputs.

Whitmire: I think there's one more thing we should say, too. That's what this conference is all about: NTP and industry interacting.

Huff: Since it's Dr. Bristol's first day on the job, maybe he hasn't heard yet, but, yes, we do plan to have outside experts help us in our system; not only when the QA program will come before our Board of Scientific Counselors, which does utilize ad hoc experts in a discipline, but, as he intimated, on a routine basis to learn.

Kristin Hoover (ARCO Chemical Company): Why do you find it necessary for the chemical manager to summarize the quality assurance report? That's obviously a high-level management decision that's been made. I would also like to know what steps you take to make sure that the chemical manager's quality assurance summary coincides exactly with what's been found in the audit report?

Whitmire: There are several things here. The reasons they do summarize it:

number one, the audit team does an audit; number two, the audit team may not have the input which we have in turn gotten from the laboratory in addition to the audit, or to the pathology support team to go back and look at various things. So, there is an interplay of what the NTP people in reviewing the audit have, what the auditors have, what the pathology support teams have in returning to the laboratory that did the work to achieve answers. This is all encompassed and one reason that the audit summary is written—the final form—by the field manager.

Bristol: It's also the chemical manager's responsibility to interpret or integrate the audit findings versus the biological response of the study, and to present to the NTP staff and peer review the conclusions that can be drawn, so that the summary of the audit findings that I've referred to in the technical report summarizes the findings from the audit report itself, but goes beyond that to indicate what the ramifications of those findings are on the interpretations given to the study.

Huff: I have a question. What would you suggest?

Hoover: I'm worried every time I see a summation. I'm worried about toxicologists who only read summaries of reports. I'm worried about quality assurance people who summarize their reports so that some important things are possibly left out. I'm worried about people who are not intimately involved with the studies making the summary. I'm worried about the peer review board not having access to the full and complete quality assurance report and possibly being encouraged to look at the summary. I would suspect that probably doesn't happen, but I would hope that the whole quality assurance report would go to the peer review board, so that they could have an idea about the study that was not biased by any summary or any other information that happened subsequent to that report.

Dan Todd (CDC): Obviously, we're beginning to focus on quality assurance now in longer-term studies, and just as the disciplines of chemistry and, more so, pharmacology have evolved into toxicology, and as toxicology, as we're realizing in this world, is evolving into risk management. How do you feel that quality assurance is going to be handled in a risk management atmosphere of longer-term studies?

Hughes: My perception of quality assurance in its relationship to risk management is part of that scientific input that is packaged and sent to the manager for administrative decision making where he can factor in nonscientific issues, societal factors, politics, and whatever else needs to be done. If someone else has a different view of quality assurance, go ahead.

Baldwin: I'd also like to add to it. When you look at all the numbers that go into risk assessment, the only real piece of hard data comes from a toxicology study. Exposure is, usually, at an estimated level and potentials are sometimes estimations or extrapolations from the toxicological data, so the only hard numbers that you really have in there are those data from toxicology studies. How hard are they? How good are those data for a hard decision? Since you only have one good piece of data to work on, you'd better make sure, at least, that piece is very good. That's where the quality assurance people are being challenged right now to make sure they've got some limits on those numbers, and that those numbers have some real meaning for use in risk assessment.

Chapter III
TOOLS OF QUALITY—PRESTUDY
ORGANIZATION

TOOLS OF QUALITY—
PRESTUDY ORGANIZATION

William H. Farland
Health Environmental Review Division
Office of Toxic Substances
U.S. Environmental Protection Agency
Washington, DC

CHAIRPERSON'S REMARKS

We have discussed some of the general aspects of the management of quality and now we want to focus more specifically on the topic of Tools of Quality. Just as any artisan has to know his tools to prepare for the job at hand, we are all responsible in various ways for activities which we might call prestudy organization. We have three speakers who will be addressing areas including the importance of the protocol, facility capability assessment and an understanding of some of the legal implications related to data acquisition. These areas roughly fall into the tools of quality and, more specifically, prestudy organization phase.

THE IMPORTANCE OF THE PROTOCOL

Ira J. Friedman
Pfizer, Inc.
New York, New York

ABSTRACT

The protocol is an essential document that enables properly skilled and trained individuals to interpret and carry out the writer's intentions. The OECD Principles of Good Laboratory Practice provide a useful guide to protocol content. Study design, protocol detail and form depend on the purpose of the study, the extent of written standard operating procedures and the experience and training of laboratory personnel. The protocol is an essential tool for management, the study director, the quality assurance unit and regulatory authorities. A well-written protocol, together with written procedures and a complete data file, bolsters confidence in the credibility and reliability of a study.

INTRODUCTION

I would no more dream of trying to learn how to run a toxicology study by simply reading a protocol than I would of trying to learn how to play a violin sonata by simply reading a sheet of music. Given some talent, education and enough practice, however, I might hope to achieve some success with either effort. A protocol is a written plan that sets forth the objectives and procedures for the conduct of a study. Like a music score, it is an essential medium of communication that enables properly skilled and trained individuals to interpret and carry out the writer's intentions. But it cannot stand alone.

I doubt that any of you really question the importance of the protocol in an abstract sense. While the various Good Laboratory Practice (GLP) regulations have formalized the requirements, the protocol has long been recognized as an essential component of the experimental approach. The real questions have to

1. Address correspondence to: Ira J. Friedman, Pfizer, Inc., 235 E. 42nd Street, New York, New York 10017.
2. Key words: OECD principles, protocol, standard operating procedures, study design.
3. Abbreviations: GLP, Good Laboratory Practice; OECD, Organization for Economic Cooperation and Development; QAU, Quality Assurance Unit; SOP, Standard Operating Procedure.

do with the content, form, and detail of a protocol, and its preparation and effective use, and these are the issues I intend to discuss with you. There are also significant differences in the importance and use of the protocol for contract versus in-house studies, which I will try to highlight.

PROTOCOL CONTENT

I'm sure you are all familiar with the Organization for Economic Cooperation and Development (OECD) Principles of GLP. This document, prepared by an international group of experts and approved by the OECD Council in May 1981, applies to the nonclinical testing of chemicals to obtain data on their properties and/or safety with respect to human health or the environment. Included in the Principles is a succinct and logical outline of what a protocol should contain. The OECD Principles require that the study plan should clearly state the nature and purpose of the study, identify the test and control substances, identify the sponsor, test facility and study director, the date of protocol approval and proposed study dates and the test methods to be used. Where applicable, it should include a description of and justification for selection of the test system, detailed information as to dose levels, route and frequency of administration, details of the experimental design and data analysis and finally, a list of the records to be retained.

While the OECD Principles are a useful guide to what topics should be addressed in a protocol, they do not answer the questions of study design and protocol detail and form.

STUDY DESIGN

It is not uncommon, particularly in a multi-discipline organization with geographically separated groups, to find that not everyone involved in a study knows what its true objective is. In one situation with which I am familiar, for example, management was hoping to obtain tissue residue data for immediate support of a regulatory submission, while the analyst was trying to validate a new analytical method not yet accepted by the authorities. The results were scientifically elegant but otherwise useless. No study should be undertaken without a clearly understood and agreed upon written statement of the objectives and the methods to be used to achieve these objectives.

If the study is intended for regulatory submission, it seems sensible to establish in advance that the proposed methods will meet regulatory guidelines, with the further unfortunate complication that guidelines vary from agency to agency and from country to country.

Management should review the proposed study design and consider whether there is a more efficient design which might yield more information. What statistical methods will be used to evaluate the results? Will the data be evaluated in the context of other studies, and if so, is the design compatible with those studies?

DETAIL

The amount of detail required in a protocol depends on the completeness of the facility's Standard Operating Procedures (SOPs), the training and experience of the laboratory staff and whether the study is conducted in-house or in an outside facility. I would not accept a study protocol without having first reviewed the SOPs relevant to that study. If the SOPs adequately describe the procedures required they need only be referenced in the protocol. Procedures unique to the study need to be described in greater detail.

But how much detail is "adequate"? The protocols and standard procedures that I have read are seldom sufficiently detailed to enable an untrained person to carry out the described tests successfully. The many essential skills and techniques have to be learned through on-the-job training and really can't be "adequately" described in writing. A necropsy procedure that instructs the technicians to sever the vena cava and aorta anterior to the liver is probably best learned through demonstration. Consequently, you must consider the training and experience of the laboratory staff in deciding how detailed the protocol must be.

If you are operating within your own testing facility, it should not be difficult to learn through your own experience how much detail is needed in your study plans. If you are a sponsor of studies in a variety of contract laboratories, however, I would suggest that you must err on the side of including more, not less, detail in your protocols.

FORM

Writing a new detailed protocol every time you run a study is time-consuming. However, much of the methodology currently used to support the safety of new pharmaceuticals has by now become rather standardized. In a typical preclinical subacute rodent or dog study, for example, perhaps 90% of the details are unlikely to vary from one drug candidate to another. In such studies it may be useful to use a standard protocol to describe fixed study elements, supplemented by fill-in-the-blank forms to describe the variable, compound-specific elements of a study. For example, the following is a partial tabulation of some fixed and variable elements of a typical one- to three-month rat study.

FIXED STUDY ELEMENTS

1. Minimum Group Size
2. Animal Housing and Preconditioning
3. Frequency of Measurements
   Body Weights
   Food Consumption
   Clinical Observations
   Clinical Pathology

4. At Necropsy
   Organs to be Weighed
   Tissues to be Examined
5. References to Relevant SOP's
6. Content of Final Report

VARIABLE STUDY ELEMENTS

1. Purpose of Study
2. Test System Description
3. Size and Number of Groups
4. Dose Levels, Route and Frequency
5. Dose Preparation and Storage
6. Specific Clinical Pathology Tests
7. Detailed Study Calendar
8. Statistical Methods
9. Safety Precautions

We have applied this concept to our preclinical drug safety testing with the result that the toxicologist is able to spend more time considering critical scientific questions and still produce a complete and acceptable protocol.

It may also be useful to include study-specific data recording forms in the protocol. If properly designed, they prompt the technical staff as to what data should be recorded and how this recording should be done, and serve as a reminder that signatures and dates as well as observations are required.

Electronic data processing systems can also serve as adjuncts to the protocol. In a typical situation, once the written protocol has been approved, it is assigned a unique identifying number and a computer study file is initiated. The basic information as to the size of each animal group, dose level, scheduled tests required and information required at necropsy is entered, and the program then prompts the technical staff at each intervention to help assure that the needed data are collected.

Having spent the time and effort to prepare a complete detailed protocol, how can we most effectively use it?

MANAGEMENT

For management, a protocol system is an essential tool for controlling and allocating resources.

Perhaps the most devastating question a manager can ask his staff is "Why on earth did you ever run that study in the first place?" Management should insist that no study be initiated without written management approval of the protocol. This applies equally to in-house as well as contract studies.

Having agreed that a study should be undertaken, management must then assure that adequate facilities and personnel are available, that scheduling conflicts do not exist or can be resolved and that sufficient test compound is available in a timely fashion.

STUDY DIRECTOR

While the study director is off attending a conference, a carefully written protocol, supported by standard procedures and training programs, provides added assurance that the technical support staff with hands-on responsibility for the study clearly understands what is supposed to be done and knows how to do it, and that the required data are being collected.

The need to be sure that the protocol is followed, however, has to be balanced by the flexibility to change study details when necessary. Minor protocol deviations should only need to be approved by the study director; major changes should be approved by management as well. In a contract study, all significant departures from the approved study plan must be reviewed with the sponsor and agreed to before, not after the fact. It might be well to define significant departures either in the protocol or in a standard operating procedure.

Finally, the protocol is an ideal vehicle for informing study personnel regarding specific health hazards, unusual safety precautions needed, compound stability and storage problems and planned departures from standard procedures.

QUALITY ASSURANCE UNIT

The Quality Assurance Unit (QAU) in a toxicology facility is responsible for ensuring that the study plan and SOPs are followed or that deviations are authorized and documented. The protocol informs the QAU that a study is planned and provides the necessary information to enable the Unit to schedule inspections, audit study records and review final reports at the proper time. Some regulatory authorities (the Food and Drug Administration, for example) require that the QAU retain copies of protocols along with other QAU records.

The QAU should be a participant in the protocol review process. In our French facility, the QAU initiates the computer data file for each new study. This assures that the Unit has an opportunity to review each study protocol for GLP compliance prior to the start of the study.

REGULATORY AUTHORITIES

The regulatory authorities most often see a study after the fact, and must consider not only the scientific issues addressed by the study but also the basic issue of credibility. Was the study really carried out the way the report says it was? The protocol alone cannot completely answer the question, but a well written protocol, together with written standard procedures, a clear and complete data file and clearly identified specimens, certainly bolsters confidence in the credibility and reliability of a study.

When the regulatory authorities inspect an ongoing study the protocol is even more critical in establishing study credibility. Is the protocol being followed?

Have the required data been collected to date? Have departures from the protocol been authorized? Do people know what they are supposed to do and are they really doing it?

In summary, the protocol is an essential document that describes the purpose and procedures to be used in conducting a study. It cannot stand alone but must be viewed in the context of written laboratory procedures and a properly trained staff. Like a piece of music, you need the protocol to do a study, but you'd better take some lessons and practice before you try it.

FACILITY CAPABILITY ASSESSMENT

John B. McCandless
Corporate Toxicology Department
Atlantic Richfield Company
Los Angeles, California

ABSTRACT

An inspection procedure has been developed to assess the capabilities of contract toxicology laboratories. This procedure has been utilized for the inspection of twenty (20) different toxicology laboratories. There are ten (10) major
areas inspected:

- Facility
- Personnel
- Operations
- Animals/Animal Care
- Standard Operating Procedures
- Quality Assurance
- Equipment
- Test Article
- Data.

Each of these areas is divided into categories with each category divided
further to specific topics. Points are assigned to each topic. The points earned by
the laboratory reflect the inspector's assessment of the laboratory's quality in
each area. Area scores are added and a percent score for the facility is calculated. This approach provided a clear distinction among the laboratories
evaluated.

This facility inspection and rating system has played an important role in
screening contract laboratories for the Atlantic Richfield Company corporate
toxicology testing program. It also highlights strengths and weaknesses of
individual laboratories.

1. Address correspondence to: John B. McCandless, Corporate Toxicology Department, Atlantic Richfield Company, 515 South Flower Street, Los Angeles, CA 90071.
2. Key words: capability assessment, contract facilities, testing laboratory.
3. Abbreviations: QAU, Quality Assurance Unit; SOPs, Standard Operating Procedures.

INTRODUCTION

The selection of a contract toxicology laboratory to conduct testing for an organization can be a very difficult task. There are many aspects of a contract laboratory that should be considered. We have developed an inspection, evaluation, and scoring system to assess many of these critical areas. This "facility capability assessment" involves the inspection and evaluation of ten (10) major areas. Each of these areas is broken down to logical categories and each category is further broken down to specific topics. Each topic has been assigned a point value. As the laboratory is inspected, each topic is evaluated and the inspector assigns a point value based on the quality of the laboratory in that topic. The points earned by the laboratory reflect a subjective assessment of the laboratory in each topic.

After the entire facility capability assessment is completed, area scores are added and a percentage score for each area as well as a total percentage score for the testing facility is calculated. We have used this inspection system to evaluate 20 different contract testing laboratories. It has provided a clear distinction among these laboratories.

When laboratories are reviewed for placing contract toxicology tests, they may be compared based on the result of this assessment. Since this gives an overall evaluation and an evaluation of the laboratory in the ten major areas, the sponsor can more clearly understand and be aware of specific strengths and weaknesses before placing test work. This knowledge can not only be applied to the selection of a contract laboratory; it can provide specific areas of investigation for pre-study visits; and it can be used to aid the sponsor in understanding some of the fundamental tasks and operations of a specific contract testing laboratory.

PROCEDURE

The Facility Inspection Procedure

Area 1 - Facility:

Area; Category; Topic	Quality Points Possible
I. Facility	(total 119)
A. Outside (describe)	
1. Access	10
2. Security	10
3. Location	5
4. Visibility	5
5. Roof	10
	Subtotal 40

B. Inside
  1. AAALAC   5
  2. Animal rooms
     a. lights   2
     b. air pressure   4
     c. condition   10
     d. walls   2
     e. ceilings   2
     f. floors (floor drains?)   2
     g. door(s)   4
     h. water pressure   4
     i. electric outlets   2
     j. sink/hose bib   2

                                 Subtotal   39

  3. HVAC
     a. heat   2
     b. water treatment, filtration   2
     c. ventilation
        (1) air changes   2
        (2) 100% fresh   4
        (3) circulation   4
            (supply/exhaust location)
        (4) clean filters, diffusers   4
     d. temperature control   1
     e. humidity control   1
     f. filtration   4
     g. central AC   1

                                 Subtotal   25

  4. Utilities
     a. electric (back-up generator)   1
     b. septic/sewerage   1
     c. water: source   1
     d. trash removal
        (1) carcasses   1
        (2) animal waste   1
        (3) paper   1
     e. incinerator: access   1

                                 Subtotal   7

  5. Maintenance
     a. in-house staff   4
     b. condition of boiler room   2
     c. relation/attitude of maintenance
        staff   2

                                 Subtotal   8

The facility area of the inspection procedure is the longest and most detailed. It covers the outside and inside of the testing laboratory and requires tours of both areas. It is important when making these tours to be in control. A floor plan of the laboratory should be requested for constant orientation. As the tour is taken, randomly ask to see animal rooms and evaluate these. Attempt to speak with employees of the laboratory. Your objectives are to understand how the physical nature of the laboratory relates to the toxicity tests that are being performed. Before the inspection, it may be advantageous to review each topic with your staff and conclude what is acceptable for maximum quality points in each topic.

Area 2 - Personnel:

Area; Category; Topic.	Quality Points Possible
II. Personnel	(total 51)
A. Organization Chart	
1. Number of Employees	
2. Attrition	
3. Expertise	
a. professionals	10
b. technical staff	4
c. support staff	4
d. consultants	4
e. subcontractors	4
4. Division of Work Force (Job Descriptions)	
a. professional duties	2
b. technical duties	2
c. support staff duties	2
	Subtotal 32
B. Training/Proficiency	
1. Skill Sheet	1
2. Certification of Proficiency	2
3. Who Trains - Who Certifies	4
4. What Animals	1
	Subtotal 8
C. Employee Cleanliness	
1. Visual	2
2. Uniforms	2
3. Attitude	1
	Subtotal 5

D. Employee Health
1. Nurse; Health Professional   1
2. Employee Physical   1
3. Employee Health Program   4

Subtotal   6

The personnel area involves gathering curriculm vitae of principal scientists, understanding the divisions of work between the study directors, the technical staff, and the support staff. It also requires an investigation into the training, cleanliness and health programs of/for the employees.

Area 3 - Test Facility Operations:

Area; Category; Topic.	Quality Points Possible
III. Test Facility Operations	(total 39)
A. Flow	
1. Animals	2
2. Test Article	2
3. Personnel	2
	Subtotal 6
B. Storage	
1. Storage	2
2. Feed Storage	5
3. Lab Supplies	2
4. Cleaning Supplies	2
	Subtotal 11
C. Cleaning/Sanitation	
1. Rooms	
a. cleaning agent	2
b. microciding agent: tests	2
2. Cages/Racks, Glassware	
a. cagewasher	
(1) temperature	2
(2) type	2
(3) appearance	4
(4) records	2
(5) numbered racks	1
3. Pest Control	1
	Subtotal 16
D. Hazardous Waste	
1. Storage	2
2. Disposal	2
3. Records	2
	Subtotal 6

Test facility operations looks into many ancillary operations which support a toxicity test. Flow patterns are looked at; storage space is investigated; and the cleaning and sanitation procedures of animal rooms are evaluated. Additionally, the procedures for handling hazardous waste are investigated in this area.

Area 4 - Animals/Animal Care:

Area; Category; Topic.	Quality Points Possible
IV. Animals/Animal Care	(total 28)
A. Receipt	
1. Sources	1
2. Method	2
Subtotal	3
B. Quarantine	
1. Where	2
2. Who's Allowed Access	2
Subtotal	4
C. Feed/Water	
1. Source	2/2
2. Analysis	2/2
Subtotal	8
D. Species Separation	2
E. Acceptable for Test	
1. By Whom	2
2. Based on What (SOP)	2
Subtotal	4
F. Housing	
1. Stainless Steel	1
2. Sizes	1
Subtotal	2
G. Animal Waste (Method of Disposal)	1
H. Necropsy/Pathology/Animal Disposal	
1. Pathology	
a. necropsy	1
b. clinical path	1
c. histopath	1
2. Carcass Disposal	1
Subtotal	4

The next area investigates the animals/animal care capabilities and practices of the testing facility. This is an area that can be evaluated best by a tour and investigation of specific facility locations. The staff veterinarian may be the best person to deal with in this area.

Area 5 - Standard Operating Procedures:

Area; Category; Topic.	Quality Points Possible
V. Standard Operating Procedures	(total 20)
A. Responsibility of:	
B. Availability	1
C. Historical File	1
D. SOP's Perused	
1. "Hazardous Waste"	4
2. "Cage Washing"	4
3. "Animal Receipt-Observations at Receipt"	4
4. "Compound Receipt"	4
E. Protocol Changes	2

The intention in this category is to get a good idea of the quality and extent of the laboratory's Standard Operating Procedures (SOPs).

We are not reviewing the SOPs to criticize the technique the lab uses in performing a task, we are reviewing the SOP to see if the topic is explained well and in sufficient detail for the tasks' repetitive performance.

Area 6 - Quality Assurance:

Area; Category; Topic.	Quality Points Possible
VI. Quality Assurance	(total 26)
A. Organizational Chart/Reporting Structure	2
B. Master Schedule (SOP)	2
C. Staff	4
D. Auditing SOPs	
1. Protocol	2
2. In-life	2
3. Path	2
4. Final Report	2
5. SOPs	2
E. Inspector Handling	2
F. Gut Feeling	6

This area of the inspection could be dealt with in more depth by a quality assurance professional; however, for the purposes of assessing the general capabilities, responsibilities, and functions of the Quality Assurance Unit (QAU), this inspection section gives an adequate appraisal.

The "gut feeling" topic is a catch-all for the intangible feeling we have concerning the ability of the laboratory's QAU to assure the quality of our studies.

Area 7 - Equipment:

Area; Category; Topic.	Quality Points Possible
VII. Equipment	(total 9)
A. Appropriate	1
B. Clean/Maintained	2
C. Calibration (SOP)	4
D. Back-up	2

Equipment should be dealt with from a toxicity testing standpoint—not analytical chemistry or clinical pathology. Animal balances, computerized data collection systems, cages, racks, etc., are the equipment of concern in this area. Equipment that may be used in our animal test room should be looked at in this area.

Area 8 - Test Article:

Area; Category; Topic.	Quality Points Possible
VIII. Test Article	(total 31)
A. Receipt	2
B. Identification/Labeling	2
C. Storage	2
D. Dispensing	1
E. Mixing	2
F. Dosing	1
G. Disposal	1
H. Diet Preparation	
1. Mixing	5
2. Scooping	5
3. Flow	10

The test article area is another tour area. Track the test article from receipt to ultimate disposal. We pay particular attention to potential problems with confidentiality, cross contamination, and poor documentation.

Area 9 - Data:

Area; Category; Topic.	Quality Points Possible
IX. Data	(total 13)
A. Flow	
1. Generation	2
2. Review	2
3. Handling	2
4. Storage	2
5. Retrieval	1
6. Disposition	2
B. Final Report	2

The flow of data from generation to final report should be looked at next. We are concerned with multiple storage places, poor accountability, and infrequent study director review of data. We also ask who writes the final report and how involved is the study director in this task.

Area 10 - Archives:

Area; Category; Topic.	Quality Points Possible
X. Archives	(total 20)
A. Location	2
B. Security	4
C. Organization (SOP)	2
D. Fire Protection	2
E. What's There	
1. Final Report	2
2. Teratology	2
3. Pathology	2
4. Tapes (computer)	2
F. Who's Responsible	2

The final inspection area is the archives. We visit these areas and take the time to understand their organization. All our test data will ultimately end up here so it is important that we be satisfied in this area.

When making these inspections, it is important to take notes to support the point value given to the lab on a specific topic. This paper has purposefully stayed away from describing what quality determines what point value. Each individual who makes these inspections for the toxicology program must determine what degree of quality is acceptable and how that equates to a point value.

DISCUSSION

After an inspection has been conducted and points assigned, a summary table can be created and diffferent laboratories compared.

Point values for each topic are summed and divided by the total point value possible for each category. This gives the percentile score for each category. The total points given are divided by the total points possible to give an overall score. The letter values may be assigned with the highest score getting an "A+" and the lowest score receiving an "F−." Eight divisions have been made from "A+" to "F−" and the percentage scores assigned appropriate letter grades. Table 1 is a summary of six different laboratories' inspection in 1982-1983.

TABLE 1
Facility Inspection Summary (1983)

Scoring

0-24%	25-40%	41-54%	55-64%	65-74%	75-84%	85-94%	95%+
F-	F	D	C	C+	B	A	A+

Laboratory	1	2	3	4	5	6

Criteria

Criteria	1	2	3	4	5	6
Facility	A	A	C	D	A+	B
Personnel	A	C+	C+	C	A+	B
Test Facility Operations	B	B	B	D	A	A
Animals/Animal Care	A+	A+	C+	A	B	A
SOP's	A+	F-	B	F	A+	A+
Quality Assurance	A	B	A	C	A+	A+
Equipment	B	A+	B	B	B	B
Test Article	B	B	A	A	A	B
Data	B	C+	A+	B	A	C+
Archives	C	C+	C	C	C+	A
Overall	A	B	C+	C	A	B

Tables 2 and 3 are similar summary tables for 12 more laboratories inspected in 1984-1985. These tables indicate the wide variability both between laboratories in certain categories, and within a given laboratory.

Table 4 summarizes the evaluation of eight laboratories capable of conducting subchronic inhalation toxicity testing. This table indicates how a sponsor can use the facility inspection and scoring process to assist in the selection of a testing laboratory.

TABLE 2
Facility Inspection Summary (1984)

Scoring

0-24% F-	25-40% F	41-54% D	55-64% C	65-74% C+	75-84% B	85-94% A	95%+ A+

Laboratory	7	8	9	10	11	12

Criteria

Criteria	7	8	9	10	11	12
Facility	A	C	F	C+	B	A+
Personnel	B	D	D	B	B	A+
Test Facility Operations	C+	D	F-	C+	B	B
Animals/ Animal Care	A	B	D	C+	B	A
SOP's	A+	F	F	C	B	C+
Quality Assurance	C+	F-	F-	F-	A	C+
Equipment	A	D	F	A	A	A
Test Article	B	F	F	A	A	A
Data	A	C	C	C+	C	A
Archives	A	F	F-	A	D	F
Overall	B	D	F	C+	B	B

135

TABLE 3
Facility Inspection Summary (1985)

Scoring

0-24% F-	25-40% F	41-54% D	55-64% C	65-74% C+	75-84% B	85-94% A	95%+ A+

Laboratory	13	14	15	16	17	18
Criteria						
Facility	A	A	A	B	A	C+
Personnel	A	A	A	A	A+	A
Test Facility Operations	B	C+	C+	C+	B	D
Animals/ Animal Care	A	A	A	A+	A+	C+
SOP's	A	C+	B	B	A	A
Quality Assurance	A	C+	A	B	A	A+
Equipment	A	A	A	A	A+	B
Test Article	B	A	A	A	A	C+
Data	A	A+	A	A	A	A
Archives	B	B	A	B	A	C+
Overall	A	A	A	B	A	C+

CONCLUSION

The inspection, evaluation and scoring system is a useful tool for evaluating and ranking contract testing laboratories in a rather quantitative fashion according to consistent criteria. The system plays an important role in our selection of contract laboratories for toxicity testing. The system provides assurance that the testing facility has the *capability* to conduct quality toxicity tests.

TABLE 4
Facility Inspection Summary, Testing Facilities Capable of Conducting Subchronic Inhalation

Scoring

0-24%	25-40%	41-54%	55-64%	65-74%	75-84%	85-94%	95%+
F-	F	D	C	C+	B	A	A+

Laboratory	I	II	III	IV	V	VI	VII
Criteria							
Facility	B	A	A+	A	A	B	A
Personnel	B	A+	A+	A	A	B	A
Test Facility Operations	B	B	B	C+	B	A	C+
Animals/ Animal Care	B	A+	A	A+	A	A	A
SOP's	B	A	C+	A+	A	A+	C+
Quality Assurance	A	A	C+	A	A	A	C+
Equipment	A	A	A	B	A	B	A
Test Article	C	A+	B	B	B	B	A
Data	C	A	A	B	A	C+	A+
Archives	D	A	F	C	B	A	B
Overall	B	A	B	A	A	B	A

PRINCIPLES OF DATA ACQUISITION

James R. Phelps
Hyman, Phelps and McNamara, P.C.
Washington, DC

ABSTRACT

This presentation will focus on the following concepts:
- legal requirements for toxicology studies;
- expectations of the regulatory authorities, and;
- mechanisms of enforcement.

In addition, methods will be described for managing to achieve compliance and avoiding regulatory involvement.

INTRODUCTION

The placement of toxicology studies in a legal context could take considerable time, especially if one tried to address all of the regulators that are applicable to studies of this type. This paper will deal primarily with the most persistent and arguably, the most difficult regulator, the Food and Drug Administration (FDA) and its impact upon toxicology testing. Even if studies are not directly regulated by FDA, there is probably at least the potential for FDA review.

BACKGROUND

There was a time when the business of toxicology testing seemed to be a matter that was removed from the highly regulated world of the product—the products being foods, drugs, devices, color additives, food additives, and other articles subject to the scrutiny of the FDA. Toxicologists did their work without much thought for the possibility of regulatory confrontation. The FDA and its interests were considered to be more or less theoretical.

Those days of innocence died in the ugliest way, publicly and with no dignity, in the Kennedy hearings in the mid-1970s. Seizing upon some examples of

1. Address correspondence to: James R. Phelps, Esq., Hyman, Phelps and McNamara, P.C., 1120 G Street, N.W., Washington, DC 20005.
2. Key words: data acquisition, enforcement mechanisms, legal requirements, regulatory authorities.
3. Abbreviations: FDA, U.S. Food and Drug Administration; GLP, Good Laboratory Practice.

villainy and more instances in which hapless people simply did not keep sufficient records to disprove fraud, the Senator painted a picture of widespread misconduct in nonclinical and clinical testing. The FDA, which was, itself, taken through the fire of adverse publicity on its role as the regulator for research, subsequently performed a study and issued a report to say that there was not widespread cheating in nonclinical and clinical research. However, by the time of this report, the die had been cast. The FDA had obtained a special appropriation of approximately $16 million in 1977 for bio-research monitoring. In addition, some 600 new jobs had been created in the agency in response to these hearings. The FDA was, thus, put permanently into the business of monitoring bio-research. Studies performed for products regulated by FDA would not be subject to close regulatory scrutiny.

REGULATORY INITIATIVES

A first step was to issue the Good Laboratory Practice (GLP) regulations. These were first proposed in 1976, and finalized in 1978. During this period, the agency was also proposing regulations for clinical investigations, including rules for protection of human subjects, institutional review boards, sponsors and clinical investigators. To date, the agency has made final the regulations for the laboratories, the GLPs, the regulations for the protection of human subjects and the institutional review board. It is curious that the agency's greatest enforcement efforts have been with the clinical investigators for whom FDA has been unable to develop final regulations for almost a decade. One cannot help but think about the King James Bible; in the days before word processors, it went from inspiration to print in about seven years. One would think that the agency would be able to finalize its regulations in that time. Perhaps they are seeking more inspiration than the translators of the King James Bible.

In terms of volume of effort, FDA has, however, made a relatively small enforcement investment in nonclinical testing. This is especially true as compared to clinical research. FDA's limited effort is no reason for toxicologists to ignore the regulator. The GLP regulations are remarkable in that they are what amounts to an official policy of distrust of research done with regulated products. The regulations articulate in minute detail the record keeping and other requirements that must be met in order for the official suspicion to be allayed. Valid research has been defined, in effect, to mean only that research for which the FDA required records was kept. Other research will be suspect— irrespective of its scientific merit. In other words, we are now in an era of regulated science.

To attempt to discuss the requirements for the performance of a good study and how these may or may not be embodied by the regulations would be outside the scope of this paper. During this conference we have heard how FDA has tried to describe a good nonclinical study; how the study should be run with directions about the protocol, facilities, equipment, handling of test animals, control and test articles, and the qualifications of personnel doing the study. For consideration of the legal situation created by the regulations, we need to examine their regulatory features.

REGULATORY IMPACT ON TOXICOLOGY STUDIES

The regulations start by firmly fixing responsibility. They require that for each study there should be a designated study director. Should anything be amiss, this is where the blame will be placed first. The regulations also require that there must be a specifically designated quality assurance unit. It is the responsibility of the quality assurance unit to monitor the study to determine that it is performed properly and that there is compliance with the regulatory requirements. The study director is expressly given the responsibility to assure that the study is properly documented. Now, by "documentation," the agency means carefully kept records, to make it possible for an inspector to follow a paper trail through the history of each study. The paper trail is central to the monitoring that the agency will perform. The regulations place considerable emphasis on the need for a clear data trail. For example, they specify that all the data entries must be in ink, not in pencil, and they must be dated and initialed. When there are any changes, the person making such changes must be clearly identified. Should a study be terminated before it is completed, the regulations require that a final report must still be written so that poor quality work is not simply dropped.

These records must be retained for inspection for at least two years and if the studies are submitted to FDA, the records must be retained for five years after the submission. In addition, if there are such items as slides, both the slides and tissue blocks must be retained. One reason this is required is that agency personnel may, if they choose, go behind the data to verify the accuracy of the report. Having created this requirement for a regulatory map on each study, the agency also wrote into the regulations that agency personnel must be given total access to these records, with the exception of the records for the quality assurance unit. Their records are very widely exempted from normal inspections in order that this group can criticize in-house work.

FDA ENFORCEMENT PRACTICES

One wonders whether there is a great amount of nonclinical research being done in this country which is first rate in its substance, but in which there is not much attention paid to the regulatory requirements. If this is the case, then some very good scientists are facing nothing short of ruin. Those who get caught in FDA's enforcement actions soon learn that there is very, very little to protect one's reputation. Reputations are gone before they can be defended. The range of enforcement powers available to FDA is impressive. To begin, the FDA uses a regulatory letter. This letter states FDA's conclusions that the standards are not being met and demands that the addressee "shape up" or face further regulatory action. This action could include injunctions, disqualification or federal prosecution.

The FDA makes these regulatory letters a matter of public record so that purported deficiencies are made a topic of discussion in the industry immediately. Of course, reputations are thereby affected. It must be recognized that there is no effective means of answering these charges to all the people who will learn of them. The GLP regulations equip FDA with a method to punish infractions. Probably the most significant method is to disqualify the testing facility from performing studies that will be recognized by FDA. Disqualification is accomplished through a hearing under Part 16 of FDA's regulations. Part 16 is a peculiar regulation. It parcels out the task of prosecutor to one FDA employee, and the task of the judge to another FDA employee who is the hearing officer. The hearing officer is not supposed to have had anything to do with the matter under consideration before his assignment. This is said to assure that the employee will be unbiased in the case. The Part 16 hearing, in fact, has few of the protections that Americans expect to find in proceedings that decide important issues. For example, the rules of the hearing establish that there will be no rules of evidence. Hearsay, rumor and nearly anything else becomes admissible, and it is up to the defending party to try to rebut this as best he can. In the recent past, these hearings have been very popular for the disqualification of clinical investigators—those folks who do not have regulations.

One of my partners has handled about five clinical disqualification proceedings representing physicians. I am pleased to be able to tell you that, notwithstanding, the Part 16 hearing rules are so poor in practice that the FDA official assigned to handle the hearings had no appetite for the kind of kangaroo court that those rules would seem to permit, and he gave our clients the chance to have an opportunity to defend themselves. After a Part 16 hearing is completed, the hearing officer makes an initial finding which is forwarded to the commissioner of the FDA, who makes a final decision. If there is a disqualification, the testing facility will be listed as unacceptable and studies from it—past, present, and future—will not be considered by the agency. The agency will also take the trouble to publicize this disqualification. Those individuals involved in nonclinical testing need to be aware of the possibility of the Part 16 hearing being used for disqualification and something about how it works. It should be recognized that it has not yet been employed for disqualification of a nonclinical testing facility because it has not been necessary. Two facilities that faced disqualification simply went out of business.

I was told by one employee of the FDA that the lawyers in the clinical investigator disqualification cases have spoiled the Part 16 hearing, making them inefficient by putting on a defense. This person, who is in a position to know, said that the Office of Scientific Investigations (those are the people who perform bio-research monitoring for the Center for Drugs) do not intend to use the Part 16 procedures as much in the future. I certainly hope this proves to be the case. It is so easy for the agency to achieve compliance with its wishes through the use or the threat of use of publicity that it is not necessary to use the formally established procedures in most instances. The only exceptions to the need to use formal procedures are for enforcement groups that consider it necessary to use written enforcement reports as an indication of their progress.

This progress, of course, is measured in terms of cases: Cases must be reported if progress is to be reported.

In egregious cases, when FDA believes there have been willful violations, the more likely regulatory action is criminal prosecution for false reports submitted to FDA. Most people would be surprised to know how easy it is to get a criminal investigation and a possible prosecution started. To illustrate how a prosecution might occur, let me share a real case.

CASE STUDY

In 1973, a client of mine worked in a testing facility. This client and two other people participated in the conduct of a toxicology study using dogs. During the study, some of the dogs started vomiting and some of these animals continued vomiting throughout the study. I understand that this is not uncommon. The client and two other people all had roles in writing the final report. This report erroneously indicated that the dogs had stopped vomiting. Later the client could not remember who had made the error because the responsibility for the error was not obvious from the way the report was written.

Shortly after this report was written, it was sent to the sponsoring company with the error. The client left the employ of this particular testing facility at about the same time and went to work elsewhere. The client's connection with the testing facility ended in 1973. This study was submitted by the sponsor in 1973 to FDA as part of a new drug application. Four years later, the study was again submitted to FDA as part of another new drug application. This time, in 1980, FDA audited the clinical aspects of the toxicology work done to support the NDA before approval. Agency personnel saw that the notes from the study showed some of the dogs had not stopped vomiting. This prompted further investigation by the agency and some eight years after working on the study and its report, my client received a 305 notice. A 305 notice is FDA's formal invitation, provided for by the Federal Food, Drug and Cosmetic Act, for one to meet with agency personnel to try to persuade them to change their decision to have one prosecuted for criminal violation. It was incumbent upon us to explain how the error occurred and what the client's involvement in that error might have been. This was not an easy task, considering the time that had passed since the event. The 305 notice did not say the misrepresentation was intentional, or even who had made the error. Obviously, the agency did not know.

It happens that FDA has wiser heads than the one who wrote that particular 305 notice. The wiser prevailed and no case was filed. Nonetheless, this example points to the hazard now faced in toxicology work and shows how long the grief begun by a mistake in reporting a study can follow the person who made the error—or a person who was unlucky enough to be around when the error was made. Those who earnestly wish to avoid the anguish of bad publicity, a possible disqualification or a possible prosecution will start with a line-by-line analysis of the GLP regulations, and a clear-eyed critique of the state of their research operations for compliance with those regulations.

MINIMIZING THE POSSIBILITY OF
CONFRONTATION WITH FDA

Most of the agency's regulatory actions are likely to begin as a consequence of information developed in an inspection. There is little in the background of persons working in nonclinical laboratories to give confidence that they will be able to handle FDA inspections properly unless special consideration and training are given. As much as we would like for them to be, these inspections are not simple exchanges of data by scientists. Inspectors are visiting to look for violations of the law or a regulation. Knowing what the inspector will want and what his tactics will be are vital. Mishandling of FDA inspections, or misunderstanding their significance, can have severe and adverse consequences. If you are in or around a regulated industry, I would hope that all of you have taken the time to read the agency's manual on methods used in inspections. I am surprised at the number of people who are regulated who have not read this little document. It is not long and it tells you what to expect. It is so much better to have read it before an inspection occurs.

If there is trouble with the agency—in fact, if a researcher has trouble with any agency—he is likely to learn quickly who his friends are. The sponsors will want to protect their research, the institutions will want to protect their reputations, and the researcher will want to save both in order to protect himself. The most valuable regulatory preparation done by testing concerns will be done prophylactically. Planning after getting into the suit is going to be of more doubtful efficacy, and planning for difficulty is not something that only a guilty party does. How to react depends upon the nature of the problems, but it is wise to have the team in place in advance to deal with problems as they arise. The worst thing to try to do is to use buzz words as a substitute for a planned response. You see this behavior when people are mindlessly told to "cooperate," or to "stonewall." Marching orders such as these should have a rabbit's foot attached because their success will depend entirely upon luck.

If there is a problem, the only thing to do is to face it and attempt to coordinate the response in a way to make it possible for the sponsor, the institution and the researcher to be part of the solution. There is not time today to cover the civil liability that a researcher might incur should regulatory problems cause a study to be unusable. It is not difficult to imagine that at the dismal end of a great expense, to be told that your study cannot be used might prompt somebody to sue. Avoiding regulatory problems is far and away the choice of survivors in this business. Under almost any circumstances, it is worth whatever is necessary to stay in compliance. If FDA's enforcement efforts regarding nonclinical research are not that intense at the moment, do not believe that this is a reason not to be vigilant. Remembering this may save your reputation and your business.

PANEL-AUDIENCE DIALOGUE
PRESTUDY ORGANIZATION

Chairperson:
William H. Farland
U.S. Environmental Protection Agency
Washington, DC

Panel:
Ira J. Friedman, John B. McCandless, James R. Phelps

Dexter Goldman (EPA): Mr. McCandless, what part within a decision to contract out a study did this pre-inspection and numerical assignment play in the corporate decision? How did your prediction, based upon this numerical sequence, pan out in terms of the performance of the laboratory?

John McCandless: (Atlantic Richfield) It played a big part. We haven't put a study at a laboratory that didn't get at least half a red circle on the bottom line. That was a combination of the facility came out well, the price was reasonable, and the people associated with the facility seemed to know what they were talking about from the scientific end of the business. As to how it turned out—we've been pretty successful. The corporate testing program at Atlantic Richfield has not been that big to date. It's expanding significantly in the next year or two. We've used four or five different laboratories and have had, I think, pretty good success. How do you assess a good study? The quality assurance comes in clean on a QA report? You get the results you wanted? It's tough to say what a good study is, but we feel that we've got our money's worth. The design of the study was proper, so that the results we got were interpretable. We got an endpoint that we were either expecting or hoping to get.

Douglas Walters (NIEHS/NTP): John, the National Fire Protection Association recommends a sprinkler system for paper type archives. This is a first-order type of approximation realizing that you may have microfiched materials as well as paper-type materials. A lot of work has been done by chemists at the National Library of Medicine and the Library of Congress on recovering water-damaged materials from libraries and other archive-type facilities. As Jerry Hardisty (the Director of E.P.L. which handles our records and pathology archives) pointed out yesterday, what's really recommended is a combination of two-hour firewalls, a sprinkler system, as well as a halon system, coupled with an alarm system, and fire and thermal smoke alarms directed to a security system. It you are going to have a sprinkler system, it's important to have it maintained and to make sure it's the right type of sprinkler system.

McCandless: I'm surprised they recommend a water sprinkler system with paper archives.

Walters: If you've ever thrown a sheaf of paper into the fireplace, it smolders and it doesn't go out. Once the halon is dumped the fire comes back, so you really need a sprinkler system that will saturate it. It will put the fire out and keep it out. There won't be a whole lot of damage that will be done, although you do have a lot of water damage. Of course, you want to make sure to use the right types of pens, anyway, in keeping with the proper QA.

John Donahue (Smith, Kline and French Labs): There seems to be potentially at least two schools of thought on the level of detail in protocols and SOPs. One is that the level of details should accommodate the training of a technician—a well-trained technician. The other is that, perhaps the level should be such that someone could come in off the street naive and actually run the procedure.

McCandless: The level of detail of a SOP depends on a number of things: the task that's going to be performed; the personnel attrition at the laboratory. If they don't have much turnover, you'll find the SOP may be somewhat brief. Again, when I look at SOP I will try and know what the task is that has to be done. Does the SOP adequately explain that for me? I prefer something a little more on the brief side than incredible text detailing every single step. I think it gets you in a lot more trouble by having too much detail in a SOP. You've got to allow the person some leeway in conducting a task to do it the way it's best for them to do it.

Donahue: Could I ask for a legal perspective on that in terms of if you had a client who was following SOPs but they were considered to be inadequate?

James Phelps (Hyman, Phelps and McNamara): I am a firm believer that lawyers cannot prescribe how protocols are to be written. They have to be written in order to be used. If the client can tell me that he can read that protocol and know what to do, then I am satisfied.

Ira Friedman (Pfizer, Inc.): I personally believe that SOPs and protocols cannot be used to teach someone from off the street how to run a study. I think that they have to have the essential details of what's important to the scientific staff but not the operational details. When we first started writing SOPs for in-house work, they were so detailed that if someone decided to change the size of the scalpel or the scissors, it was a SOP violation. We very soon got away from that, fortunately.

We don't do much contract work. Generally, I would say these SOPs would not be sufficiently detailed for contract studies.

McCandless: In a contract situation, unless you deal with a lab consistently—

146

if you have to go through the bidding process, you want to make sure that everybody's bidding apples for apples—the protocol will have to be significantly more detailed.

Bill Farland (EPA): From our perspective, the scientific staff in our organization are interested in seeing detail that they can deal with. They don't expect to see so much detail that they could go in and run the study in a lab that they have never been in before, obviously, but it needs to be scientifically complete.

Andrew Tegeris (Tegeris Laboratories): Ira Friedman, you said that you have yet to read the protocols that an untrained person would understand. I really think we should try to distinguish between executing an official protocol and teaching. I think official protocols should be addressed to experienced personnel; in other words, I think we should not try to make a protocol so detailed that it ties down the investigator without any leeway to make an intelligent decision. I think we should really address more the spirit of the law than the letter of the law in these matters.

Steve Harris (Independent Consultant): What is your impression on the two-corridor system or the barrier facility based upon cost effectiveness?

McCandless: I've seen both run well, and I have seen both run poorly. I don't think it costs that much from a construction standpoint to go to a clean/dirty two-corridor system; operationally, it's a nightmare, and I think the people here who are involved in management may disagree, but I think it's a lot more difficult than a single-corridor system. And it's not just the technical people, it's the maintenance people; it's everybody else who's getting things in and out of that room, getting through it—if you violate it, what happens? I think the bio-clean rooms are a step in the right direction. Charcoal's not cheap, filters aren't cheap, but I think a lot of it has to do with what comes into the facility. What kind of shape is it in? How clean is it? How healthy are your animals when they come in? Do you autoclave anything? What type of hygiene measures do you take? The purpose of the clean/dirty system is to cut down on transmitting disease and also cross-contamination of test articles. I think if you have good procedures in-house, you have well-trained people who enjoy what they're doing, who take a personal interest in what you're doing then you can get away with a single-corridor system and have a successful study.

Harris: Does someone evaluate your assessment of these laboratories within ARCO when it comes to contracting?

McCandless: No, people have come with me on these things, and I try to help, or teach, and they'll ask questions as we go.

Farland: Have you shared the results of these assessments with the laboratories?

McCandless: I won't give them a copy of the form or a copy of my results, but I will debrief them on what I have found. These are my personal observations, and who am I to say what's really right, and what's really wrong? They have a business to run, and they can agree with me or disagree with me on these things, and that's well within their bailiwick. They've changed my mind on some things, too. Because a lot of times what you find is that you directed your question to the wrong person.

Phelps: That's why regulatory inspections should be very carefully planned. You'd be surprised how much grief comes from the wrong person being asked a question and unintentionally giving uninformed answers.

Didar Hothi (Dynamac Corporation): How long should the laboratories continue using the surplus animals to replace animals dying during the initial phase of the study? According to my experience, laboratories do replace some of the animals during the initial phase of the study. Are they considered in addition to the original number or are they considered just a replacement for the previous one, with no account for the previous animals which have already died? Also, do they always document when the surplus animals were discarded, and how they were discarded—during necropsy, or without necropsy?

McCandless: Obviously, it depends on how early in the study they are replaced. I think most protocols that I'm familiar with allow this to happen: The animals are replaced only up to two or three weeks into the study. I'm not familiar with any protocol that will allow you to replace an animal further than that. The end stays the same. You do not increase the number of total animals on the study. You document that the first ones were removed—however, you continue on with your 50 per sex per group.

My personal opinion is that it is absolutely necessary that it be documented when animals are discarded. There should be a necropsy to find out why they died. It could be something endemic.

Tegeris: I think when you start a study, if you are going to replace animals, you have to have all animals being exposed to the test agent from the very beginning. Therefore, if the study calls for 50 on the test to start with, and five of them die within a week, and you replace them with five more, then these five more, in order to come into the program, must have been taking the same compound from the very beginning. The proper thing to do is to ask your statistician how many animals should you end up with to have data which can be statistically meaningful, and that's the number you should start out with. Those animals stay on test and those that die—they just die.

Hothi: How do those leading laboratories document their day-to-day disposal of the chemical? Where is that chemical stored? Is it in a central place, or is it in the same animal room where the animals are kept? What is the probability of misdosing the animals with the different compounds?

McCandless: I've found that it depends on the laboratory as to how they dispose of the test article, and it depends on the corporation sponsoring the study on how they want them to dispose of the test article. We tell people what we want them to do with it—send it back to us, pour it down the drain, that type of thing. In most cases, the laboratories will have an SOP that leaves it up to the sponsor, or they will decide it themselves. As far as storage of the test article, again, it depends on the specific test article. The better laboratories have very good storage and documentation. They'll have refrigeration, freezers, explosion-proof cabinets. As far as storing the test article in the animal room, my personal opinion is that it depends on the duration of the study. I don't think it's a good idea in general; it depends on the type of the study. In some skin painting studies; it's advantageous to do that. I'm not that familiar with misdosing, but to detect a misdosing would be very, very difficult, unless you analyzed what you were giving the animals the minute you were giving it to them. As to a misdosing from a different material standpoint, I don't recommend having more than one study in a given room.

Doug Bristol (NIEHS/NTP): Would you as a panel consisting of a toxicologist responsible for monitoring studies, a director of quality assurance, and a legal expert speak to the issue of the utilization of quality assurance unit reports on studies that are performed under contract? As the sponsor for the study, you're paying for the reports, and you would like to see that the quality assurance unit is truly performing properly; on the other hand, you don't want to interfere with the confidentiality of the process that's involved in reporting the findings of quality assurance inspections and audits.

McCandless: I'm not going to get involved in the management of your operation but I want to see what QA is finding.

Friedman: I certainly want to see what the QA function has found in a contract facility. The contract labs that we've dealt with has been willing to share this after first saying, "No, we won't"; then they say, "Well, maybe we will"; then finally they share things with us. I think it's important, and I would certainly consider it carefully in my choice of a laboratory.

Phelps: The legal implications of sharing the quality assurance unit's work with the regulator are significantly different from sharing between two private parties who have contractual obligations. I see no legal problems in sharing the data between two private parties.

Jack Polidoro (Toxicol Laboratories): John, did your report include European laboratories? Does your form include any mechanical things that would cover European regulations that don't apply to the U.S.?

McCandless: No European labs were included. I'm totally naive when it comes to European regulations. If I were to go to a European laboratory, I would really like to sit down and understand those regulations with those people.

Polidoro: On a scale of the ten items that you present, are the points that are given for each of the categories equal? Also, under your category for animal usage you might want to back up and consider the source of the animals, and their surveillance prior to the receipt. There's no use starting a study that doesn't have quality in it.

McCandless: The facility has the greatest number of points, and I believe the equipment has the least number. The source of the animal is part of the inspection form.

Kathryn Hackett-Fields (Product Safety Labs): Ira, I was really interested in your detail on the deviations from SOPs and protocols—what you would consider significant. Who might determine things like that? Would it be a statistical decision or is it based on experience? I'm primarily concerned with studies that are two weeks and under in length. What might you consider to be deviations that are significant in areas like temperature and humidity when you're talking about such short-term work?

Friedman: I was talking about such things as changing the dose levels without consulting a study director or sponsor; moving the animals from one room to another in the midst of a study without consulting the sponsor; someone deciding that since the compound seemed to be rather slow in dissolving, they might put the solution on steam bath to speed things up. Those are very significant departures from a protocol that I think should not be carried out without some careful discussion with the study director or sponsor. Departures from temperature and humidity conditions ought to be well documented, but usually you can't do anything about it. It's happened; it's beyond the control of people; you have to decide whether the study has been flawed, or whether it's been affected by it.

Donahue: Under the current law, what is the potential for disqualification of individual study directors and/or even medical monitors?

Phelps: The agency wrote its good laboratory manufacturing practices regulations with facilities in mind. They have acted with clinical investigators in mind. I am not aware of any effort to disqualify any individual study director. There is not express provision for it in the regulations. Since the regulations are entirely made up by FDA as to what they're going to consider as acceptable work or acceptable people, I'm sure that they would consider it to be within their power to disqualify such people.

Goldman: I look at SOPs with this question in mind: If you brought in another technician—not somebody naive—with basically the same training, would they be able to follow that particular SOP? James, it seems to me that you used a rather broad brush on the question of government regulation of science. I interpreted your saying that this was government involvement in science with a capital "S" and I wonder if you meant it to be that broad? I think you could even argue that the NIH study sections and grant award mechanism is government regulation of science. The other thing is that you're looking at the regulation of applied science that is used to come up with risk benefit evaluations that people and society are involved with. There are no regulations comparable to that within basic and developmental research.

Phelps: In the context in which I spoke, I did not mean it, but in fact there is government involvement in science with a capital "S." You've described some of it. Obviously, the source from which the money flow will have some impact upon the activities that take place.

150

Chapter IV
ANIMAL QUALITY

ANIMAL QUALITY

Stephen H. Weisbroth
AnMed Laboratories
Rockville, Maryland

CHAIRPERSON'S REMARKS

In 1964 when I entered the world of laboratory animal science, the life span of the laboratory rat was 14 to 16 months. Today, about 30 months is closer to current projections. We have, in a sense, more than doubled the life span of the rats in the laboratory in a mere 20 years. If you will bear with me for a bit of history, it is probably difficult for most of you to appreciate the profound effect of disease on laboratory rodents in the 1950s and '60s. In study after study, the experimental effects were overridden by the symptomatologic and physiologic effects of disease burdens. How much scientific data collected in that era were synergized or generated by disease is unknown but acknowledged as substantial.

This adverse impact was the primary reason for seeking practical methods for large-scale production of rodents free of infectious disease. The solution lay in harnessing the principles of gnotobiology, a process by which starter colonies of desired stocks and strains are derived by hysterectomy and reared behind barriers from which disease agents are excluded. The strategy was enormously successful, particularly with primary bacterial, mycoplasmal, and parasitic agents. By the mid 1970s, routine provision of so-called specific pathogen-free (SPF) animals was readily available.

Why then is there so much recent concern about rodent viruses and environmental variables? If these agents existed 10 years ago, why weren't they causing problems then? There are at least three reasons why viral agents and environmental variables were not recognized as problems a decade ago. First of all, it was only after primary disease burdens had been lifted from laboratory rodents that the effect of many of the viral agents and environmental variables could even be recognized and determined. Many of these agents are clinically silent and it is in only recent years that the significance of these conditions has been appreciated. Secondly, the precision of modern experimentation, much of it at the interface of in vivo and in vitro systems, the use of immunologically compromised animal models, and the kinds of studies collectively embraced by the term biotechnology are often profoundly affected by viral agents and environmental processes that remain clinically silent in random bred, normal, intact rodents.

Thirdly, it is often true that whether a problem is recognized as being a problem depends on who is affected. Overt clinical infection promptly becomes a problem for the animal care director or the animal supplier. On the other hand, clinically silent infections, particularly in the past, were not a problem for the animal care office, but may well have been for the animal user. Thus, a degree of apathy attended detection of so-called latent or silent agents and processes until the primary disease burdens were lifted and the effects of these more subliminal agents recognized. Only in the last several years has the knowledge of the biological cycles of viral agents even been correlated with antibody tracking systems.

Suffice it to say that in the last several years, as we have begun to consolidate the knowledge of these subliminal and silent infections and environmental conditions, there has been a gradual redefinition of the concept of what constitutes a disease or an undesirable condition. In a sense, there has been a redefinition of the experimental substrate animal. The study strategy involves recognition that extraneous microbial forms and environmental variables may perturb the physiologic reactions of substrate animals in ways that may or may not be clinically apparent. The present goal is to emphasize the stability of the substrate animal by excluding all known indigenous viral agents and by providing a known, stabilized environment so that the physiologic effects of treatment may be recognized as such with our contribution by disease or milieu. The nature of this strategy is the basis for the presentations of our next two speakers.

ANIMAL HEALTH IN TOXICOLOGICAL RESEARCH: AN APPRAISAL OF PAST PERFORMANCE AND FUTURE PROSPECTS

J. Russell Lindsey, Donald B. Casebolt and Gail H. Cassell
Departments of Comparative Medicine and Microbiology
Schools of Medicine and Dentistry
University of Alabama at Birmingham
and The Birmingham Veterans Administration Medical Center
Birmingham, Alabama

ABSTRACT

In recent times, regulatory, economic and scientific pressures have focused an unprecedented amount of attention on animal health as an important determinant of data quality in toxicological research and testing. Largely in response to the Good Laboratory Practices Act of 1979, many governmental agencies, industrial firms and contract laboratories established programs of animal health quality assurance. A general appraisal of the effectiveness of those programs is made, and significant weaknesses in current programmatic approaches and practices are identified. A series of model programs are outlined for use in achievement of much higher and more consistent health standards in the future.

INTRODUCTION

Animal health in toxicological research is a very large topic. In the broadest sense it could include all of the genetic and environmental factors known to affect the "normal" well being of research animals and/or their "normal" biologic responses to experimental treatments (Baker et al., 1979; Pakes et al., 1984). However, this presentation will be limited to indigenous infectious agents

1. Address correspondence to: Dr. J. Russell Lindsey, Department of Comparative Medicine, Schools of Medicine and Dentistry, University of Alabama at Birmingham, Birmingham, AL 35294.
2. Key words: animal health, barrier programs, health monitoring, microbiological status, pathogen status, rodent diseases.
3. Abbreviation: MRM, murine respiratory mycoplasmosis.

of rats and mice, many of which are known to affect host health and/or biologic responses in toxicological investigations. Since several authoritative publications on this subject have appeared recently (Bhatt and Murphy, 1986; Fox, 1977; Fox et al., 1979; Hamm, 1983, 1986; Jacoby and Barthold, 1981), our presentation will concentrate on an appraisal of past performance in control of these agents and practical approaches to future improvements.

TERMINOLOGY OF MICROBIOLOGICAL STATUS

The development of gnotobiotic methodology during the 1940s and 1950s (Luckey, 1963) provided the foundations for the high standards of health possible in contemporary laboratory animals. The use of cesarean derivation as a means of promptly eliminating the majority of pathogens (Van Hoosier et al., 1966) and the development of improved diets (Wostmann, 1959) adequate for gnotobiotic life were major milestones. However, introduction of the Trexler type plastic film isolator (Trexler and Reynolds, 1957; Trexler, 1963) revolutionized the field as this innovation made the methodology economically and technologically feasible for widespread use by breeders beginning in the early 1960s. Following these developments came a bewildering array of terms for the designation of different levels of research animal quality based on microbiological status. Three examples of such schemes are given in Fig. 1.

Although no effort will be made to describe all of the nuances of each term given in Fig. 1, it is important that the essential meaning of the three examples be given. One should first appreciate the fact that each of the systems is unidirectional. "*Axenic*" or "*germfree*" (these terms are actually misnomers as all animals probably have endogenous viruses) animals are first obtained by cesarean derivation. While being maintained continuously in an isolator, one or more organisms may be introduced (*gnotobiotic, defined microbially associated, or defined flora*) and maintained indefinitely as flora of the animals. Defined flora animals are usually given "cocktails" consisting of several nonpathogenic bacteria to reduce cecal size and make the animals more or less physiologically "normal" (Dubos et al., 1965). An absolute requirement is that animals designated as axenic, germfree, gnotobiotic, defined microbially associated, or defined flora be maintained continuously in isolators and by gnotobiotic methods with regular monitoring (Newton, 1965; Wostmann, 1970).

The second major grouping of terms is that which begins with animals from any of the former isolator maintained types followed by housing under so-called "barrier maintenance" conditions. These terms are *barrier maintained, pathogen free, specific pathogen free (SPF)*, and *virus antibody free* (Fig. 1). There are serious problems with these terms. They have been abused and misused to the extent that most of them are meaningless. The reason is that the terms themselves are elusive, nonspecific labels which have different meanings to different people. "Barrier-maintained" falls short as few people appreciate the meaning of "barrier." The usual concept is that a barrier is merely a facility with a clean corridor-dirty corridor design. "A *barrier* is a system that combines construction features, equipment, and operating methods to stabilize the enclosed

156

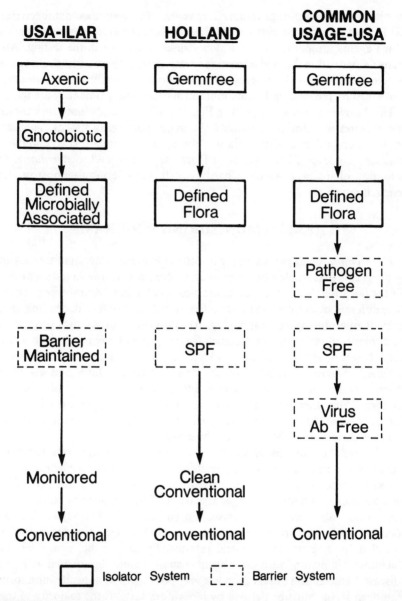

FIGURE 1. Terminology of microbiological status. The three schemes from left to right are: USA-ILAR (Jonas, 1976a), Holland (Solleveld, 1978), and the one in common usage in the United States presently.

environment and to minimize the probability that pathogens or other undesirable organisms will contact or infect the enclosed animal population" (Jonas, 1976a). In other words, a true barrier is a comprehensive preventive medical program that must be supported without interruption by management of the physical plant, strict operational and husbandry practices, and regular health monitoring to determine program effectiveness. Terms such as "pathogen free," "SPF," and "virus antibody free" fall short as there is no universal agreement on which agents are pathogens or which viruses to include in the testing. Also, many individuals in the field learned very early on that these terms could be used with total impunity as long as no testing was done at all. All of these terms must be defined by reliable, up to date monitoring data every time they are used.

The third level of health quality in Fig. 1 (*monitored* and *clean conventional*) also requires monitoring to identify the major pathogens present. The terms imply a standard of quality without defining what standard is acceptable. In practice, this level differs very little from the fourth level, *conventional* (no definition of quality), which is hardly worth considering for most modern research purposes.

HEALTH MONITORING PROGRAMS

Health monitoring programs (or health surveillance programs) are diagnostic programs that employ batteries of laboratory procedures in testing animals for the purpose of defining their microbiological status. Monitoring programs have different objectives and utilize different batteries of tests depending on the level of microbiological status (Fig. 1). Programs for axenic, germfree or gnotobiotic animals must be designed for detection of any microbial contaminant (Newton, 1965; Wostmann, 1970). Those for defined flora animals are designed to detect organisms of the desired bacterial flora and assure the absence of unwanted contaminants. Indigenous "pathogens" are the chief concern in the other types of animals listed in Fig. 1 (i.e., pathogen free, SPF, barrier maintained, etc.) and procedures for their detection are included in the health monitoring test batteries for those animals.

Published lists of "pathogens" for laboratory mice and rats sometimes include more than 25 viruses, 25 bacteria, 7 fungi (dermatophytes), and 25 parasites (protozoa, nematodes, tapeworms, and ectoparasites). Such lists include agents representing a wide spectrum of pathogenicity—strong pathogens, weak pathogens, opportunists and commensals. Although a few (e.g., sialodacryoadenitis virus) regularly produce clinical signs, the vast majority of so-called "pathogens" in mice and rats usually cause subclinical infections. Therefore, "infection" with these agents usually cannot be equated with overt "disease," and clinical observation is a very poor method of health monitoring. Pathogen status must be defined by laboratory tests. If the majority of these agents do not produce overt disease, then what is the definition of the word "pathogen?" In the context of laboratory rodents, a *pathogen* is best defined as an agent that can cause disease and/or alter biologic response(s) during experimentation. This broad definition allows for the numerous and often subtle interactions of subclinical infections with experimental treatments.

What "pathogens" should be tested for in test batteries for mice and rats? One approach is to select tests for only those agents deemed most likely to interfere with a specific research project. For example, an investigator whose research concerns the respiratory system might decide to intensively monitor his animals for respiratory pathogens while ignoring agents affecting other systems. Unfortunately, it is not possible to reliably predict which agent(s) will compromise the results of a given study or series of studies involving an organ system. A second approach is to select tests for a larger list of agents likely to affect research being done by individuals in a large community of investigators with related research interests, e.g., the National Toxicology Program (Thigpen and Tortorich, 1980). This approach too has merit but there is considerable diversity of opinion as to which agents should be included for different communities of investigators (Fox et al., 1979; Hamm, 1983; Hsu et al., 1980; Iwai et al., 1980; Jacoby and Barthold, 1980; Small, 1984; Thigpen and Tortorich, 1980).

There is no single group of agents universally accepted as most important by all laboratories. Similarly, there is little agreement on the actual test procedures that should be used. Some laboratories insist that comprehensive test batteries (virus serology, mycoplasma, ELISAs, bacterial cultures, parasitologic examinations, and histopathology of all major organs) are most cost effective while some recommend a much narrower approach, e.g., virus serologies alone. Pathogen status must be defined by the actual monitoring procedures used (battery of specific tests done) and the date of testing as results have finite reliability and usefulness (i.e., microbial status can change). Thus, timely data are required for their definition. Also, one must avoid any lapses in maintenance of barrier conditions. Monitoring animals shipped directly from a breeding facility in cartons protected by bacterial filter media and tested immediately upon arrival gives data which accurately reflect the microbial status of the breeding population, whereas monitoring data on animals shipped in open cartons and housed in open cages within a multipurpose facility for two weeks has limited value in establishing the source of contaminant(s).

Clearly there is need for greater objectivity in rodent health monitoring. The selection of agents to be included depends on numerous considerations such as the original microbiological status of the population(s) to be tested, housing background and current practices, and agents most likely to interfere with the program of research. In other words, there needs to be justification for each agent to be included. The test procedures to be used should have proven reliability, high sensitivity and specificity, and be reasonable in cost. Sampling of animals for testing should be by a system of randomization and sample sizes should be according to statistically determined confidence limits (Hsu et al., 1980; Jonas, 1976a, b; Small, 1984). Frequency of sampling should take into account the relative risks of contamination from nearby rodent populations. The ages of animals to be sampled should be based on the ages most likely to give positive test results. Perhaps these principles can be best summarized by saying that design and operation of health monitoring programs, performance of all tests, interpretation of test results, and development of recommendations for corrective action when necessary, are tasks for competent specialists.

PREVALENCE OF PATHOGENS IN CONTEMPORARY LABORATORY RODENTS

After briefly summarizing some of the terminology and methodology used in producing animals of high quality based on microbiological status, we should now ask the question, how effective have these efforts been?

It is difficult to obtain meaningful data on such a large number of diverse rodent populations as currently exist in the United States. However, 65% of the mice and 81% of the rats used for research in the United States are produced by commercial breeding facilities. The data from our laboratory (UAB) given in Tables 1, 2 and 3 are for mice and rats from many of the larger commercial "barrier" facilities in the country. They were shipped to our laboratory and tested within 24 hours using a large battery of accepted, standard procedures (necropsy, serology, bacterial cultures, parasite examinations, and histopathology). We believe the results are representative of contemporary mice and rats produced in commercial "barriers" in the United States (Lindsey, 1986).

Table 1 shows the prevalence of viral pathogens based on our data as well as those of Parker (1980). For the mouse, Sendai virus, mouse hepatitis virus (MHV) and minute virus of mice (MVM) are best described as ubiquitous, and pneumonia virus of mice (PVM), Theiler's poliomyelitis and reovirus 3 were quite common. Adenovirus was found in 19% of mice by histologic methods at UAB. In rats, rat coronaviruses (SDA/RCV), Kilham rat virus (KRV), Sendai virus, PVM, and Toolan H-1 virus were common, and many colonies had reovirus 3 and adenovirus. The interpretation of serologic positives for Theiler's virus in rats is unknown.

TABLE 1
Prevalence of Viral Pathogens in Mice and Rats in the United States

	Mice % Colonies Positive[a]		Rats % Colonies Positive[a]	
Virus	UAB[b]	Parker[c]	UAB[b]	Parker[c]
PVM	36	95	44	64
Sendai	73	86	61	52
MHV	83	81		
MVM	73	81		
Theiler's	5	62		44
Reo 3	14	52	6	44
Polyoma	0	5		
Adenovirus	19[d]	0	6[d]	36
Mousepox	0	0		
LCM	0	0		
SDA/RCV			44	68
KRV			44	71
Toolan H-1			1152	52

[a]Results are based on serologic testing except for UAB adenovirus results (see below).

[b]Data compiled in our laboratory at the University of Alabama at Birmingham during the period 1980-1982. The populations sampled were exclusively commercial "barrier" breeding facilities. Mice (n = 2,811) were from 77 rooms in 13 facilities; rats (n = 1,034) were from 18 rooms in 9 facilities.

[c]From Parker (1980). Data include results from both commercial breeding colonies and user colonies, 1965-1978.

[d]Diagnosis was based on finding typical intranuclear inclusions in intestinal epithelium (Luethans and Wagner, 1983). All animals were serologically negative for adenovirus.

TABLE 2
Prevalence of Bacterial Pathogens in Mice and Rats in the United States[a]

Bacteria	% Colonies Positive[b]	
	Mice	Rats
Mycoplasma ELISA	91	78
Mycoplasma pulmonis	19	17
Mycoplasma arthritidis	3	6
Pseudomonas sp.	57	50
Pasteurella pneumotropica	18	33
Salmonella enteritidis	6	0
Mycobacterium avium	1	0
Citrobacter freundii (4280)	1	0
Corynebacterium kutscheri	0	0
Streptococcus pneumoniae	0	0
Bacillus piliformis	0	0
Streptobacillus moniliformis	0	0

[a]Data compiled in our laboratory during the period 1980-1982. The populations sampled were exclusively commercial "barrier" breeding facilities. Mice (n = 2,811) were from 77 rooms in 13 facilities; rats (n = 1,034) were from 18 rooms in 9 facilities.

[b]All results are based on cultural isolations except for the mycoplasma ELISA (enzyme-linked immunosorbent assay), which was performed by the method of Horowitz and Cassell (1978).

Table 2 gives data on prevalence of bacterial pathogens in mice and rats of commercial "barrier" breeding facilities. *Pseudomonas sp.* and *Pasteurella pneumotropica* are opportunists that rarely cause significant disease. Thus, mycoplasmas are the most prevalent and important bacterial agents in commercial "barriers." *Mycoplasma pulmonis* was isolated by cultural methods from 19% of mice and 17% of rats, respectively. Since cultural methods are insensitive for detection of this agent unless active disease is present, these

TABLE 3
Prevalence of Parasitic Infections or Infestations in Mice and Rats in the United States[a]

Parasite	% Colonies Positive	
	Mice	Rats
Entamoeba muris	51	24
Spironucleus muris	42	17
Syphacia sp.	38	17
Mites	29	0
Tritrichomonas sp.	26	17
Giardia sp.	12	11
Hymenolepis sp.	4	0
Eimeria sp.	1	0

[a]Data compiled in our laboratory during the period 1980-1982. The populations sampled were exclusively commercial "barrier" breeding facilities. Mice (n = 2,811) were from 77 rooms in 13 facilities; rats (n = 1,034) were from 18 rooms in 9 facilities.

figures are undoubtedly very conservative. *Mycoplasma arthritidis* characteristically produces latent infections which are notoriously difficult to demonstrate by culture, but this agent is presently thought to be ubiquitous in mice and rats in the United States. Both *M. pulmonis* and *M. arthritidis* are considered responsible for the high prevalence of mycoplasma ELISA positives, 91% in mice and 78% in rats (Cassell et al., 1986; Lindsey et al., 1986).

Table 3 gives the prevalence of parasites in commercial "barriers." *Entamoeba muris, Spironucleus muris, Syphacia sp.*, mite infestations, and *Tritrichomonas sp.* were rather common. *Giardia sp., Hymenolepis sp.*, and *Eimeria sp.* were encountered infrequently.

In response to our question about effectiveness of gnotobiotic methods and "barrier" programs in this country, the answer should by now be quite obvious. Such programs have thus far achieved only limited success. In fact, it appears that certain agents such as MHV, Sendai virus, MVM, PVM, KRV, and SDA/RCV are particularly well adapted epizootiologically for the intensive production currently being practiced. It should be emphasized that the UAB data above apply only to breeding facilities. This probably means that prevalence of pathogens would be even higher in user facilities which usually receive animals from several breeding populations. The data of Parker (1980) in Table 1 include results from both breeding and user populations and, indeed, the prevalence rates are often much higher than the rates in the UAB data.

EFFECTS OF INFECTIOUS AGENTS ON RESEARCH RESULTS

A number of recent publications have listed many of the known effects of infectious agents on specific research endpoints (Bhatt and Murphy, 1986; Hsu et al., 1980; Jacoby and Barthold, 1980). Therefore, we have chosen to discuss only a few of the more prevalent agents as possible prototypes of the effects infectious agents can have on toxicological research.

MHV has an extremely high prevalence among mouse populations in the United States (Table 1). Clinical disease due to MHV is seldom seen, but research results may be significantly altered by subclinical infection (Barthold, 1986). MHV infection results in immune depression or immune stimulation during the course of the infection (Virelizier et al., 1976). Infection decreases phagocytic function (Gledhill et al., 1965; Williams and DiLuzzio, 1980), but increases the tumoricidal activity of peritoneal macrophages (Boorman et al., 1982). MHV infection also alters hepatic enzyme activity (Budillon et al., 1973; Caccitore and Antoniella, 1971; Carter et al., 1977; Paradisi et al., 1972; Ruebner and Hirano, 1965), and results in slower repair following partial hepatectomy (Carthew, 1981). Subclinical MHV infection may be converted to clinical disease with mortality by treatment with immunosuppressants such as cortisone (Taylor et al., 1981), cyclophosphamide (Willenborg et al., 1973), or other chemotherapeutic agents (Braunsteiner and Friend, 1954).

Sendai virus has a high prevalence among populations of both rats and mice in the United States (Table 1); the effects of this virus in toxicologic research have been discussed by Parker (1980), Hamm (1983), and Hall et al. (1986). Each of these authors cited the study by Henry et al. (1981) in which BC3F1/Cum mice treated with 3-methylcholanthrene had shortened lifespans if infected with Sendai virus. Infected mice also had low probabilities of lung tumor development because they did not live long enough for tumors to arise. Subsequent experiments with mice vaccinated against Sendai and maintained under barrier conditions to eliminate other pathogens showed that (a) mice lived for over 80 weeks of treatment versus 45 weeks for infected animals, and (b) the incidence of lung tumors was greatly increased. Peck et al. (1983) reported that enzootic Sendai infection in their strain A mice reduced the number of 10-chloromethyl-9-chloranthracene induced pulmonary adenomas, and increase the number of 7,12-dimethylbenz(a)anthracene induced adenomas. A third example of an effect of Sendai virus on pulmonary carcinogenesis was that reported by Nettesheim et al. (1974, 1981), who studied squamous cell metaplasia and neoplasia in the lungs of mice exposed to smoke and viral respiratory infections. They concluded that Sendai virus was responsible for many of the pulmonary changes seen previously and mistaken for toxic effects. The studies of Richter (1970, 1973) demonstrated squamous metaplastic changes due to Sendai infection alone.

Murine respiratory mycoplasmosis (MRM) is a chronic disease of rats and mice caused by infection with *Mycoplasma pulmonis*. There are multiple agent, host, and environmental factors which influence the expression of MRM. In general, *M. pulmonis* infection is subclinical, but the disease may result in morbidity and mortality in long term studies, particularly in rats (Lindsey et al., 1971, 1982, 1986). As with Sendai virus, this effect alone might significantly affect long term studies by decreasing the life span of infected animals. Several respiratory toxins have been shown to increase the expression of MRM. These include ammonia (Broderson et al., 1976; Saito et al., 1982; Schoeb et al., 1982); tobacco smoke (Wynder et al., 1968), and hexamethylphosphoramide (Lee and Trochimowitz, 1982a, b; Overcash et al., 1976). Hexamethylphosphoramide is a particularly relevant example for this conference as it is the most potent promoter of *M. pulmonis* disease expression known, and it seems likely that MRM will be found to complicate toxicological studies of other compounds in a similar manner. In addition, MRM alters the effects of respiratory carcinogens. Schreiber et al. (1972) found that the incidence of lung tumors induced by a cyclic nitrosamine was significantly increased in rats with active MRM when compared with "specific pathogen free" rats.

These examples are by no means an exhaustive listing of the effects these three agents have been reported to have on experimental results, and many other agents are known to have similar effects. The important points with regard to the effects of infectious agents on research results are: (a) these pathogens, like many others, rarely produce clinical disease, so their effects are often insidious and undetected unless results are compared with those from barrier maintained animals known to be free of infection, (b) alterations of experimental results may be indirect, such as decreased longevity of infected animals leading to a decreased apparent tumor incidence, (c) pathogens may confound experimental results in many ways, causing increases and/or decreases in one or several endpoints.

OUTLOOK FOR FUTURE IMPROVEMENT

The foregoing review of past performance strongly suggests that one should be pessimistic about future prospects for improvement. On the contrary, we believe there are reasons for optimism. First, there are finally sufficient reliable data available (Tables 1, 2 and 3) to bring some objectivity to the evaluation of current quality control practices. Secondly, investigators, institutional administrators, funding agencies, and rodent breeders in the United States seem to be increasingly aware of past quality control failures and interested in the possibilities for improvement. What is needed to bring about significant improvements? *Genuine commitment* (on the part of investigators, administrators, funding agencies and breeders) to preventing indigenous infections throughout the life of the rodent is the single most important need but others are important as well. Key requirements for success[a] include:

(a) The investigator must be strongly committed.

(b) The investigator and the support personnel must understand the terminology and principles involved.

(c) There must be availability and use of appropriate facilities and equipment.

(d) Housing practices must assure physical separation and avoidance of cross contamination between different animal populations throughout life.

(e) Reliable health monitoring must be maintained to identify breeding populations free of pathogens, and to redefine the microbiological status of the animals at regular intervals after receipt in the user facility until completion of each study.

(f) Written standard operating practices must be developed and followed without interruption; clear objectives must be defined in advance along with detailed procedures for reaching those objectives.

Many investigators would like to improve the health status of their animals but are not aware of some of the practical alternatives available for accomplishing their objectives. The following is the range of optional approaches which should be considered in meeting the needs of each investigator (or institution).

Option 1

| Unmonitored animals from many breeding facilities | → | Transported in open cartons | → | Housed in a conventional multipurpose research facility |

---

[a]From a consensus developed during the seminar entitled "Barrier Maintenance of Rodents in Multipurpose Facilities," 36th Annual Session, American Association of Laboratory Animal Science, Baltimore, MD. Seminar participants: J. Russell Lindsey (Leader), G. L. Van Hoosier, Jr., D. B. Casebolt, J. G. Fox, R. O. Jacoby, and T. E. Hamm, Jr.

This option was the standard many years ago and is still surprisingly common today. In essence, this is the animal procurement and use system devoid of any quality control. The animals generally look healthy but nearly always harbor an assortment of subclinical pathogens.

Option 2

| Unmonitored animals from "barrier" breeding facilities | → | Containment transport | → | Housing in a barrier room in a multipurpose research facility |

In Option 2 there is no user monitoring of the so-called "barrier" breeding facility; chances of obtaining animals from a room with one or more indigenous pathogens are very good (Tables 1, 2, and 3). Some so-called "barrier" breeding facilities have some rooms free of pathogens and others that are contaminated, but only one shipping room. Therefore, animals may exchange pathogens before being placed in filter protected cartons for shipping. Even though housed in a "barrier room" in the user facility, chances of arrival with active infection are incubating other infections are excellent. Also, since the research facility is multipurpose (i.e., houses animals of different pathogen status, from many sources, for many different research programs), the chances of cross-contamination between animal subpopulations are excellent despite efforts to protect animals within a given room by a barrier program.

Option 3

| User monitored, vendor monitored, protected, barrier breeding facility | → | Containment transport | → | Remote quarantine | → | Barrier facility, barrier rooms |

Option 3 utilizes animals from a barrier facility that is regularly monitored by the user institution and by the vendor, and all subpopulations found to be consistently negative on both test batteries. One of the most positive developments in recent times has been the new policy of several commercial breeders to make their monitoring data (including subpopulation identification, numbers of animals tested, a listing of tests actually done, and the latest test date) available either upon request or with every shipment of animals. A few breeders also promptly notify users in the event an unexpected pathogen is detected in the breeding facility. In option 3 the vendor also has made a commitment to protect the *entire* facility from pathogens by immediately eliminating any subpopulation diagnosed as having any pathogen on a predetermined list of agents (most producers are unwilling to do this). Animals are shipped in filter-protected cartons, and received at a quarantine facility remote from the research facility. There they are quarantined in a separate barrier room (for 3 to 6 weeks), then monitored and found to be free of all pathogens, then transferred by filtered cartons to a barrier room in the research facility. The value of a remote quarantine facility has been demonstrated over many years by the Jackson Laboratory (Parker and Richter, 1982).

165

		a. Barrier facility
		b. Barrier room
		c. Barrier room with
User controlled,		filter cages and
monitored, and		laminar flow
protected barrier	Containment	change station
breeding facility →	transfer →	d. Trexler isolators

Option 4 offers the greatest protection for the investigator (or institution) genuinely committed to the production and use of animals definitely free of pathogens. All aspects of the barrier breeding program, containment transfer to the user facility, housing conditions in the user facility, and the health monitoring program are controlled by the user (or institution). There is a commitment to eliminate breeding populations immediately if they become contaminated with any of a predetermined list of agents. Many laboratories maintain small numbers of germfree or pathogen free "seed stocks" of each of their valuable lines in plastic isolators for use in the event their regular breeding stocks become contaminated. Option 4 allows for a range of containment systems to be used in the user facility, depending on the needs of the research program. The entire facility may be operated as a barrier (barrier at facility level) where an entire community of investigators is fully committed to such a program. Alternatively, individual investigators may house their animals in barrier rooms (barrier at the room level). An increasingly popular approach is the filter cage system (barrier at the cage level) used with a laminar flow unit for changing cages (Kraft et al., 1964; Sedlacek et al., 1981). Another alternative is to house the animals in Trexler type plastic film isolators (barrier at the isolator level). With either of these containment systems (institution, room, cage, or isolator), it is mandatory that detailed written protocols be followed and that regular health monitoring be done to evaluate effectiveness of the program.

Options 1 through 4 above are not intended to illustrate four entirely separate systems of procuring and maintaining rodents. Instead, they represent, from 1 through 4, general systems of increasing effectiveness in preventing pathogen contamination of rodent populations. The individual investigator (or institution) must select the combination(s) of these components most appropriate for their research needs, resources, geographic location, and other requirements.

SUMMARY AND CONCLUSIONS

The importance of animal health and animal health quality assurance in toxicological research has been recognized for many years. However, an objective appraisal of past performance in excluding pathogens from experimental rodent populations in the United States leads to the conclusions that these efforts have had only limited success. The outlook for future improvement will depend largely on the level of commitment made by investigators, institutional administrators, funding agencies, and animal breeders, as the basic methodology and technology for major improvements have been available for many years.

ACKNOWLEDGEMENTS

Supported in part by contract NO1-ES-95616 from the National Institute of Environmental Health Sciences, NIH; grants RR00463, RR00959, and RR07003 from the Animal Resources Branch, Division of Research Resources, NIH; HL19741 from the National Heart, Lung, and Blood Institute; and the Research Service of the Veterans Administration.

REFERENCES

BAKER, H. J., LINDSEY, J. R. and WEISBROTH, S. H. (1979). Housing to control research variables. In: *The Laboratory Rat* (H. J. Baker, J. R. Lindsey and S. H. Weisbroth, eds.) Vol. I, pp. 169–192. Academic Press, New York.

BARTHOLD, S. W. (1986). Research complications and state of knowledge of rodent coronaviruses. In: *Complications of Viral and Mycoplasmal Infections in Rodents to Toxicology Research and Testing* (T. E. Hamm, Jr., ed.) pp. 53–89. Hemisphere Press, Washington, DC.

BHATT, P. N. and MURPHY, F. A., eds. (1986). *Viral and Mycoplasma Infections of Laboratory Rodents.* (In press).

BONATH, K., ed. (1983). *Schwerpunkte der Infektionsuberwachung in Versuchstierbestanden (Principal Problems of Infectious Disease Surveillance in Laboratory Animal Colonies).* 79 p., Paul Parey Verlag, Berlin.

BOORMAN, G. A., LUSTER, M. I., DEAN, J. H., CAMPBELL, M. L., LAUER, L. A., TALLEY, F. A., WILSON, R. E. and COLLINS, M. J. (1982). Peritoneal macrophage alterations caused by naturally occurring mouse hepatitis virus. Am. J. Pathol. **106**:110–117.

BRAUNSTEINER, H. and FRIEND, C. (1954). Viral hepatitis associated with transplantable mouse leukemia. J. Exp. Med. **100**:665–676.

BRODERSON, J. R., LINDSEY, J. R. and CRAWFORD, J. (1976). Role of environmental ammonia in respiratory mycoplasmosis of the rat. Am. J. Pathol. **85**:115–130.

BUDILLON, G., CARELLA, M., DEMARCO, F. and MAZZACCA, G. (1973). Effect of phenobarbital on MHV-3 viral hepatitis of the mouse. Pathol. Microbiol. **39**:461–466.

CACCIATORE, L. and ANTONIELLO, S. (1971). Arginase activity of mouse serum and liver tissue in some conditions of experimental liver damage. Enzymologia **41**:112–120.

CARTER, E. A., WANDS, J. R. and ISSELBACHER, K. J. (1977). Effect of acute murine hepatitis (MHV-1-59) on ethanol oxidation *in vivo.* Gastroenterol. **73**: 321–326.

CARTHEW, P. (1981). Inhibition of the mitotic response in regenerating mouse liver during viral hepatitis. Infect. Immun. **33**:641–642.

CASSELL, G. H., COX, N. R., DAVIS, J. K., BROWN, M. B., MINION, F. C. and LINDSEY, J. R. (1986). State of the art detection methods for rodent mycoplasmas. In: *Complications of Viral and Mycoplasmal Infections in Rodents to Toxicology Research and Testing* (T. E. Hamm, Jr., ed.), pp. 143–160. Hemisphere Press, Washington, DC.

167

DUBOS, R. J., SCHAEDLER, R. W., COSTELLO, R. and HOET, P. (1965). Indigenous, normal and autochthonus flora of the gastrointestinal tract. J. Exp. Med. **122**:67–82.

FOX, J. G. (1977). Clinical assessment of laboratory rodents on long term bioassay studies. J. Environ. Pathol. Toxicol. **1**:199–226.

FOX, J. G., THIBERT, P., ARNOLD, D. L., KREWSKI, D. R. and GRICE, H. C. (1979). Toxicology studies. II. The laboratory animals. Food Cosmet. Toxicol. **17**:661–675.

GANNON, J. and CARTHEW, P. (1980). Prevalence of indigenous viruses in laboratory animal colonies in the United Kingdom 1978–1979. Lab. Anim. **14**:309–311.

GLEDHILL, A. W., BILBEY, D. L. J. and NIVEN, J. S. F. (1965). Effect of certain murine pathogens on phagocytic activity. Brit. J. Exp. Pathol. **46**:433–442.

HALL, W. C., LUBET, R. A., HENRY, C. J. and COLLINS, M. J., JR. (1986). Sendai virus-disease processes and research complications. In: *Complications of Viral and Mycoplasmal Infections in Rodents to Toxicology Research and Testing* (T. E. Hamm, Jr., ed.), pp. 25–52. Hemisphere Press, Washington, DC.

HAMM, T. E., JR. (1983). The effects of health and health monitoring on oncology studies. In: *The Importance of Laboratory Animal Genetics, Health and the Environment in Biomedical Research* (E. C. Melby, Jr. and M. W. Balk, eds.), pp. 45–60. Academic Press, New York.

HAMM, T. E., JR., ed. (1986). *Complications of Viral and Mycoplasmal Infections in Rodents to Toxicology Research and Testing*, 191 p. Hemisphere Press, Washington, DC.

HENRY, C. J., BILLUPS, L. H., AVERY, M. D., RUDE, T. H., DANSIE, D. R., SASS, B., WHITMIRE, C. E. and KOURI, R. E. (1981). Lung cancer model system using 3-methylcholanthrene in inbred strains of mice. Cancer Res. **41**: 5027–5032.

HOAG, W. G. (1964). Animal health control for inbred mouse colonies of the Jackson Laboratory. Lab. Anim. Care **14**:253–259.

HOROWITZ, S. A. and CASSELL, G. H. (1978). Enzyme-linked immunosorbent assay for detection of *Mycoplasma pulmonis* antibodies. Infect. Immun. **22**:161–170.

HSU, C.-K., NEW, A. E. and MAYO, J. G. (1980). Quality assurance of rodent models. In: *Animal Quality and Models in Biomedical Research*. (A. Spiegel, S. Erichsen, and H. A. Solleveld, eds.), pp. 17–28. Gustav Fischer Verlag, New York.

IWAI, H., ITOH, T., NAGIYAMA, N. and NOMURA, T. (1980). Monitoring of murine infections in facilities for animal experimentation. In: *Animal Quality and Models in Biomedical Research* (A. Spiegel, S. Erichsen, and H. A. Solleveld, eds.), pp. 219–222. Gustav Fischer Verlag, New York.

JACOBY, R. O. and BARTHOLD, S. W. (1981). Quality assurance for rodents used in toxicological research and testing. In: *Scientific Considerations in Monitoring and Evaluating Toxicological Research* (E. J. Gralla, ed.), pp. 27–55. Hemisphere Press, Washington, DC.

JONAS, A. M., Chmn. (1976a). Long-term holding of laboratory rodents. ILAR News **19**:L1–L25.

JONAS, A. M. (1976b). The research animal and the significance of a health monitoring program. Lab. Anim. Sci. **26**:339–344.

KRAFT, L. M., PARDY, R. F., PARDY, D. A. and ZWICKEL, H. (1964). Practical control of diarrheal disease in a commercial mouse colony. Lab. Anim. Care **14**:16–20.

LEE, K. P. and TROCHIMOWITZ, H. J. (1982a). Pulmonary response to inhaled hexamethylphosphoramide in rats. Toxicol. Appl. Pharmacol. **62**:90–103.

LEE, K. P. and TROCHIMOWITZ, H. J. (1982b). Induction of nasal tumors in rats exposed to hexamethylphosphoramide by inhalation. J. Natl. Cancer Inst. **68**: 157–171.

LINDSEY, J. R. (1986). Prevalence of viral and mycoplasmal infections in laboratory rodents. In: *Viral and Mycoplasmal Infections of Laboratory Rodents*. (P. N. Bhatt and F. A. Murphy, eds.) (In press).

LINDSEY, J. R., BAKER, H. J., OVERCASH, R. G., CASSELL, G. H. and HUNT, C. E. (1971). Murine chronic respiratory disease. Significance as a research complication and experimental production with *Mycoplasma pulmonis*. Am. J. Pathol. **64**:675–716.

LINDSEY, J. R., CASSELL, G. H., DAVIS, J. K. and DAVIDSON, M. K. (1982). Mycoplasmal and other bacterial diseases of the respiratory system. In: *The Mouse in Biomedical Research* (H. L. Foster, J. D. Small, and J. G. Fox, eds.) Vol. II, pp. 21–41. Academic Press, New York.

LINDSEY, J. R., DAVIDSON, M. K., SCHOEB, T. R. and CASSELL, G. H. (1986). Murine mycoplasmal infections. In: *Complications of Viral and Mycoplasmal Infections in Rodents to Toxicology Research and Testing* (T. E. Hamm, Jr., ed.) pp. 91–121. Hemisphere Press, Washington, DC.

LOEW, F. M. and FOX, J. G. (1983). Animal health surveillance and health delivery systems. In: *The Mouse in Biomedical Research* (H. L. Foster, J. D. Small, and J. G. Fox, eds.) Vol. III, pp. 69–82. Academic Press, New York.

LUCKEY, T. D. (1963). *Germfree Life and Gnotobiotics*, 512 p. Academic Press, New York.

LUETHANS, T. N. and WAGNER, J. E. (1983). A naturally occurring intestinal mouse adenovirus infection associated with negative serologic findings. Lab. Anim. Sci. **33**:270–272.

MCGARRITY, G. J. and CORRIELL, L. L. (1973). Mass air flow cabinet for control of airborne infection of laboratory rodents. Appl. Microbiol. **26**:167–172.

NETTESHEIM, P., SCHREIBER, H., CRESIA, D. A. and RICHTER, C. B. (1974). Respiratory infections in the pathogenesis of lung cancer. Recent results. Cancer Res. **44**:138–157.

NETTESHEIM, P., TOPPING, D. C. and JAMBASI, R. (1981). Host and environmental factors enhancing carcinogenesis in the respiratory tract. Ann. Rev. Pharmacol. Toxicol. **21**:133–163.

NEWTON, W. L. (1965). Methods in germfree animal research. In: *Methods of Experimentation* (W. I. Gay, ed.) Vol. I, pp. 215–273. Academic Press, New York.

OVERCASH, R. G., LINDSEY, J. R., CASSELL, G. H. and BAKER, H. J. (1976). Enhancement of natural and experimental respiratory mycoplasmosis in rats by hexamethylphosphoramide. Am. J. Pathol. **82**:171–189.

PAKES, S. P., LU, Y.-S. and MEUNIER, P. C. (1984). Factors that complicate animal research. In: *Laboratory Animal Medicine* (J. G. Fox, B. J. Cohen, and F. M. Loew, eds.), pp. 649–665. Academic Press, New York.

PARADISI, F., GRAZIANO, L. and MAIO, G. (1972). Histochemistry of glutamicoxaloacetic transaminase in mouse liver during MHV3 infection. Experientia **28**:551–552.

PARKER, J. C. (1980). The possibilities and limitations of virus control in laboratory animals. In: *Animal Quality and Models in Biomedical Research* (A. Spiegel, S. Erichsen, and H. A. Solleveld, eds.), pp. 161–172. Gustav Fischer Verlag, New York.

PARKER, J. C. and RICHTER, C. B. (1982). Viral diseases of the respiratory system. In: *The Mouse in Biomedical Research* (H. L. Foster, J. D. Small, and J. G. Fox, eds.) Vol. II, p. 133. Academic Press, New York.

PECK, R. M., EATON, G. J., PECK, E. B. and LITWIN, S. (1983). Influence of Sendai virus on carcinogenesis in strain A mice. Lab. Anim. Sci. 33:154–156.

RICHTER, C. G. (1970). Application of infectious agents to the study of lung cancer: Studies on the etiology and morphogenesis of metaplastic lung lesions in mice. U. S. Atomic Energy Commission Symposium Series 21:365–382.

RICHTER, C. B. (1973). Experimental pathology of Sendai virus infection in mice. J. Am. Vet. Med. Assoc. 163:1204.

RUEBNER, B. H. and HIRANO, T. (1965). Viral hepatitis in mice. Changes in oxidative enzymes and phosphatases after murine hepatitis virus (MHV3) infection. Lab. Invest. 14:157–168.

SAITO, M., NAKAYAMA, K., MUTO, T. and NAKAGAWA, M. (1982). Effects of gaseous ammonia on Mycoplasma pulmonis infection in mice and rats. Exp. Anim. 31:203–206.

SEDLACEK, R. S., ORCUTT, R. P., SUIT, H. D. and ROSE, E. F. (1981). A flexible barrier at cage level for existing colonies: Production and maintenance of a limited stable anaerobic flora in a closed inbred mouse colony. In: Recent Advances in Germfree Research (S. Sasaki, A. Ozawa, and K. Hashimoto, eds.), pp. 65–69. Tokai Univ. Press, Tokyo.

SCHOEB, T. R., DAVIDSON, M. K. and LINDSEY, J. R. (1982). Intracage ammonia promotes growth of Mycoplasma pulmonis in the respiratory tract of rats. Infect. Immun. 38:212–217.

SCHREIBER, H., NETTESHEIM, P., LIJINSKY, W., RICHTER, C. B. and WALBURG, H. E. (1972). Induction of lung cancer in germ free, specific pathogen free and infected rats by N-nitroso-heptamethyleneimine: Enhancement of respiratory infection. J. Natl. Cancer Inst. 4:1107–1114.

SMALL, J. D. (1984). Rodent and lagomorph health surveillance—quality assurance. In: Laboratory Animal Medicine (J. G. Fox, B. J. Cohen, and F. M. Loew, eds.), pp. 709–723. Academic Press, New York.

SOLLEVELD, H. A. (1978). Types and quality of animals in cancer research. Acta Zool. Pathol. Antverpiensia 72:5–18.

TAYLOR, C. E., WEISSER, W. Y. and BANG, F. B. (1982). In vitro macrophage manifestation of cortisone-induced decrease in resistance to mouse hepatitis virus. J. Exp. Med. 153:732–737.

THIGPEN, J. E. and TORTORICH, J. A. (1980). Recommended goals for microbiological quality control for laboratory animals used in the National Toxicology Program (NTP). In: Animal Quality and Models in Biomedical Research. (A. Spiegel, S. Erichsen, and H. A. Solleveld, eds.), pp. 229–233. Gustav Fischer Verlag, New York.

TREXLER, P. C. and REYNOLDS, L. I. (1957). Flexible film apparatus for the rearing and use of germfree animals. Appl. Microbiol. 5:406–412.

TREXLER, P. C. (1963). An isolator system for the control of contamination. Lab. Anim. Care 13:572–581.

TREXLER, P. C. (1983). Gnotobiotics. In: The Mouse in Biomedical Research. (H. L. Foster, J. D. Small, and J. G. Fox, eds.) Vol. III, pp. 1–16. Academic Press, New York.

VAN HOOSIER, G. L., JR., TRENTIN, J. J., SHIELDS, J., STEPHENS, K., STENBACK, W. A. and PARKER, J. C. (1966). Effect of cesarean derivation, gnotobiote foster nursing and barrier maintenance of an inbred mouse colony on enzootic virus status. Lab. Anim. Sci. 16:119–128.

VIRELIZIER, J. L., VIRELIZIER, A. M. and ALLISON, A. C. (1976). The role of circulating interferon in the modifications of immune responsiveness by mouse hepatitis virus (MHV3). J. Immunol. **117**:748–753.

WEISBROTH, S. H. (1984). The impact of infectious disease on rodent genetic stocks. Lab. Anim. **13**:25–33.

WILLENBORG, D. O., SHAH, K. V. and BANG, F. B. (1973). Effect of cyclophosphamide on the genetic resistance of C3H mice to mouse hepatitis virus. Proc. Soc. Exp. Biol. Med. **142**:762–766.

WILLIAMS, D. L. and DILUZZIO, N. R. (1980). Glucan-induced modification of murine viral hepatitis. Science **208**:67–69.

WOSTMANN, B. S. (1959). Nutrition of the germfree mammal. Ann. N.Y. Acad. Sci. **78**:175–182.

WOSTMANN, B. S., Chmn. (1970). Gnotobiotes: *Standards and Guidelines for the Breeding, Care and Management of Laboratory Animals.* National Research Council, National Academy of Sciences, 52 p., Washington, DC.

WYNDER, E. L., TAGUCHI, K. T., BADEN, V. and HOFFMAN, D. (1968). Tobacco carcinogenesis. IX. Effect of cigarette smoke on respiratory tract of mice after passive inhalation. Cancer 21:134–153.

SIGNIFICANCE OF ENVIRONMENTAL FACTORS ON THE TEST SYSTEM

Ghanta N. Rao
National Toxicology Program
National Institute of Environmental Health Sciences
Research Triangle Park, North Carolina

ABSTRACT

Animals inherit genetically controlled response patterns, the genotype, and its variation can be modified by selective breeding. Much of the variation between animals and between experiments is a product of genetic and environmental factors. However, with genetically defined inbred or hybrid strains, most of the variability is due to environmental factors. Environmental factors can be physical factors such as light, temperature, relative humidity, ventilation, air flow, water, bedding, diet and biological factors such as infections, diseases, group composition and group compatibility of the animals in the experiments. The duration, intensity and quality of light will influence many functions of the animal. Photoperiodicity is the most important factor in synchronization of inherent circadian rhythms that determine most, if not all physiological parameters and reactions. In addition, light may cause eye lesions and influence body weight, survival and tumor incidences. Temperature and relative humidity can influence the severity, duration and variability of toxic responses to chemicals by influencing the physiology of the animal and metabolism and disposition of the chemical. Ventilation will effect the air quality with regard to gaseous and particulate contamination of the animal room environment as well as the microenvironment of the animal. The gasses such as ammonia and particles containing microbial, inorganic and organic components will influence the susceptibility of animals to infections, their health status, survival and incidence of lesions in various tissues. Chemical contaminants of the feed, bedding and

---

1. Address correspondence to: Dr. G. N. Rao, NIEHS/NTP MD C2-12, P. O. Box 12233, Research Triangle Park, NC 27709.

2. Key words: biological factors, housing, light, physical factors, temperature.

3. Abbreviations: B6C3F1, (C57BL/6N X C3H/HeN MTV-)F1 hybrid; ILAR, Institute of Laboratory Animal Resources; MTD, Maximum Tolerated Dose; NCTR, National Center for Toxicological Research; NIH, National Institutes of Health; NTP, National Toxicology Program; R. H., Relative Humidity.

4. Unit of measure: 1 ft. candle = approx. 10.8 Lux.

water, vitamin and mineral deficiencies of the diet, type and concentration of fat, protein and carbohydrates in the diet can markedly influence the metabolism of test chemicals and tissue susceptibility of the animals for chemical toxicity. The basic functions of the animals such as food and water consumption and locomotor activity are strongly influenced by relatively less defined factors such as barometric pressure and ionicity of the air. It is necessary to control these environmental factors so that one can determine the pharmacologic and toxicologic activity of the chemical on the biologic system, rather than the effect of environmental factors on the biologic activity of the test chemical.

INTRODUCTION

Animals inherit genetically controlled response patterns called the genotype. This is the reason why some species are more sensitive to certain classes of chemicals than others. The genotype is also responsible for differences in the response between strains, such as the inbred and hybrid strains within a given species. One can select species and strains to enhance the pharmacologic or toxicologic responses of chemicals. However, when genetically homogeneous (inbred and hybrid) strains or species are used, the genetically determined response will be relatively uniform, but the environmental and experimental factors will influence or modify the response and increase the variability between experiments and between animals of an experimental group. The purpose of this review is to discuss the effects of environmental factors on experimental animals, especially the rodents in biomedical research with special emphasis on pharmacology and toxicology.

ENVIRONMENTAL FACTORS

Various factors that may influence the normal physiologic functions of experimental animals, especially the mouse, are presented in Figure 1. The environmental variables could be physical factors or biological factors and some of these factors are listed in Table 1. All biologic systems, especially the intact animal, have some reserve capacity to withstand insult or stress due to variable environments and maintain normal physiologic functions. Such reserve capacity will be diminished or exhausted by chemical treatment at a dose such as the Maximum Tolerated Dose (MTD). Since the animals treated with chemicals may have diminished capacity to maintain homeostasis in a changing environment, it is necessary to control the environmental variables in a narrower range so that one can determine the biologic effects of the test chemical rather than the effect of the environmental factors on the biologic activity of the test chemical. This concept is illustrated in Figure 2.

PHYSICAL FACTORS

Light: This is the most important environmental factor for animals, espe-

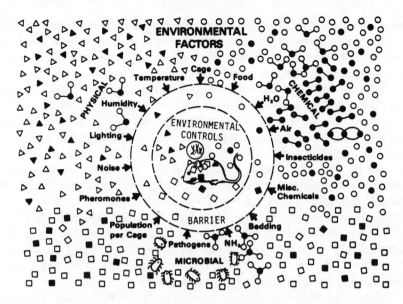

FIGURE 1. Environmental factors influencing the responses of the test system (mouse). Adapted from a concept, courtesty of Dr. J. David Small, NIEHS, NIH.

TABLE 1
Environmental Factors Influencing the Biologic
Response of the Test Animals

A. Physical factors

- Light
  Intensity
  Duration
  Quality

- Temperature

- Relative Humidity

- Ventilation
  Air quality
  Air velocity

- Atmospheric conditions
  Barometric pressure
  Altitude
  Ionicity of the air

- Noise

- Diet
  Nutrients
  Contaminants

- Bedding
  Endogenous hydrocarbons
  Contaminants

B. Biological factors

- Group compatibility
- Group composition
- Infections
- Diseases

175

cially the rodents. Since rodents are nocturnal animals, light will influence the circadian rhythm, endocrine functions and reproductive processes. Due to its profound effect on the endocrine system, light will have a marked effect on the physiology and, in turn, on the pharmocologic and toxicologic responses of rodents to chemicals. The light intensity of 75 to 125 ft. candles (807-1345 lux) at approximately 3 ft. from the floor—common in the animal rooms of most animal facilities—is designed for the convenience and comfort of the people and not the experimental animals, especially the rodents. The Canadian Council on Animal Care (1980) and the NIH Guide for the Care and Use of Laboratory Animals (ILAR, 1985), acknowledged that the above light intensity is not appropriate for rodents. Light intensity of 2-19 ft. candles has been shown to be adequate (Clough, 1982; Canadian Council on Animal Care, 1980) for the normal physiologic processes of rodents. Light intensity of approximately 30 ft. candles at about 3 ft. from the floor as the normal lighting (Bellhorn, 1980; Clough, 1982), with provision to increase to 50-75 ft. candles for detailed observation of the animals, controlled by a two stage lighting system, should be seriously considered for animal rooms with rodents.

High light intensity may cause eye lesions in the albino rodents on chronic studies. In the NTP studies, Fischer-344 rats housed in the top rows and side columns of racks, where they were exposed to more light than the rats in other cages, developed opacity of the eyes. This is due to inflammation of the anterior structures of the eye (except cornea) as a result of irritation by high intensity light. This lesion later led to generalized inflammation of the eye (panophthal-

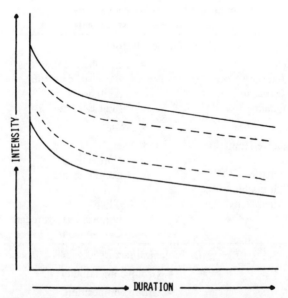

FIGURE 2. Concept of tolerance ranges of environmental factors for normal and stressed animals. Range between solid lines (——) is for normal or control animals and range between broken lines (----) is for animals stressed with chemical treatment.

176

mitis) with cataract formation. Greenman et al. (1982) reported light intensity related incidence of retinal degeneration in the BALB/c mice of the EDO1 study at NCTR. Approximately 30% of the BALB/c mice in the top row of cages that were exposed to 2000 lux and 12% of the animals in the next row, exposed to 335 lux, developed retinal degeneration. By contrast, the animals in the lower rows exposed to 85-224 lux had < 1.0% incidence of retinal degeneration. It is not unusual to see a high incidence of retinal degeneration in albino rats of 2-year or lifetime studies, if the light intensity is too high (Bellhorn, 1980). In the EDO1 study at NCTR, there was a significant delay in the onset of spontaneous tumors in the BALB/c mice on the top row (Greenman et al., 1984), and this delay may be related to the high light intensity in the top row. There are reports indicating that the incidence of skin tumors in dermal carcinogenicity studies may be different in the animals on the top shelf of cages compared to those in the lower shelves. These data indicate that high light intensity may influence the induction and development of tumors. For these reasons, the rodents in the NTP 2-year studies are rotated from top to bottom of a rack within the same cage column at 1 to 2 week intervals, so that all the animals in a study will be exposed to similar light intensities over the 2-year period. Light intensity has an effect on the estrous cycles and reproductive processes of rodents. The duration of the estrous cycles will be longer at light intensities higher or lower than 18 lux (Clough, 1982).

The normal light cycle in most of the animal facilities is 12 hours light and 12 hours dark. This cycle is in use to accommodate the workdays and work schedules. Rodents can tolerate one to two hours more or less of this photoperiod without detectable changes in physiology. However, marked change in the length of the light cycle will affect the physiology of the rodents. In Sprague-Dawley rats at 12 hour light period, the duration of estrous cycle was 4 days; however, at 16 hour light period, the estrous cycles were ≥ 5 days (Hoffman, 1973). If there is a marked increase in the light cycle, the length of gestation in the rat increases to 24 days. In toxicology studies, if the lights stay on just one weekend due to malfunction of the light controlling timers, the rodents—especially the mice—will have discharge from the eyes with marked loss of body weight. To avoid these problems, it is useful to examine the light controlling timers frequently, preferably 3 to 4 times a week.

Rodents can not see color *per se* (monkeys and perhaps cats have color vision), but they respond differently to different wavelengths of light. They show high activity in dark and red light, medium activity in yellow light and low activity in blue, green and daylight. The cool white and daylight fluorescent lamps will be satisfactory for rodents.

Temperature and Relative Humidity (R. H.): Ranges of temperature and relative humidity recommended for rodents are given in Table 2. These ranges are for normal, healthy and unstressed animals for growth, breeding and lactation. In these ranges the healthy animals can adapt and maintain homeostasis. The tail, ear and paw of rodents are involved in thermoregulation; therefore, the ambient temperature during the growth of the rodents will affect the length or size of these appendages. Length of the rat tail was 15 cm at 5° C, 17

TABLE 2
Recommended Temperature and Relative Humidity Ranges for Rodents

Rodent	Temperature (°F)			R. H. (%)	
	Comfort Range[a]	ILAR[b]	GUIDE[c]	ILAR	GUIDE
Rat	75–84	65–75	64.4–78.8	45–55	40–70
Mouse	79–98	68–75	64.4–78.8	50–60	40–70
Hamster	70–79	68–75	64.4–78.8	40–55	40–70

[a]Weihe (1971)
[b]ILAR (1976)
[c]ILAR (1985)

cm at 20° C, and 20 cm at 30° C (Chevillard et al., 1963). As illustrated in Figure 2, animals treated with high doses of chemicals will have diminished capacity to adapt to wider ranges of temperature (Table 2) and maintain homeostasis, so it is necessary to control the temperature and R. H. in a narrow range to decrease the influence of these environmental factors on toxic responses.

Temperature can influence severity, duration, nature and variance of the toxic response (Ellis, 1967; Weihe, 1973). The influence of temperature on the potency of toxic response to most chemicals may follow one of three patterns (Fuhrman and Fuhrman, 1961). These patterns are shown in Figure 3. A U-shaped response curve (Figure 3A) is the most common type. Minimum toxicity is in the optimum temperature range (Table 2) and increasing toxicity is at temperatures above and below. Examples of chemicals showing U-shaped potency of acute toxicity with change in ambient temperature are given in Table 3 (Keplinger et al., 1959). The second pattern is a straight line response (Figure 3B), in which toxicity increases continuously with increasing temperature. In the third type of response, the toxicity remains constant over a wide range of temperature up to the optimum temperature (Table 2) and then increases with increasing temperature (Figure 3C). Examples of chemicals with the second and the third pattern of response are given in Table 3. Some striking effects of temperature on the potency of chemical toxicity (Ellis, 1967) are: insulin is 80 times more toxic to mice at 40° C than at 20° C and methadone in rats and mice was twice as toxic at 29° C than at 18° C.

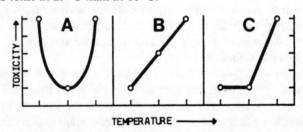

FIGURE 3. Possible patterns of toxic responses of rodents to chemicals with changing ambient temperature.

TABLE 3
Effect of Room Temperature on the LD100 of Chemicals Given Intraperitoneally to Albino Rats[a]

Chemical[b]	Room Temperature		
	8C	26C	36C
PATTERN A[c]			
Acetylsalicylic Acid	80	420	55
Atropine	280	420	55
Benezene	500	1150	225
Carbon Tetrachloride	1400	7100	940
Kerosene	2100	10,700	940
Pentobarbital	55	80	10
Chlorpromazine	12	210	62
Strychnine	0.25	1.5	0.25
PATTERN B[c]			
Diphenhydramine	180	80	16
Ephedrine	420	180	120
Pentachlorophenol	620	420	120
Quinidine Sulfate	210	140	94
PATTERN C[c]			
Caffeine	280	280	55
DDT	940	940	120
Procaine	280	280	80
Promethazine	140	140	42

[a]Keiplinger et al. (1959)
[b]mg/kg body weight
[c]See Figure 3

Temperature also influences the duration of toxic responses. For example, barbiturate induced duration of sleep decreases with increasing temperatures above 26°C. The nature of the toxic response is also affected by the animal room temperature and a few examples are given below. Chlorpromazine at 20 to 25°C causes CNS depression and ataxia, but at 30°C it will cause the opposite effects such as nervousness, convulsions and death. Reserpine at 4 to 12°C causes sedation but no sedative effect at 30 to 36°C. Temperature may affect not only the potency but also the variability of the toxic response in a group of rodents.

In animals not subjected to stress the feed consumption, hematology and serum chemistry values may not be significantly affected between 20 and 26°C (Yamauchi et al., 1981). However, for the animals stressed by chemical treatment, such as MTD, the temperature range to maintain homeostasis could be much narrower (22 to 24°C) as shown in Figure 2. The environmental temperature could affect the normal body functions so that the rate of absorption, diffusion, distribution and metabolism of chemicals could be altered with changes in pharmacologic and toxicologic responses. So, it is necessary to control the ambient temperature of animals in pharmacology and toxicology

179

studies in a narrow range to decrease the variability in potency, duration and type of toxic response.

Both R. H. and temperature are important for thermoregulation. If R. H. is high, the temperature could be low (or vice versa) for the animal to adapt and maintain homeostasis. However, in practice both will increase or decrease and cause stress to the animals on study. Relative humidity will affect feed consumption, behavior, disease susceptibility and chemical effects. Rats at 21°C and 35% R. H. consumed 5% more diet than the animals at 21°C and 75% R. H. Mice were more active at low R. H. than at high R. H. (Clough, 1982). These activities appear to be related to increased heat loss at low R. H. Since R. H. influences activity, fluctuations in R. H. will influence the behavior of animals and results of behavior studies.

Ring tail was reported in some strains of young rats and mice when the R. H. was less than 40%. High R. H. promotes ammonia production in the cages and a high concentration of ammonia increases the susceptibility of animals to infections, especially with the respiratory pathogens. Transmission of viral infections may be high at both low and high R. H., and a R. H. around 50% appears to be optimal to decrease the spread of viral infections.

Ventilation: Ventilation includes air quality and air velocity in the animal room and in the animal cage. A 30g mouse at 22°C may eat only 4 to 5g of feed, but will breathe in 30 to 40 liters of air daily. Since the animal will be exposed to a large volume of air, even low concentrations of toxic gasses, dusts, microorganisms and other pollutants will affect the physiology of the animal and increase the susceptibility of the upper respiratory tract and lungs to infections. Microorganisms and dust from bedding will cause lesions in the respiratory tract. Thus, the air quality is important in maintaining the health of the experimental animals. Effect of air velocity on food consumption of hairless mice (Weihe, 1971b) is shown in Figure 4. The feed consumption increases with increases in air velocity even in a cage with solid sides, solid bottom and bedding. The feed consumption will be 20 to 40% higher if the animals are housed in a screen cage (Figure 4) than in a solid bottom cage with bedding. Increasing air velocity increases the heat loss of the animals, so the animals will eat more food to compensate for the heat (energy) loss and to maintain homeostasis. In studies where the test chemical is administered by the feed (dosed feed), increasing air velocity increases the chemical consumption, rate of metabolism and possibly the toxic effects of the test chemical. Thus, the air velocity in the animal rooms should be low and constant to reduce the varibility of toxic responses to the test chemical.

Atmospheric conditions: Sprott (1967) reported the effects of barometric pressure fluctuations on the activity of laboratory mice. Wheel turning activity and frequency of licking a small tube to receive sweetened condensed milk were higher after increases in barometric pressure than they were after decreases of barometric pressure. When the barometric pressure was relatively stable, intermediate levels of activity were observed. Thus, variable barometric pressure may influence the physiology and toxic responses. Mori-Chavez (1958) evaluated the effects of altitude on the incidence of spontaneous leukemia in C58

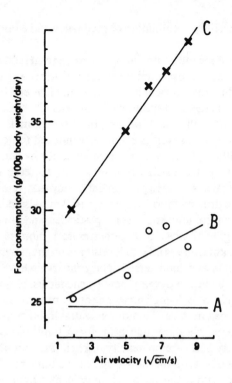

FIGURE 4. Effect of air velocity and the type of cage on food consumption by hairless mice (Weihe, 1971b). A. Mice in plastic cages with solid bottoms, solid sides and bedding, in still air. B. Mice in plastic cages with bedding and exposed to the air movements. C. Mice in wire mesh cages without bedding and exposed to air movements.

mice. One group was maintained at 14,900 ft., and another group was housed at sea level. Both groups were maintained at the same temperature and R. H. and were given the same diet and water. A statistically significant decrease in the incidence of spontaneous leukemia was observed in the male mice at the high altitude. There are negative and positive ions in the air. Passing the air through metal ducts may cause imbalance of the ions. Ion depleted air and air with low density of either charge may increase the activity of animals and their susceptibility to infections (Clough, 1982). Thus the barometric pressure, altitude and ionicity of the air may affect the toxic responses to chemicals by influencing the physiology of the animals.

Noise: In man the visual system is well developed, whereas in laboratory animals the auditory system is well developed. Sounds commonly encountered in animal facilities can trigger audiogenic seizures in sensitive species and strains of laboratory animals. Extraneous sound stimuli may cause hypertension, cardiac hypertrophy and changes in electrolyte metabolism in rats, and reduction in body weight, changes in immune response and tumor resistance in mice. Adverse effects of sound on reproductive functions include changes in estrous cycles, decrease in fertility, termination of pregnancy and embryonic abnormalities (Clough, 1982).

Diet: Diet is one of the most important environmental factors with which the laboratory animals have most intimate contact. Conner and Newberne (1984) recently reviewed the drug-nutrient interactions and Everett (1984) reviewed the effect of diet on the incidence of spontaneous tumors. Diet restriction and lower caloric content of diet will retard the growth of the animals and decrease the incidence of spontaneous as well as chemically induced tumors (Tannenbaum and Silverstone, 1957). Dietary protein concentrations within the range to support growth did not consistently decrease or increase the carcinogenic responses of all chemicals. Severe protein deficiency may retard tumor growth and depress hepatic drug metabolizing enzymes. Animals on high protein diets are less sensitive to the toxic effects of some pesticides, and low dietary protein is associated with higher toxicity to cholinesterase inhibitors and chlorinated hydrocarbons (Shakman, 1974). High levels of protein may markedly increase kidney lesions in rats and hamsters. Dietary fat levels have not consistently increased or decreased tumor development by chemicals. However, ingestion of high fat diet is associated with high incidence of spontaneous mammary tumors in rats and hepatomas in mice. The four essential lipotropic methyl-donating nutrients (methionine, choline, folic acid and vitamin B12) of rodents will influence the toxicity and carcinogenicity of chemicals but not in a consistent pattern. Consistent effects on the induction or development of tumors have not been demonstrated within the range of vitamin and mineral concentrations sufficient to maintain growth. However, marked deficiency of selenium, vitamin A, B12 and E, or several fold higher than the normal requirements of these micro-nutrients, may markedly influence the tumor induction and growth by some chemicals.

The presence of chemical contaminants and extraneous materials in diets can markedly influence the biological response of experimental animals used in toxicology studies. The natural ingredient diets may contain varying concentrations of chemical contaminants. The contaminants of concern in the toxicology studies include nitrosamines, heavy metals, mycotoxins, pesticide residues, halogenated polycyclic hydrocarbons and estrogens. These contaminants may change the physiology of animals, induce chemical metabolizing enzymes and may influence the pharmacologic and toxicologic effects of chemicals. Thus the nutrient and contaminant concentrations of diets may influence the physiology of the animals and possibly the animals' response to chemicals. Therefore, the quality of the diet for toxicology studies should be defined and standardized.

Bedding: Endogenous volatile hydrocarbons (e.g., cedrene and cedrol) may be present in beddings manufactured from coniferous softwoods such as cedar and pine. These chemicals induce increased activity of hepatic microsomal enzymes, which in turn may affect the pharmacologic and toxicologic responses to chemicals. Contact bedding may also contain bacteria and molds which may be pathogenic to the rodents in the toxicology studies. Heat treated hardwood (beech, birch and maple) bedding will help to decrease the variabilities associated with contact bedding. Contact bedding may contain chemical contaminants such as mycotoxins, pesticide residues, halogenated polycyclic hydrocarbons and heavy metals. The drinking water may be contaminated with pesticide residues, hydrocarbon solvents and heavy metals. These contaminants may influence the physiology of the animals, metabolism of chemicals by the animals and, thus, the pharmacologic and toxicologic responses to chemicals.

BIOLOGICAL FACTORS

Group Compatibility and Composition: Rodents for toxicology studies may be caged individually or in groups. Survival of individually caged and group housed (4-5 per cage) B6C3F1 mice and Fischer-344 rats at the end of two-year studies are presented in Table 4. The survival of male mice was higher when they were individually housed. The lower survival in group caged male mice was due to fighting, resulting in early mortality. Survival of group caged female mice appears to be higher than that of individually caged mice. The reason for this difference is not known, but may be related to the social behavior of female mice. There were no consistent and marked differences in the survival of group housed and individually caged rats. Consistent differences in the incidence of spontaneous tumors in mice were not observed in studies investigating the effects of group housing vs. individual caging (Everett, 1984). However, toxic responses to some chemicals may differ depending on the density of animals in a cage. The effect of ambient temperature and housing conditions on the acute toxicity of ephedrine sulfate in Swiss-Webster male mice is given in Table 5 (Peterson and Harginge, 1967). There was no marked difference in toxicity at temperatures of 18 and 22°C. At 26 and 30°C the toxicity of ephedrine sulfate

TABLE 4
Survival (%) of B6C3F1 Mice and F-344 Rats in Two-Year Studies

Species	Sex	Group Housing[a]	Individual Housing
Mice	Male	65	78
		69	82
		74	85
	Female	73	64
		79	73
Rats	Male	79	81
		54	47
	Female	78	73
		64	57

[a]4-5 animals per cage

TABLE 5
**The Effect of Ambient Temperature and Housing Conditions on the LD50 Values
of Intraperitoneally Administered Ephedrine Sulfate[a]**

| Temperature (°C) | LD50 Value (mg/kg) | |
	Group Housed[b]	Individually Housed[c]
18	360	325
22	350	385
26	257	380
30	55	273
34	13.5	14

[a]Peterson and Harginge (1967).
[b]10 Swiss-Webster male mice at each temperature point.
[c]10 mice per cage at each temperature point.

was higher in group housed mice than in the individually housed mice. The increased toxicity in the group housed mice at higher temperatures may be due to an adverse effect on the thermoregulation of the mice resulting from excessive heat accumulation in the cage and decreased heat dissipation from the animals.

Infections and Diseases: Viral and mycoplasmal infections common to the rodents may influence the host defense mechanisms, immune functions, chemical metabolism and possibly the toxic and pathological responses to chemicals (Hall et al., 1986; Barthold, 1986; Lindsey et al., 1986). These infections, which show no overt clinical symptoms, may predispose the animals to secondary infections with bacteria and mycotic organisms. Bacterial, viral and mycoplasmal diseases will cause anorexia, dehydration, weight loss and increased mortality. Marked changes in reproductive processes such as estrous cycles, decreased fertility and termination of pregnancy may be observed in recovered animals. The common viral and mycoplasmal infections may cause lesions in the liver, lungs, eyes and the upper respiratory tract. These lesions will complicate the interpretation of chemically induced pathologic changes. To obtain reproducible pharmacologic and toxicologic effects to chemicals, it is necessary to use disease and infection free animals and maintain them free of diseases and infections throughout the course of the study.

Stress is an important modulator of pharmocologic, toxicologic and carcinogenic responses. Various environmental factors discussed in this review, if not properly controlled, will cause stress and influence the animals' response to chemicals. It is necessary to control these environmental factors to conduct reliable and reproducible studies and to determine the pharmacologic and toxicologic effects of the chemical on the biologic system rather than the effect of environmental factors on the biologic activity of the test chemical.

ACKNOWLEDGEMENT

The author gratefully acknowledges the help of Ms. Phyllis Duff for typing the manuscript.

REFERENCES

BARTHOLD, S.W. (1986). Research complications and state of knowledge of rodent corona viruses. In: *Complications of Viral and Mycoplasmal Infections in Rodents to Toxicology Research and Testing* (T. E. Hamm Jr., ed.) pp. 53–89. Hemisphere Publishing, Washington.

BELLHORN, R. W. (1980). Lighting in the animal environment. Lab. Anim. Sci. 30:440–450.

CANADIAN COUNCIL ON ANIMAL CARE. (1980). Guide to the Care and Use of Experimental Animals. Vol. I, p. 16. Ottawa.

CHEVILLARD, L., PORTET, R. and CADOT, M. (1963). Growth of rats born and reared at 5°C and 30°C. Fed. Proc. 22:669–703.

CLOUGH, G. (1982). Environmental effects on animals used in biomedical research. Biol. Rev. 57:487–523.

CONNER, W. M. and NEWBERNE, P. M. (1984). Drug-nutrient interactions and their implications in safety evaluations. Fundam. Appl. Toxicol. 4:S341–S356.

ELLIS, M. T. (1967). Environmental influences on drug responses in laboratory animals. In: *Husbandry of Laboratory Animals* (M. L. Conally, ed.) pp. 569–588. Academic Press. New York.

EVERETT, R. (1984). Factors affecting the spontaneous tumor incidence rates in mice: A literature review. CRC Crit. Rev. Toxicol. 13:105–113.

FUHRMAN, G. J. and FUHRMAN, F..A. (1961). Effects of temperature on action of drugs. Ann. Rev. Pharmacol. 1:65–78.

GREENMAN, D. L., BRYANT, P., KODELL, R. L. and SHELDON, W. (1982). Influence of cage shelf level on retinal atrophy in mice. Lab. Anim. Sci. 32:353–356.

GREENMAN, D. L., KODELL, R. L. and SHELDON, W. G. (1984). Association between cage shelf level and spontaneous and induced neoplasms in mice. J. Natl. Cancer Inst. 73:107–113.

HALL, W. C., LUBET, R. A., HENRY, C. J. and COLLINS, M. J. Jr. (1986). Sendai virus-disease process and research complications. In: *Complications of Viral and Mycoplasmal Infection in Rodents to Toxicology Research and Testing* (T. E. Hamm, Jr., ed.) pp. 25–52. Hemisphere Publishing, Washington.

HOFFMAN, J. C. (1973). The influence of photoperiods on reproductive functions in female mammals. In: *Endocrinology II. Handbook of Physiology,* Section 7, pp. 57–77. American Physiological Society, Washington.

ILAR, NRC. (1976). Long term holding of laboratory rodents. ILAR News, 19:L13.

ILAR, NRC. (1985). Guide for the Care and Use of Laboratory Animals, pp. 20–21. NIH Publication No. 85–23, Washington.

KEPLINGER, M. L., LANIER, G. E. and DIECHMANN, W. B. (1959). Effects of environmental temperature on the acute toxicity of a number of compounds in rats. Toxicol. Appl. Pharmacol. 1:156–161.

LINDSEY, J. R., DAVIDSON, M. K., SCHOEB, T. R. and CASSELL, G. H. (1986). Murine mycoplasmal infections. In: *Complications of Viral and Mycoplasmal Infections in Rodents to Toxicology Research and Testing* (T. E. Hamm, Jr., ed.) pp. 91–121. Hemisphere Publishing, Washington.

MORI-CHAVEZ, P. (1958). Spontaneous leukemia at high altitudes in C58 mice. J. Natl. Cancer Inst. 21:985–988.

PETERSON, D. and HARGINGE, M. (1967). The effect of various environmental factors on cocaine and ephedrine toxicity. J. Pharm. Pharmacol. 19:810–814.

SANVORDEKER, D. R. and LAMBERT, H. J. (1974). Environmental modifications of mammalian drug metabolism and biological response. Drug Metab. Rev. 3:201-229.

SHAKMAN, R. A. (1974). Nutritional influences on the toxicity of environmental pollutants. Arch. Environ. Health 28:105-113.

SPROTT, R. L. (1967). Barometric pressure fluctuations: Effects on the activity of laboratory mice. Science 157:1206-1207.

TANNENBAUM, A. and SILVERSTONE, H. (1957). Nutrition and the genesis of tumors. In: *Cancer* (R. W. Raven, ed.) Vol. I, pp. 306-334. Butterworth, London.

WEIHE, W. H. (1971a). The significance of physical environment for the health and state of adaptation of laboratory animals. In: *Defining the Laboratory Animal* (Inst. Lab. Anim. Resour.) pp. 353-378. Natl. Acad. Sci., Washington.

WEIHE, W. H. (1971b). The effect of temperature on the action of drugs. In: *Pharmacology of Thermoregulation* (P. Lomax and E. Schonbaum, eds.) pp. 409-425. Karger, Basel.

YAMAUCHI, C., FUJITA, S., OBARA, T. and UEDA, T. (1981). Effect of room temperature on reproduction, body and organ weights, food and water intake and hematology in rats. Lab. Anim. Sci. 31:251-258.

PANEL-AUDIENCE DIALOGUE
ANIMAL QUALITY

Chairperson:
Stephen H. Weisbroth
AnMed Laboratories
Rockville, Maryland

Panel:
J. Russell Lindsey, Ghanta N. Rao

Dorothy Brach (University of Wisconsin): Were those figures regarding viral and mycoplasma infections based on actual recovery of the viruses, or just evidence of viral infection?

Russell Lindsey (University of Alabama): The viruses were based on serologic tests and the figures for mycoplasma were actual recoveries of *M. pulmonis,* so it is a mixture of different techniques to cover all those different agents.

Brach: If both your treated animals and controls came down with the same infection during a toxicological study, could you go ahead and use the results of the study anyway?

Lindsey: One must very carefully weigh the aspects of the science involved, the project, the objectives, and so forth, and then make a value judgment. Ideally, one would not like that situation to arise and I think the problem in the past was that very few people focused up front to prevent the problems. We need to shift our efforts more up front, working to build the problems out, and then we don't have to make that decision.

Gene McConnell (NIEHS/NTP): You gave two examples of chemicals which exacerbated infectious disease. Do you have examples of infectious diseases that exacerbate the effect of a chemical in regard to carcinogenesis?

Lindsey: There is a study that came out of Philadelphia—Fox Chase Cancer Center—with Sendai virus where the response went both ways. With one chemical there were more cancers than the control levels, and with another one, it went the opposite way. Most of the examples we have are examples that people have stumbled on and took the time to describe.

187

McConnell: If you saw an obvious or unequivocal response in the lung with that colony, you did see titers to Sendai, or an equivocal response in the liver, but in that colony or study you saw M.H.V., how would you interpret that carcinogenic response if you were a regulator?

Lindsey: Very cautiously. I would not go beyond what I could find hard facts to support. So much of the evidence has been generated out of studies that really weren't well-controlled. There are many areas where there are not hard data. The regulators should be basing their judgments on facts.

Stephen Weisbroth (AnMed Laboratories): Presumably, it's a controlled study with internal controls, not only treated animals—and they should guide the interpretations.

Andrew Tegeris (Tegeris Laboratories): I was impressed by the slide showing the protective effect of immunizing rats against Sendai virus. There is the tendency in this country to run experiments using VAF animals. Would we not be better off using animals which are viral antibody positive?

Lindsey: That question comes up very often. Why not use the garden variety animal that has everything because that simulates man better than virus antibody free animals. I take the position that the scientific method is really a sacred trust which tells me that I must keep things simple and build out every variable I can, so as to keep the results as crisp as possible. These systems are so enormously complicated that there will still be a lot of variables around that I won't know about. I think that in departing from that guidance of rigid adherence to the scientific principle, one is likely to run into trouble. That is a very idealistic approach. I think the key here is that we always have to make value judgments in such situations. We should recognize the ideal and proceed just as far toward the ideal as we can, and then, when necessary, make those value judgments based on hard data that we can find in the literature.

Lloyd Hazleton: I want to add a little bit to Dr. Weisbroth's statement about 14 to 16 months as the average age of rats in 1964. I can assure you that in the late 1940s, and even in the late 1930s with individually housed Carworth Farm rats, it was routine for us to get 90 percent or more survival at two years. For the sake of history, and not debating your data, rats were doing a whole lot better than that in 1964.

Garoom Singh (EPA): Do you know anything about synergistic or antagonistic effects of any carcinogens with SDA virus?

Lindsey: With SDAV, I don't. I can tell you that it's doing more than we normally think. Dr. Schoeb of the University of Alabama has some studies showing that SDAV will also promote mycoplasmosis. I think there is evidence from the people at Yale and from those studies that it is attacking a lot of cells in the respiratory tract in addition to those tissues that we normally think of; so, I think the opportunity is there to alter some results in all those tissues. The Yale group has recently reported that the immuno-suppressive drugs neither enhance nor delay the clinical cycle, so that gives you some information that the virus has

188

an effect to exert and may not be greatly affected by chemicals. On the other hand, SDAV is an example of one of the acute agents that makes rats sick. When they're sick they don't eat and drink, and that in turn affects compound intake, body weight, food consumption—all the parameters that you're measuring during the episode.

Elizabeth Feussner (Argus Research): The large number of 2-year mouse studies are being conducted with mice in group housing. It seems that no consideration is being given to the antisocial behavior of male mice, which fight with each other rather savagely. They inflict skin wounds which progress frequently to skin abscesses, systemic infections and death. It seems that the investigators are either not aware of or don't care about this effect in the group housing of mice for these long-term carcinogenicity studies.

Ghanta Rao (NIEHS): Effective January 1, 1984, all mice are being individually housed for new studies within the National Toxicology Program. Especially with the male mice, there is the problem of territorial behavior, fighting, injuries, and mortality in long-term studies.

John Sagartz (Veritas Laboratories): Should the approach to genetic monitoring be to ascertain whether, for instance, the B6C3F1 mouse is genetically a B6C3F1 mouse when it gets to the laboratory?

Weisbroth: The genetic integrity of the animal substrate, particularly with inbred strains, is a critical element in conducting studies for comparability from study to study. Inbred animals are less variable. The genetic integrity of the substrate strain is one of the important aspects of defining the research model, equally as important as defining the microbial composition, the diets, the waters, the environmental background—all the other equipment and components of conducting a study.

Rao: I cannot speak for industry, but in NTP we monitor the animals. Genetic monitoring of the inbred rodents is done in the production colonies by biochemical monitoring as well as skin grafts. I'd say one major question is: Are you sure that what you're getting in the testing facilities is the same as you ship? To answer that, for the last three years we have selected 10 B6C3F1 mice from the shipments received at the testing facilities and the kidneys have been collected and shipped to the genetic monitoring lab to make sure the shipment received is genetically the same as what was shipped from the production colony. So we are monitoring, even to the extent that they are going into the animal rooms.

Chapter V
STUDY CONDUCT QUALITY

STUDY CONDUCT QUALITY

Desmond L. H. Robinson
United Kingdom Good Laboratory Practice Monitoring Unit
Department of Health and Social Security
London, England

CHAIRPERSON'S REMARKS

Ladies and Gentlemen, we have been talking about the tools that are needed in the generation of a toxicology study and we moved on to the question of the quality of the animals that we should use. In this session we now move to the subject of the involvement of the human animals and the pressures put on them to actually maintain study conduct quality. Although management provides the facilities, the equipment, and the personnel, including people experienced and competent to maintain study quality, there are still many problems to be tackled to achieve and maintain acceptable study quality and to comply with GLP principles.

It would be naive for those involved in regulatory matters, in particular GLP monitoring, to pretend that they are unaware that problems do exist. They commonly recur during GLP monitoring. The first item for this session is a fairly common one, the provision of physical-chemical data. The second presentation deals with quality control in the field of clinical chemistry. The third subject covered by two of our speakers, from different standpoints, is that of the study director. The role of the study director always forms a good discussion item, whether it is in a formal meeting like this or on a GLP inspection. I very much doubt that we shall resolve the controversy regarding how much the QA Unit should audit a particular study.

These are rather brief introductory remarks. Allow me to emphasize something that the UK delegates have heard me say on many occasions: The personnel who are involved in regulatory affairs, especially those responsible for GLP Monitoring, must as an absolute necessity be aware of the practical problems involved during the generation of high quality toxicological data. I need hardly add, as a postscript, that there is no place for the checklist approach.

TEST ARTICLE CHARACTERIZATION—
INDUSTRIAL VIEWPOINT

James P. Dux
Independent Consultant
Lancaster, Pennsylvania

ABSTRACT

Laboratories involved in chemical analysis and microbiological testing sometimes encounter problems in interpreting Good Laboratory Practice (GLP) regulations. Difficulties may involve operational procedures or physical limitations of the facility. Technical personnel may lack an adequate understanding of how to apply these regulations. Practical solutions to these problems will be addressed.

INTRODUCTION

The GLPs define the test article as "any food additive, color additive, drug, biological product, electronic product, or medical device for human use, or any other article subject to regulation under this act (Federal Food, Drug and Cosmetic Act) or subject to regulation under Sections 351 and 354-360F of the Public Health Service Act." This paper will consider GLP compliance problems with regard to chemical analyses and microbiological tests which involve the test article and the various matrices with which it may be combined. In general, these matrices will be animal feeds, water, bedding, or pharmaceutical preparations.

GLP COMPLIANCE ISSUES

The GLPs were obviously written with a particular type of testing facility in mind, the type in which both toxicological tests and chemical and/or microbiological analyses are performed in the same testing facility by personnel under the supervision of only one or a very few managers. In other words, they apply to

1. Address correspondence to: James P. Dux, Ph.D., 2152 New Holland Pike, Lancaster, PA 17601.
2. Key words: chemical analysis, Good Laboratory Practices, quality assurance.
3. Abbreviations: FDA, Food and Drug Administration; GLP, Good Laboratory Practice; QA, quality assurance; SOPs, Standard Operating Procedures.

the type of facility usually encountered in government or academic laboratories. In many industrial situations, this is not the case. Toxicological laboratories and analytical chemical laboratories may be geographically separated and under different supervisory personnel who may or may not report to the same manager. The reason for this is that toxicology, analytical chemistry and microbiology are different scientific disciplines and it is often inefficient to attempt to accommodate all three disciplines in the same facility, especially if there are preexisting facilities for these disciplines. The laboratories for chemical analysis and microbiological tests may be serving many other clients besides the toxicology laboratory.

In addition to the separation which occurs "in-house" when all three disciplines are available within the same corporate organization, there are many companies which "contract out" the necessary chemical or microbiological analyses to a commercial, independent laboratory. This may be done for many reasons, such as lower cost, more rapid turnaround times, or lack of instrumentation or experienced personnel in the sponsor's organization.

Many commercial laboratories cannot afford to run their laboratories across the board in compliance with GLPs. GLP compliance is costly and may not be justifiable to those clients who do not require compliance for the uses to which the data may be put. Therefore, it is necessary for the sponsor of the study to inform laboratory management that the work they are requesting must be done in compliance with the GLPs. Indeed, paragraph 58.10 of the FDA GLPs specifically mandates this.

Another difficulty with the GLPs is that requirements for compliance are rather loosely defined in many cases, but very rigid in others. For example, it is required that the Quality Assurance (QA) unit of the testing facility conduct periodic inspections or audits to verify data integrity. Paragraph 58.35(b)(3) states that the phase or segment of the study shall be indicated in the report of the inspection. However, it is not clear what is meant by a phase or segment of the study. Is the entire analytical process a phase? Is sample log-in or handling a phase? Is proper notebook data acquisition a phase? Should the audit comprise inspection for conformance to the written analytical method or general conformance to QA Standard Operating Procedures (SOPs)?

For this reason and because of other problems encountered in interpretation, it is recommended that the study director discuss with laboratory supervision what their interpretation is with regard to GLP compliance. In addition, it is recommended that this interpretation be submitted in writing after discussion and agreement on what is required. Laboratory supervisors should insist on this type of requirement documentation before agreeing to perform the work and before preparing any cost estimates of the work to be done.

REQUIRED OPERATIONS AND MANAGEMENT PRACTICES

Compliance with the GLPs requires certain specific operations and management practices which may not be in place in the average analytical or biological testing laboratory, but which must be instituted if the laboratory is to do this kind of work. In the remainder of this paper I shall discuss some of these requirements.

Under paragraph 58.29 (Personnel) of the Food and Drug Administration (FDA) GLP regulations, we read that personnel training records are required for all personnel engaged in testing work. In many laboratories personnel training is "on the job" training which is carried out rather casually. For good quality assurance, it is necessary that this training be documented and records kept of the dates on which personnel were judged capable of performing specific tests. In addition, this capability is preferably documented by "hard data," that is, results obtained on standard materials, or comparison of results obtained on samples with results obtained by an experienced analyst. Training records should be signed by the analyst's supervisor and always recorded in ink.

Paragraph 58.35 deals with the quality assurance unit. One of the requirements is that the QA personnel be separate from, and independent of, the personnel directing and performing the testing. Unfortunately, this requirement is not realized in many laboratories. All too often, the laboratory supervisor is charged with responsibility for QA. The possibility of "conflict of interest" is obvious, necessitating an independent QA manager and staff. This requirement may be especially difficult to implement in the smaller laboratory, since personnel with the necessary technical background cannot be spared for QA management. If the laboratory is organized by department, it may be possible to choose an analyst in department A as QA manager for department B, and vice versa.

Another requirement of this section of the GLPs is that a *written* quality assurance program must be available. Although an obvious requirement for good QA, there are many laboratories even today which do not have a QA manual. Unfortunately, the GLPs offer little guidance about what the contents of the written manual should include.

With regard to facilities, there are two requirements which must be met by the analytical or microbiological laboratory. First, provision must be made for storage space for samples after receipt and prior to analysis. This storage area must be appropriate to the type of sample, i.e., refrigeration or freezing may need to be available if this is required to maintain sample integrity.

The second requirement is for an "archive" area. The archives referred to in the GLPs is the area in which raw data, calculated results, data, and, in general, all information relating to a study is kept. The archive area should be of limited access, i.e., only open to designated personnel (the keeper of the Archives, and his/her alternate) who are authorized to deposit and remove documents. Such deposit and removal should also be documented so that tight control over document location is achieved and loss of documents prevented.

Since long-term storage of paper in the archives is necessary, the choice of the archive area is important. The area should be cool, dry and free of laboratory fumes, dust and gases. Documents should be stored where they are not exposed to excessive light, moisture or heat. In other words, they should be kept away from windows, radiators, steam pipes, damp basements or hot attics.

Documentation is the key to good quality assurance, providing the ability to assure others, such as the FDA or clients, that the laboratory is practicing good quality control and generating quality data. To this end, the GLPs contain many requirements for documenting operations and results. These include:

- A written Quality Assurance manual as described previously.
- Written analytical methods.
- Written sampling methods, if sampling is performed by laboratory personnel.
- Documentation of sample receipt and distribution.
- Documentation of results of quality assurance inspections or audits and any resulting action to correct any defects found.
- Written procedures for calibration, maintenance, testing, cleaning, and standardization of instruments and auxiliary equipment.
- Documentation of results of calibration, maintenance, inspection, etc. of instruments and auxiliary equipment.
- A master schedule sheet which is maintained for all nonclinical studies being conducted in the laboratory.
- Current personnel training records as described previously.
- Labels on all reagents and reagent solutions containing date of preparation, identity and concentration of active ingredients, storage requirements and date of expiration.
- A historical file of all analytical methods, both current and obsolete, with date of issuance and dates of revisions.

Many other documents are required to be kept as part of a nonclinical study, but the above is a summary of those relating to test article characterization. There are requirements regarding the length of time such records must be kept, e.g., five years after results are submitted to FDA for an application for a research or marketing permit, or ten years as required by the Environmental Protection Agency. In view of the fact that many years may elapse before application is made, it is recommended that the laboratory keep all records for at least 10 years, and more if possible.

AVOIDING PITFALLS IN CLINICAL CHEMISTRY—QUALITY CONTROL IS NOT QUALITY ASSURANCE

Morrow B. Thompson
Toxicology Research Testing Program
National Institute of Environmental Health Sciences
Research Triangle Park, North Carolina

ABSTRACT

If reliable interpretations are to be made from clinical laboratory data concerning the medical status of laboratory animals, the results must be consistent, precise and accurate. In attempting to achieve this objective, laboratories adopt and follow a quality control program. In the clinical laboratory, two visible aspects of such a program are the analysis of quality control materials and animal samples and participation in a proficiency testing service. The quality control materials, which must be obtained in quantities that will last for an extended period, are repeatedly analyzed and mean values and standard deviations are established for various components and analytes. Through adherence to established procedures, short- and long-term deviations in an analysis can be detected and, hopefully, knowledgeable decisions can be made about an assay and about the acceptability of the data. Proficiency testing programs allow a laboratory to compare its performance in the analysis of unknown samples with that of other participating laboratories. All such services are designed for the analysis of human samples.

Unfortunately, results can be consistent, precise and accurate and still not be reliable. Numerous factors, in addition to the actual analysis of a sample, affect the final results. These include the manipulation and preparation of the animals prior to sampling, collection and handling of the sample and reporting of the data. Examples of how these different phases of animal, sample and data handling can affect the final results will be given. For present consideration, one example is presented. Through a recent statistical analysis of hematology data from control animals in more than 60 subchronic studies, significant differences

1. Address correspondence to: Morrow B. Thompson, D.V.M., Ph.D., Toxicology Research and Testing Program, NIEHS, P.O. Box 12233, Research Triangle Park, NC 27709.
2. Key words: clinical chemistry, quality assurance, quality control.
3. Abbreviation: NTP, National Toxicology Program.

were present between laboratories for all determinations. Up to 50% of the variability was related to the use of different bleeding sites and anesthetics. In addition to the use of different sites and anesthetics by different laboratories, various combinations are used by a laboratory within the same study. Although all assays performed on these samples may be accurate, the use of different sampling techniques can have profound effects on the data. To ensure the proper interpretation of data and to develop a historic data base within the program, differences between and within laboratories in the generation of clinical laboratory data must be minimized.

INTRODUCTION

Clinical laboratory investigations are frequently performed in subchronic (90 day) studies conducted for the National Toxicology Program (NTP). These investigations are scheduled at the end and often at multiple time points during the study. To have confidence in the findings and the resulting interpretation, factors or variables that can affect the results of clinical laboratory studies must be recognized and, if appropriate or possible, removed or controlled. Laboratories that conduct clinical studies for the NTP subscribe to proficiency testing services and maintain quality control programs. Both functions help monitor the analytical phase of testing. Sample analysis, however, is only one of a series of interdependent stages in a toxicologic study (Figure 1). The integrity of each stage depends upon the integrity of those that precede it. Because there are factors at any stage that can introduce variability and bias into a study, researchers must be aware of the sources and of the potential effects on the data.

VARIATION IN CLINICAL CHEMISTRY DETERMINATIONS

Within studies there are inherent and external sources of variation. The former cannot be eliminated but can be changed by selections or decisions that must be made. By selecting animals that are a specific age, strain and sex, that are fed a certain diet and kept in specific conditions, bias has been introduced into the data (Ringler and Reed, 1979). Furthermore, the use of an anesthetic, the selection of a bleeding site and the analysis of the sample in a specific laboratory are considered inherent factors because some combination of these must be used if a sample is to be collected and analyzed. In an experiment in our laboratory at NIEHS, there were marked differences in specific analytes in blood collected from various bleeding sites using different anesthetics (Table 1). White blood cell counts in blood from the heart were significantly lower than counts in samples from the retroorbital sinus or inferior vena cava, regardless of the anesthetic that was used. In 8 of 9 comparisons, anesthesia with phenobarbital produced lower counts than carbon dioxide, methoxyflurane, or ketamine-xylazine. Differences between groups, which are summarized in Table 2, were not confined to hematology variables. The activity of creatine kinase in blood (serum) collected from the retroorbital sinus was significantly higher than that from the vena cava or heart. Also, the use of pentobarbital and, to a lesser

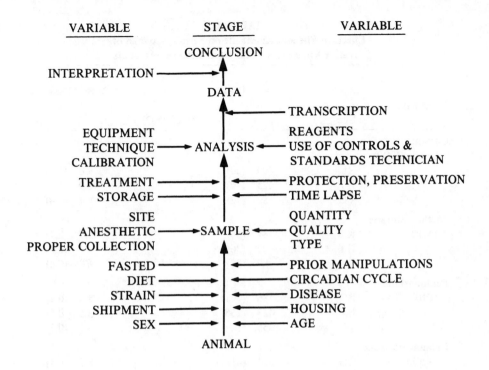

VARIABLE	STAGE	VARIABLE

CONCLUSION

INTERPRETATION ——————→

DATA

——— TRANSCRIPTION

EQUIPMENT | REAGENTS
TECHNIQUE ———→ ANALYSIS ←——— USE OF CONTROLS &
CALIBRATION | STANDARDS TECHNICIAN

TREATMENT ———————→ | ←——— PROTECTION, PRESERVATION
STORAGE ———————→ | ←——— TIME LAPSE

SITE | QUANTITY
ANESTHETIC ———→ SAMPLE ←——— QUALITY
PROPER COLLECTION | TYPE

FASTED ———————→ | ←——— PRIOR MANIPULATIONS
DIET ———————→ | ←——— CIRCADIAN CYCLE
STRAIN ———————→ | ←——— DISEASE
SHIPMENT ———————→ | ←——— HOUSING
SEX ———————→ | ←——— AGE

ANIMAL

FIGURE 1. Stages in a study and variables that affect clinical laboratory data

extent, ketamine-xylazine, resulted in increased creatine kinase activities compared to those in samples collected from animals anesthetized with carbon dioxide or methoxyflurane. Reasons for these differences can be proposed, but the important point is that data from samples collected using various techniques are not comparable.

In a recent statistical analysis of hematology data from control rats in a group of subchronic studies (NTP), significant differences were identified within and between laboratories. One purpose of this analysis was to examine the effects of various bleeding sites and anesthetics on data from control animals. Because numerous combinations of sites and anesthetics had been used in these studies, there were few combinations with sufficient data to permit comparisons of one component (That is, site, anesthetic or laboratory) while the others were held constant. For those few comparisons that could be made, however, the laboratory and the combination of bleeding site and anesthetic were identified as factors contributing to differences in control data. The selection of bleeding site and anesthetic must be controlled if consistent data are to be produced within and between studies.

EXTERNAL FACTORS

External factors also must be recognized and controlled if clinical laboratory studies are to be reliable, and an accurate interpretation of the data is to be

TABLE 1
**Effects of Site and Anesthetic on Serum Activities of
Creatine Kinase and Total White Blood Cell Counts**

Anesthetic	Site	CK (IU/L)		WBC (1000/ul)	
			Assay		
			Mean (SD)		
Carbon dioxide (CO2)					
	RO	100	(20)	9.0	(1.3)
	HT	125	(40)	6.9	(1.1)
	VC	86	(12)	8.7	(0.4)
Methoxyflurane (MF)					
	RO	184	(54)	5.7	(0.7)
	HT	102	(36)	4.1	(0.5)
	VC	89	(38)	6.0	(0.4)
Pentobarbital (PB)					
	RO	536	(198)	5.9	(0.9)
	HT	423	(236)	3.6	(0.5)
	VC	455	(149)	5.1	(0.7)
Ketaminexylazine (KX)					
	RO	224	(41)	6.5	(0.4)
	HT	160	(86)	(5.5	(0.9)
	VC	169	(85)	7.1	(0.8)

made. Examples of such factors and their effects are numerous.

Fasting. Fasting animals the night before blood samples are collected can affect the concentrations or activities of some serum constituents. In rats, fasting can decrease the serum activity of alkaline phosphatase and concentration of albumin (Jenkins and Robinson, 1975) and increase concentrations of bilirubin (Blanckaert and Schmid, 1982), free fatty acids (Bortz and Steele, 1973) and bile acids. In a study of human patients, a moderate meal several hours before the collection of a blood sample produced only mild increases in glucose and no significant changes in 14 other analytes (Annino and Relman, 1959). The preference to animals the evening before blood samples are collected may induce changes comparable to or greater than those resulting from feeding. At all times within the study, the pretreatment of animals (for example, access to feed, water and collection of samples at similar time periods during the day) must be identical.

Sequencing. Sequencing is the placement of two or more procedures in a study with consideration of the possible effects that one may have upon another. The sequence in which procedures are performed that are close together in time can affect clinical data. In an experiment with rats in our laboratory at NIEHS, total white cell counts decreased significantly from one tube to the next in three samples of blood collected in rapid succession from the right side of the heart of each animal. If, during a sampling point in an

TABLE 2

Statistical analysis of data for creatine kinase and white blood cell counts
from bleeding site-anesthetic study

Creatine kinase		Sites and Anesthetics[b]			
	anesthetic	CO2	MF	PB	KX
	site	VC		HT	RO
WBC					
	anesthetic	CO2	MF	PB	KX
	site	VC	RO		HT

[a]Data analyzed by 2-way ANOVA. Anesthetics and sites different for CK and WBC at significance level of $p < 0.001$.

[b]Individual comparisons made with Newman-Keuls multiple test. Variables not connected by line are different at significance level of $p < 0.01$.

experiment, two or more tubes of blood were collected from each rat and the order in which the tubes were filled was not consistent, increased variability and possibly differences in hematology data between groups could be produced. Other examples in which the lack of sequencing could affect data can be proposed: the collection of a blood sample from rats (frequently the removal of 15 to 20% of blood volume) after which the animals are placed in metabolism cages for the collection of urine (decreased urine production related to decreased blood volume); the frequent collection of blood from rats after which a qualitative and quantitative evaluation is made of bone marrow (hematopoiesis stimulated by prior bleedings); and the collection of a blood sample from the heart for coagulation studies immediately after a sample was collected from the retroorbital sinus for hematology and chemistry determinations (effect, if any, uncertain, but possible alteration of coagulation studies by volume depletion and release of tissue fluids into blood). To prevent the introduction of artifacts into data by previous manipulations, careful consideration of the potential effects of one procedure upon another is necessary.

Sample quality. Hemolysis (Frank et al., 1978; Chin et al., 1979), lipemia (Thompson and Kunze, 1984), icterus (Statland and Winkel, 1979) and clotting (in an anticoagulated blood sample) are examples of factors that can alter the results of specific assays. Regardless of the causes (pathologic or artifactual), uniform, consistent methods of measuring and reporting these factors must be used in a laboratory. By doing this, the effects, which are spurious, can be distinguished from true changes and the data can be accurately interpreted. Sample quality also depends upon selection of the proper sampling technique and its proper use. While poor technique can produce obvious artifacts (hemolysis, clotting), other more subtle effects can occur. For example, the excessive addition of an anticoagulant to a blood sample prior to performing coagulation tests can produce prolonged times. This can occur during the collection of samples from small animals if, because of blood volume limitations, the anticoagulant has to be measured and added to a small syringe. Additionally, the use of an improper collection tube or the inadequate filling of a tube which contains a pre-measured amount of an anticoagulant can preclude or alter specific measurements (Pickard, 1984).

Sampling Handling—Time Lapse and Storage. The distinction between time lapse and storage may be arbitrary, but for the sake of discussion, if a sample is analyzed the same day it is collected, the period between collection and analysis is the time lapse. If a sample is analyzed the next day or later, it has been stored. The extent of time lapse is critical for some procedures and measurements. Methemoglobin should be measured within 30 minutes of sample collection if decreases in concentration are to be avoided (Fairbanks, 1976). Bone marrow preparations for cytologic examination should be made immediately after an animal has died to avoid subtle to marked degenerative changes in cellular morphology. Other time lapse considerations include the recommendation to determine coagulation times within 6 hours (Koepke et al., 1975), to prepare smears and perform routine hematology measurements on blood samples held at room temperature within 2 and 6 hours, respectively (Nelson, 1979) and to quickly remove serum from the blood clot to avoid artifactual changes in certain variables. Increases in the activities of lactate dehydrogenase, aspartate aminotransferase, malic dehydrogenase (Korsrud and Trick, 1973) and creatine kinase (Shibata and Kobayashi, 1978) can occur within 1 hour in rat serum (compared to plasma) if it is not separated from the blood clot. To minimize such effects, uncoagulated blood should be centrifuged within 30 minutes of collection and the serum promptly removed. For most analytes in serum or plasma, sealing the sample and storing it at 4°C for 24 hours produces no adverse effects (Wilding et al., 1977; Ezigbo and Storey, 1980; Colombo, 1981; Hohnadel, 1984). For storage beyond 24 hours, the samples should be deep frozen, but with the realization that the activities or concentrations of some constituents will not remain constant or tolerate thawing.

Protection. In addition to keeping a sample cool, other precautions are necessary to ensure its integrity. For example, blood samples should be protected from excessive vibrations during transportation (Pickard, 1984). Damage to red cell membranes can release electrolytes and enzymes into plasma. If bilirubin is to be measured, the blood sample must be protected from light (Sherwin and Overnote, 1984). The exposure of a blood sample for 2 hours can decrease the concentration of bilirubin by 50% (Wilding et al., 1977) and thereby invalidate the measurement of this constituent. Serious consequences also can result from the evaporation of serum or plasma water (Burtis et al., 1975). Serum samples that are transferred to reservoir cups for pipetting prior to analysis can be exposed to ambient conditions for several hours. Evaporation from some unprotected cups can exceed 25% within 2 hours. A similar and very common problem can occur with urine samples that are being collected from rats and mice. During collection periods of 16 to 24 hours, there can be significant evaporation from unprotected samples. Failure to prevent such volume losses results in significant increases in analyte concentrations and activities.

204

CONCLUSION

In conclusion, clinical laboratory tests are conducted during toxicology studies in order that hematologic and biochemical effects of a specific treatment can be evaluated. The resulting data must be reliable if sound interpretations and conclusions are to be made. In addition to performing routine quality control measurements and participating in a proficiency testing service, laboratory personnel must have an overall awareness of the interdependency of all phases of a toxicology study and of the numerous factors that can affect the data at any stage of the study. Procedures must be standardized if comparable data are to be produced at different time points within a study, between studies within a laboratory and between laboratories within the NTP. While, by their nature, all factors cannot be controlled or eliminated, all reasonable efforts to do so should be made to ensure confidence in the quality of clinical laboratory studies.

REFERENCES

BLANCKAERT, N. and SCHMIDT, R. (1982). Physiology and pathophysiology of bilirubin metabolism. In: Hapeatology: A Textbook of Liver Disease (D. Zakim and T. D. Boyer, eds.) pp. 246–296, W. B. Saunders Co., Philadelphia.

BORTZ, W. M. and STEELE, L. A. (1973). Synchronization of hepatic cholesterol synthesis, cholesterol and bile acid content, fatty acid synthesis, and plasma free fatty acid levels in the fed and fasted rat. Biochem. Biophys. Acta 306:85–94.

CHIN, B. H., TYLER, T. R. and KOZBELT, S. J. (1979). The interfering effects of hemolyzed blood on rat serum chemistry. Toxicologic Path. 7:19–22.

COLOMBO, J. P. (1981). Collection of blood. In: Clinical Chemistry: Theory, Practice and Interpretation (R. Richterich and J. P. Colombo, eds.) pp. 94–109, John Wiley and Sons, New York.

EZIGBO, J. C. and STOREY, D. M. (1980). Effect of storage at various temperatures on the activity of cotton rat serum enzymes. Indian J. Exp. Biol. 18:96–97.

FAIRBANKS, V. F. (1976). Hemoglobin, hemoglobin derivatives and myoglobin. In: Fundamentals of Clinical Chemistry (N. W. Tietz, ed.) pp. 401–454, W. B. Saunders Co., Philadelphia.

FRANK, J. J., BERMES, E. W., BICKEL, M. J. and WATKINS, B. F. (1978). Effect of in vitro hemolysis on chemical values for serum. Clin. Chem. 24:1966–1970.

HOHNADEL, D. C. (1984). Enzymes. In: Clinical Chemistry: Theory, Analysis and Correlation (L. A. Kaplan and A. J. Pesce, eds.) pp. 927–952, C. V. Mosby Co., St. Louis.

JENKINS, F. P. and ROBINSON, J. A. (1975). Serum biochemical changes in rats deprived of food or water for 24 h. Proc. Nutr. Soc. 34:37A.

KOEPKE, J. A., RODGERS, J. L. and OLLIVIER, M. J. (1975). Pre-instrument variables in coagulation testing. Am. J. Clin. Pathol. 64:591–596.

KORSRUD, G. O. and TRICK, K. D. (1973). Activities of several enzymes in serum and heparinized plasma from rats. Clin. Chim. Acta 48:311–315.

NELSON, D. A. (1979). Basic methodology. In: Clinical Diagnosis and Management by Laboratory Methods (J. B. Henry, ed.) pp. 858–917, W. B. Saunders Co., Philadelphia.

PICKARD, N. A. (1984). Collection and handling of patient specimens. In: Clinical Chemistry: Theory, Analysis and Correlation (L. A. Kaplan and A. J. Pesce, eds.) pp. 43–50, C. V. Mosby Co., St. Louis.

RINGLER, D. H. AND DABICH, L. (1979). Hematology and clinical biochemistry. In: The Laboratory Rat (H. J. Baker, J. R. Lindsey, and S. H. Weisbroth, eds.). pp 105–121, Academic Press, New York.

SHERWIN, J. E. (1984). Liver function. In: Clinical Chemistry: Theory, Analysis and Correlation (L. A. Kaplan and A. J. Pesce, eds.) pp. 420–438, C. V. Mosby Co., St. Louis.

SHIBATA, S. and KOBAYASHI, B. (1978). Blood platelets as a possible source of creatine kinase in rat plasma and serum. Thrombos. Haemostas. 39:701–706.

STATLAND, B. E. and WINKEL, P. (1979). Sources of variation in laboratory measurements. In: Clinical Diagnosis and Management by Laboratory Methods (J. B. Henry, ed.) pp. 3–28, W. B. Saunders Co., Philadelphia.

THOMPSON, M. B. and KUNZE, D. J. (1984). Polyethylene glycol-6000 as a clearing agent for lipemic serum samples from dogs and the effects on 13 serum assays. Am. J. Vet. Res. 45:2154–2157.

WILDING, P., ZILVA, J. F. and WILDE, C. E. (1977). Transport of specimens for clinical chemistry analysis. Ann. Clin. Biochem. 14:301–306.

THE ROLE OF THE STUDY DIRECTOR AS SEEN BY THE SPONSOR

Marshall Steinberg
Hazleton Laboratories America, Inc.
Vienna, Virginia

ABSTRACT

There are differences among sponsors regarding what is expected to the study director. These differences often relate to the sophistication of the sponsor and to the industry represented by the sponsor. The advent of the GLPs has affected what the study sponsor expects of the study director and governs, to a great extent, the relationship between the two. The study director's role is to ensure that the sponsor's protocol and the resultant study meet the requirements of the regulatory agency to which the data are to be submitted. It is also the study director's responsibility to see that the reports are generated on time, and that the scientific content and format are acceptable and meet the requirements of the regulator. The study director is responsible for presenting to his management the comments, questions and even the impressions of the sponsor. He must work to develop a rapport with the sponsor and also be in the position to caution the sponsor. But primarily, the function of the study sponsor is to serve as the arbitrator of data acceptance criteria in the scientific, rather than the GLP sense. The development of these criteria is usually not a formalized, systemtic endeavor and is certainly not institutionalized. The sponsor may regard the study sponsor as his ombudsman, proxy scientist and, ultimately, the person who ensures that the study report is consistent with the protocol.

INTRODUCTION

The role of the study director as seen by the sponsor is subject to a variety of factors ranging from the personalities involved, corporate policies, nature of the study, potential market value of the chemical agent, past experiences, outside pressures from the regulators, advocacy groups, and other matters which also may include how the sponsor views the role of the laboratory. This view has

---

1. Address correspondence to: Dr. Marshall Steinberg, Hazleton Laboratories America, Inc., 9200 Leesburg Turnpike, Vienna, VA 22180.
2. Key words: regulatory agency, study director, study sponsor.
3. Abbreviation: GLPs, Good Laboratory Practices.

study conduct, relationship and potential legal implications, depending upon how the laboratory reciprocates the view. The laboratory may be viewed as an independent operation, employed to provide a critical independent assessment. The view of the laboratory as an extension of the sponsor's organization is an alternative view and implies a subtle connotation, particularly if the work is to be presented by a client to a regulatory agency.

In the case of the former view, all concerned parties understand that the laboratory is operating as a free agent, providing its own view of the action of the candidate test material, without implied prejudice from the sponsor. Indeed, often the sponsor withholds data garnered from previous studies in order to obtain an unbiased opinion. The interpretation of results of the testing laboratory is not subject to change by the sponsor. If there is a difference of opinion, the sponsor is free to provide his view along with that of the laboratory, but not in place of that provided by the study director or the supporting scientists. This relationship is the prevailing one between study directors and commercial clients, particularly when the report is to be submitted to a regulator.

The laboratory extension view generally applies to studies not destined for the regulator. It often also applies to research being conducted for the government. In this instance, the report may not require recommendations and conclusions from the study director, although individual support scientists may render opinions through their diagnoses. These reports are often the subject of a review procedure by scientific boards, which may have a direct impact upon the final interpretation in the final report, which may be written by the sponsor.

INCREASED REGULATION AND THE ROLE
OF THE STUDY DIRECTOR

The role of the study director has changed dramatically over the past twenty years. Twenty years ago, there were very few regulatory guidelines and a great deal was left to the discretion of the study director when designing, conducting and reporting a study. The role of the study director since that time has been greatly impacted by the advent of the Good Laboratory Practices (GLPs), the institution of test guidelines by a variety of regulatory agencies—some of which did not even exist at that time—and changes in the art and science of toxicology. The relationship between study director and study sponsor is considerably more formalized now then it was before the advent of GLPs. The GLPs impose certain legal constraints and responsibilities on both parties. There are more checks and balances on the sponsor/director relationship that are directly related to these constraints and responsibilities. There are minimum requirements that must be met irrespective of the nature of the science and each party implies that it will meet these requirements while the other party introduces systems to verify that they have been met. Also, the high cost of developing new chemicals, increased competition for markets, and heightened public concern and skepticism regarding the safety of the chemicals have had their influence.

While test guidelines instruct us about protocol requirements and the types of data desired by regulatory agencies and Good Laboratory Practices provide for an auditable trail for these data, and the National Institutes of Health and National Academy of Sciences provide us with guidance about how the animals should be housed and in some instances treated, nowhere in these guidelines is the quality of the science from which these data are drawn covered. We still speak of that undefinable gray area called "state-of-the-art," and therein lies one of the most critical aspects of the study director's role.

The study director has the paramount role of overviewing and ensuring the quality of the science. While good laboratory practices address the data trail and provide some assurance that the data are what they say they are, they address the quality of the science only in a tangential manner. The study director, when implementing data acceptance criteria, must make judgments regarding the quality of the science. This is not to be confused with GLP requirements, but in its purest form may require differentiation of biological from statistical significance. The sponsor's expectations regarding this aspect are a function of the sponsor's knowledge and experience in toxicology.

There is no question that one of the roles of the study director is to ensure that the sponsor's protocol meets the requirements of the regulatory agency to whom the data are to be submitted. It is also the study director's responsibility to see to it that the reports are not only generated on time, but that the format is also acceptable in scientific presentation and meets the regulator's demands. It is also the study director's role to present to his management the comments, questions, and even the impressions garnered from his contact with the sponsor. The study director must be sensitive to the nuances, as well as the direct communications, of the sponsor. He must work to develop a rapport with the sponsor and must also be in the position to caution the sponsor when the sponsor is moving into an area that may be correct but possibly improper with respect to what the regulator or other adjudicators may require or desire. Sponsors vary in their sophistication about toxicology. Some sponsors have well-qualified staffs of professionals thoroughly familiar with regulatory requirements. Others use consultants and other professionals. Some are completely naive about regulatory demands and depend entirely upon the contractor for guidance and interface with the regulators.

Data from a toxicology study may be divided into two areas. The first comprises volatile data and represents those data which must be collected at a given point in time. The opportunity to duplicate those data will not exist again. For example, the body weight of an animal on Friday will not be the same as the body weight of the animal on Wednesday. The weights may approximate one another and similar conclusions may be drawn, but the data will not be the same. This is true of every measurement taken during the in-life phase of a study. On the other hand, pathology data usually represent non-volatile data. There is a certain volatility to gross pathology, since formalization of tissue changes its color and some other characteristics. Once the tissue processing has been completed and the tissue slice stained and coverslipped on a slide, one may return to view that slide repeatedly. Therefore, the anatomic pathologist tends to deal with non-volatile data, while the study director is concerned with both.

INTERPRETATION AND ACCEPTANCE OF DATA

The study director either must himself develop criteria for acceptance of data or must, in concert with others, develop such criteria. Developing these criteria may not necessarily be a formalized systematic endeavor, and in the majority of instances is certainly not institutionalized. However, there must be an implicit set of criteria which defines the acceptability of data. There must be a hierarchy established regarding the importance of specific sets of data. Some findings, such as organ changes, are more important than others, such as water consumption, in evaluating a toxic effect. Others may assume a new importance when related to other findings, as with food consumption and lethargy. The ability to establish acceptance criteria, coupled with a capability to interpret these data, is often referred to as experience.

The study director reviews the data to ensure that the different components fit. Once he has established that all of the components are acceptable, he then interprets the data. This interpretation is not done in all instances, since for some studies the sponsor has established other systems for reviewing and interpreting the data.

The sponsor may not request that all studies be conducted under GLPs. However, most laboratories make no distinction between studies conducted and those not conducted under GLPs. Having two standards of performance criteria leads to confusion and errors in the laboratory. The only difference usually applied to studies conducted under, and not under, GLPs, is the frequency of data and report review by the QA unit. However, irrespective of this, the study director is responsible for reviewing the data for their quality. It is his responsibility to ensure that the data meet established standards of quality.

The study director may delegate the data acquisition and interpretations, as in the case of clinical pathology data, to the clinical pathologist who has systems in place for monitoring data quality. If the study director is not a pathologist, he certainly delegates responsibility to a pathologist to ensure that the slides are of sufficient quality to permit an accurate diagnosis. To a certain extent, he also delegates responsibility to the technician in the laboratory, who actually collects the bulk of the data used in any given study. However, it is ultimately the study director's responsibility to ensure that his delegates have performed their duties in an acceptable manner.

The study director wears many hats. He obviously has responsibilities to the company for which he works and from which he collects his pay. In addition, he may serve as an ombudsman for the sponsor, ensuring to the best of his ability and circumstances that the interests of the client are met when there are differences of opinion. He has a legal responsibility incurred as a result of GLPs and he has a responsibility to himself that what he is doing is proper, correct and done to the best of his ability. His responsibility to the sponsor not only includes the quality of the science and of the data trail but is also involved with the timely delivery of a usable product, the report, in such a manner that it may be used by the sponsor.

Overlaying the delivery of the report is the supposition that the sponsor's project leader has made commitments to his superiors that the product will be delivered on time so that delivery dates to regulatory agencies may be met. Schedules that include marketing, manufacturing, packaging and a host of other activities are involved. The commitment is made by virtue of what the study director has told the sponsor's representative. Failure to deliver on time may initiate a domino effect that for some sponsors may approximate the old saying, "for want of a nail, the shoe was lost." This is often why the evaluation of the performance of the study director and the performing laboratory is based not only on the quality of the report, but also on its timeliness, even though some of the controlling factors are completely out of the study director's hands. In those instances in which deliveries cannot be met and/or there are problems with the conduct of the study, it is the study director's responsibility to ensure that the sponsor is kept apprised of any schedule changes. The eleventh commandment for a contract laboratory is "Thou shall not surprise the sponsor." The surprise to the sponsor can be worse than the bad news being delivered.

CONCLUSION

In conclusion, the sponsor may regard the study director as his ombudsman, proxy scientist, sometime confidant, and person to whom to communicate his needs, likes and dislikes. Ultimately he is the person responsible for ensuring that the sponsor places additional studies with the laboratory.

THE ROLE OF THE STUDY DIRECTOR IN ASSURING QUALITY— REGULATORY VIEW

Dexter S. Goldman
Laboratory Data Integrity Program, Office of Compliance Monitoring
U.S. Environmental Protection Agency
Washington, DC

ABSTRACT

The Study Director is the interface between management and science. Compliance with the Good Laboratory Practice Regulations in no way assures the quality of a test. Test quality is a function of the agreed-upon protocol which is signed off by the Study Director. Both Quality Assurance and Good Laboratory Practices are management tools and, when properly utilized by the Study Director, can assure management that the test protocol represents both good science and good management.

INTRODUCTION

From the regulatory point of view, both the Study Director and the Quality Assurance Unit (QAU) are basic requirements of both the Good Laboratory Practice (GLP) regulations in this country and of the GLP guidelines in many of the member countries of the Organization for Economic Cooperation and Development (OECD). Among the other basic requirements built into all GLP regulations are proper facilities, proper personnel and proper record keeping and archiving.

VARIOUS APPROACHES

After visiting many laboratories and discussing the role of various professionals in relation to the QAU and its operations, it is possible to classify

---

1. Address correspondence to: Dexter S. Goldman, Laboratory Data Integrity Program, Office of Compliance Monitoring, Environmental Protection Agency, Washington, DC 20460.

2. Key words: compliance, management tools, regulation, study director.

3. Abbreviations: EPA, U.S. Environmental Protection Agency; FDA, Food and Drug Administration; GLP, Good Laboratory Practice; OECD, Organization for Economic Cooperation and Development; QAU, Quality Assurance Unit; SOPs, Standard Operating Procedures.

scientists in terms of art rather than science. There may be those among you who feel that this is entirely appropriate, in any event.

Minimalist Approach. The QAU is a nuisance to which I am obliged to pay some degree of attention and I intend to keep this to a minimum. Management takes care of facilities, Personnel takes care of hiring people, I will put up with the Safety Officer, QA takes care of the archives so leave me alone to get my work done as I have too much to do and why did the Sales Manager take on so many contracts in the first place? If the QAU wants to inspect the laboratory, do it in such a way that QA technicians don't interfere with my work schedule.

Abstract Approach. Ignore reality, maybe it will go away.

Impressionistic Approach. QA is here to make a good impression on the clients and on these nosy government inspectors who keep on insisting they have to inspect laboratories. The result of my work is the only thing that counts; everything else is designed to make an impression on visitors.

Old Masters' Approach. I have been in this business of toxicity testing longer than anyone else around here and I know the best way to get things done. SOPs are for the new kids to follow. I remember precisely how I did things 30 years ago and it is still the best way to do them.

Old Realism. There were some bad actors in the field of toxicity testing. I remember meeting some of these people now accused of wrongdoing and it is hard to believe they did terrible things like making up results or putting the same table of weights into four different final reports or making an educated guess on how the results should come out and then making sure they did. However, thanks to the swift actions of the FDA, such things are of the past and everything today is fine, especially in the laboratory where I work.

Neuvo-Realism. QA is part of overhead, public confidence in testing results is absent and I had better behave because management says I have to and besides I just made a down payment on a new house.

Of course, I jest. Study Directors can't be categorized in such a fashion and regulations covering laboratory practices and procedures aren't absolutely necessary any more.

Perhaps we should face reality. GLPs are not a scientific tool. Adherence to GLPs will not assure the scientific quality of a study. GLP regulations are universally accepted as a management tool and should be recognized for that value. Adherence to GLP regulations is a management, a supervisory tool and attitude, and as a manager and as a supervisor the Study Director is deeply involved in the assurance of quality of testing, the validity of the data, and whether he likes it or not the Study Director will have to sign the final report statement of content and quality.

The Study Director is a manager and a supervisor. He or she makes decisions that will affect the protocol of a test under contract, makes decisions on the adequacy and background of new personnel, sets up training programs for new employees, supervises the work of others according to written and accepted procedures and has to accept both credit and blame for studies conducted under his or her supervision. These are all decisions that affect the reputation and profitability of the company. The Study Director cannot delegate these responsibilities. He may have the supervisory technicians check notebooks and calculations but he is the one who has to sign off on the study. Other professionals and specialists report to him on their participation in the study, not the other way around.

The role of the Study Director in QA operations is simple and direct. Both the Study Director and the QAU report to management, although usually along different routes. It is the Study Director's responsibility to assure that all work conducted under his control is in full compliance with both the regulations and the protocols and at the same time meets the needs of the QAU. The QAU is management's mechanism for checking on the conduct of the study, not the science of the study. The QAU is management's mechanism for assuring that the QA statement required to accompany the study can be signed off for both accuracy and procedure. The QAU is management's mechanism for finding areas that lack compliance with the regulations and attending to them either directly or through the Study Director. The Study Director ignores the regulations and the actions of the QAU at his own peril.

The EPA inspectors focus their attention on the QAU and on the Study Director, for these are the individuals who will guide the inspectors in their work and provide the materials and the answers needed. Data improperly recorded or archived is brought to the attention of these individuals, and the SOPs are used as the references to find out the origin of the problems and to suggest their solution. The Study Director who is a good supervisor and a good manager will have no problems coming through a compliance inspection. There is no such thing as a study that is free of compliance issues but that is a far cry from studies in which management obviously has little interest and does not take its role seriously.

The GLP regulations were written in such a way as to be an enforceable document. The EPA is committed to enforcement and, as many of you know from firsthand experience, will use its legal authority when necessary. The EPA is committed to compliance and enforcement for one basic and simple reason—a regulatory agency, in following its legal mandate, must base its decisions on data of the highest caliber and validity. The public deserves no less. I make no claim that we always realize this goal but we try.

TOXICOLOGISTS' EXPECTATIONS OF QUALITY ASSURANCE

Glenn S. Simon
Rhone-Poulenc Inc.
Monmouth Junction, New Jersey

ABSTRACT

The sponsoring toxicologist can utilize the expertise of Quality Assurance (QA) personnel in several ways. The contract laboratory's own QA practices can determine whether procedures are conducted reasonably within the laboratory's Standard Operating Procedures (SOPs). Data audits can be conducted on a third party basis by QA personnel, both prospectively and retrospectively. These audits should allow the toxicologist to determine whether the materials used in the study are accurately documented, that all of the results are presented in the final report, and that they are presented accurately. An additional benefit that QA can provide which often is not recognized is the ability to highlight events and occurrences which could be considered by the laboratory to be insignificant and perhaps not worthy of mention, but which could have great impact on the study's usefulness. An example of such an occurrence might be that animals in a particular study come from more than one shipment, or that some had a particular abnormal physical sign during quarantine which could obscure a potential, early treatment-related effect.

INTRODUCTION

The domain of toxicology is at once increasingly expanding and yet restrictively limited. Each day newspapers and news broadcasts contain stories about good and bad sides of the profession. Technological advancements, lay recognition of toxicology as a bona fide science, the insidious threat of cancer, birth defects and environmental catastrophe have placed the toxicologist in an influential position. Toxicologists appear regularly on television and radio shows, write newspaper columns and books, and are considered a necessary (if necessarily evil) professional in many companies that concern themselves with chemical and physical agents. Yet, the often competing realities of regulatory requirements, business interests, public pressure, personal convictions, economic feasibilities and time limitations can lead our lofty aspirations for toxicological advances to equivocal, ambiguous or even invalid results. In his/her efforts to cope with these realities, the toxicologist has come to utilize the services and expertise of others. QA personnel are among these experts. Regulatory guidelines have recommended that QA departments in laboratories be

1. Address correspondence to: Dr. Glenn S. Simon, Rhone-Poulenc Inc., P.O. Box 125, Monmouth Junction, NJ 08852.

2. Key words: audits, data integrity, data verification, quality assurance, toxicology.

3. Abbreviations: EPA, United States Environmental Protection Agency; GLPs, Good Laboratory Practices; QA, Quality Assurance, SOPs, Standard Operating Procedures.

independent of the laboratory's Toxicology Departments, and increasingly, this independence is finding favor in sponsoring organizations as well, though for different reasons.

In the ensuing discussion, when the term "toxicologist" is mentioned, the intention is to refer to a corporate "consulting" toxicologist who is not directly involved in the conduct of a toxicological study. The situations and examples presented in this paper may not apply directly to an academician, a toxicologist in an industrial or contract laboratory, or a toxicologist working for the government.

The sponsor's toxicologist responsible for a study conducted in an independent contract laboratory conducts QA for his company's own internal use and to satisfy himself/herself as to the integrity of the data. Although there is no legal requirement for sponsors to quality assure studies conducted in outside laboratories, the EPA GLPs require that the sponsor provide a signed statement specifying the degree of compliance with the GLP regulations. Therefore, it is clearly in the interest of the sponsoring toxicologist that determinations of compliance be properly conducted.

The toxicologist who has elected to subject a study to QA monitoring or auditing must decide whether to conduct the QA procedures himself/herself, utilize another toxicologist, or utilize a specialist in QA. It is not the purpose of this paper to suggest one means over another; rather, its purpose is to demonstrate the usefulness of the different approaches taken during QA monitoring visits versus toxicological monitoring.

BENEFITS

Most toxicologists are trained and gain experience in the design, conduct and interpretation of single research programs, although today most corporate toxicologists find themselves designing, administering or monitoring many complex study programs simultaneously. The burden of maintaining continuing familiarity with each program can become too great to bear when the toxicologist must not only put together the technical pieces of a scientific deduction, but also be concerned with ascertaining the authenticity and completeness of the data being considered. This problem is especially acute when both toxicological and QA reviews must be conducted simultaneously.

Of all the raw data generated in a study, those with the greatest significance to the toxicologist are the data which would commonly be found in the "results" section of most technical publications. There can be a tendency for the toxicologist reviewing a study to pay relatively little attention to the vast amount of ancillary data generated during the course of a study, or to whether the methodology stipulated in the study protocol was adhered to strictly.

Normally, the toxicologist is intimately familiar with the study protocol, because he/she was prominent in its design. The toxicologist is likely to be far less familiar with the SOPs of the laboratory conducting a specific study. Also, during a routine toxicological review visit to a laboratory, the toxicologist is not likely to review specific laboratory SOPs. However, the way a particular procedure is conducted may be significantly different from that which is considered usual to the toxicologist. Fortunately, it is quite common for routine QA audits to include review of pertinent SOPs. The QA auditor can utilize this review to ask technical questions of the laboratory staff and inform the toxicologist about the adequacy and details of certain procedures. Currently, in some companies, the QA auditor is only expected to question the adequacy of the *documentation* of a particular procedure, not its actual conduct.

For example, when collection of blood samples is called for, several methods of collection are commonly employed. Venipuncture, retroorbital sinus puncture, tail clipping and cardiac puncture are all commonly used methods for collection of blood from rodents. They can differ, however, in several important respects. Some are more likely to lead to hemolysis; others allow the potential for contamination of the blood sample with other body fluids. Some provide venous blood and others arterial. Cardiac puncture can increase the levels of serum enzymes due to damage of cardiac muscle. The gauge of needle or capillary tube used can significantly affect the degree of hemolysis incurred, as can the amount of negative pressure exerted on the collection device. Some of these specifics might not be described in the protocol. The toxicologist might imagine that methods he has experience using are identical to the laboratory's SOPs. The QA auditor can prepare an SOP review checklist for the toxicologist even before the study has begun. This checklist would inform the toxicologist of the details of each critical practice. Regular communication between the toxicologist and QA auditor, plus experience, will allow for rapid establishment of this SOP review checklist. If the toxicologist wishes to change a procedural practice, it would certainly be advantageous to change any planned procedure prior to study commencement. Once a study has begun, if a procedure is being performed in a somewhat less than preferred manner, changing the procedure entails technical improvement (presumably) but procedural inconsistency. The ultimate effect of this inconsistency on the study's outcome may never be discerned.

One practice commonly utilized by study sponsors involves reading a final report and comparing the report's methodology section with the study protocol plus amendments originally signed. This task, commonly referred to as protocol compliance verification, can be performed by the QA auditor reviewing the final report, or by the toxicologist. However, SOP compliance verification is not likely to be performed at all by the toxicologist. Some laboratories list pertinent SOPs in their protocols; others list them in their final reports. Still others list pertinent SOPs at both opportunities. These SOPs can be reviewed for adequacy of detail and documentation, but only a prospective audit (an audit conducted during the course of the study) can determine whether the SOPs are being strictly carried out. The toxicologist is likely only to discern gross technical flaws while observing procedural operations during a laboratory site visit, and not likely to have familiarized himself/herself with the laboratory's SOPs prior to the visit. The QA auditor is better suited to making that evaluation since he/she will have routinely been monitoring changes to SOPs and reviewing them for adequacy of description.

Data authenticity verification is probably the most recognized function of QA. Whiteouts, write-overs, erasures and pencil entries have all but disappeared from our current experiences. Instead, today we are faced with mechanization, computerization and other means by which the appearance of well organized and compiled data is provided. In an effort to decrease the amount of time required for entering data, conventions have been established by which to satisfy GLP requirements and yet save time. This can allow the laboratory to exist with a smaller staff or to take on a greater workload. One common convention is to record data by exception. For example, all animals in a cage (or a rack, or a treatment group, or in a study) are declared normal unless a particular animal or animals have abnormal signs recorded for them. The task of determining that data trails are able to be followed, and are accurate, is perceived to be the prime domain of QA.

During the course of routine data audits, the QA auditor may discover information about a study that, while it might not indicate a violation of GLPs or SOPs, could have a great impact on the study's usefulness. For example, could the presence of a mild, transient abnormal sign during quarantine ultimately mask or be mistakenly considered the cause of an early, treatment-related abnormal sign? Could a faulty automatic watering device terminally overburden the kidneys of animals whose kidneys' ability to concentrate had been impaired by the test compound? Once such information has been discovered, where should it be documented: in the raw data? in the final report? At times, the laboratory staff may not know the potential significance of a seemingly insignificant event. The trained QA auditor can bring these occurrences to the attention of the toxicologist.

The toxicologist expects that during the audit of a final report, the QA auditor verifies the accuracy of the data contained therein, presumably by comparing those data with the raw data. Of equal concern should be whether *all* of the pertinent raw data are accurately reflected in the final report. This is an important place where close interaction between the toxicologist (who can determine the significance of data, but may not know of their existence) and the QA auditor (who knows what data exist but may not fully appreciate their significance) is essential. Otherwise, final reports may omit significant data or be so overburdened with insignificant data as to render the report unreadable.

QUALITY ASSURANCE VERSUS PEER REVIEW

A relatively recent question that has arisen concerns how to ascertain the integrity of data contained in and supporting manuscripts submitted for publication to peer-reviewed toxicology journals. Scientific publications can influence the direction and intensity of research at other laboratories. Results of some publications are reported by the lay press. Still others can favorably or adversely affect the future of a company's chemical or drug, even when the company had not been aware that the research was being conducted. As a result of these concerns, the toxicology community has been pursuing a means by which to verify the authenticity and validity of data submitted to journals for publication. Although these concerns exist for data obtained from the laboratories at major industrial and commercial entities, they pertain especially to manuscripts describing work conducted at academic laboratories where no QA unit may exist. Oftentimes, manuscripts do not contain sufficient data to allow a determination of whether mean values presented are accurate. Thus, manuscript reviewers must comment on the soundness of conclusions based on the abbreviated data presented in a manuscript, but not on the integrity and quality of data supporting the manuscript.

One proposed solution would have a peer review panel available to review supporting data, and issue an "approval" to the journal's editor. There are at least two problems with this approach:

1. The peer review panel can only review data provided to them. They have no knowledge of the total database that may exist, nor do they have the authority to demand to review it.
2. The panel will be faced with the necessity to decide on a study's integrity without the ability to site-visit a laboratory, review SOPs or review protocols.

It is in this case that the toxicologist must rely on QA most heavily. All laboratories should maintain active QA groups, regardless of whether studies being conducted are projected to have regulatory or commercial impact. These groups should be required to certify the authenticity and integrity of the data *supporting* the manuscript as well as the data presented in it. In this way, the toxicology community as a whole can derive some degree of comfort from knowing that all data submitted for publication will have been verified. Then, the toxicologist can draw his/her own conclusions from the results.

CONCLUSION

In summary, toxicologists ought to expect that QA personnel provide them not only with a determination of data integrity and protocol adherence, but also that they offer technical insight by virtue of their privileged access to the most intimate study occurrences and practices. This access is easier, greater and more frequent than most toxicologists have the opportunity to utilize.

STATISTICAL APPROACHES TO AUDITING

Richard M. Siconolfi
Sherex Chemical Company, Inc.
Dublin, Ohio

ABSTRACT

Statistical approaches to auditing began over five years ago with the modification of a procedure used in the manufacturing and defense industries for more than 25 years. The basis of this modification comes from the international military standards, British Standards 6000 and 6001, and MTL-STD 105D. Statistically based auditing (SBA) was the result of this research and development. Prior to this, validation of toxicology reports was limited to two methods: 100% and *ad hoc* type inspections. The former diverts the responsibility for quality from the Study Director to the Quality Assurance Unit (QAU). However, the QAU has no means of inserting quality into a study if the Study Director has not already done so. Thus, the result of 100% inspection is hard work, high costs and poor quality. The *ad hoc* inspection method is not any better, because it leads to uncalculated and unjustified high risks. Furthermore, it does not provide any criteria for the acceptance or rejection of data tables or appendices being inspected. The SBA procedure is based on the theory of probability and has one disadvantage: only a statistically significant part of each table or appendix will be inspected. However, this risk can be precisely calculated and puts the responsibility of quality where it belongs, with the Study Director. The proper use of the SBA procedure leads to less inspection work, lower costs and a high quality final report. The criteria to establish an acceptable SBA procedure involves the risks the laboratory and sponsor are willing to take. The laboratory's risk is the decision to reject a table when it should be accepted and the sponsor's risk is the decision to accept a table when it should be rejected. The risks can be identified. What error rate and acceptable quality

1. Address correspondence to: Richard M. Siconolfi, Sherex Chemical Co., Inc., P.O. Box 646, Dublin, OH 43017.
2. Key words: BS 6000 and 6001, MIL-STD 105D, quality assurance, statistically based auditing, team auditing.
3. API, American Petroleum Institute; AQL, Acceptable Quality Limit; OC, Operating Characteristic; QAU, Quality Assurance Unit; SBA, Statistically Based Auditing; SOP, Standard Operating Procedure.

limit (AQL) are the laboratory and sponsor willing to accept? What percentage of tables in a report can be expected to be accepted? These risks can be discussed, adjusted and established prior to study conduct. Previously conducted team audits have found that a 1% error rate, an AQL of 1.0 and a 95% expected table acceptance rate appear to satisfactorily evaluate the validity of reported toxicology studies. This paper will present the background, provide the basis for use and discuss the results of the SBA procedure.

INTRODUCTION

Industry, government agencies, and contract testing facilities have been auditing toxicology studies for ten years. Some have developed efficient, simple and reliable auditing methods, while others have not. Those that have such procedures started their program with criteria designed to encompass the entire Quality Assurance area. One part of this program should include statistically based auditing (SBA). Many Quality Assurance professionals have had this as part of their repertoire for over half a decade. Auditing is an art involving a number of key items. Figure 1 shows the relation between these components, namely: protocol, raw data, standard operating procedures (SOPs), and report. Each interacts with the other and is essential for the study conduct, and evaluation and preparation of the final product, the Report. Although SBA is used for report validation and evaluation, it uses each one of these key items. Early experience and participation in Team Audits with peers have shown that SBA provides Quality Assurance professionals with the criteria to accept or reject tables and appendices submitted with the draft report.

AIM

The toxicology laboratory can be compared to a sophisticated manufacturing process, where the main concern is the final product. A product that is well

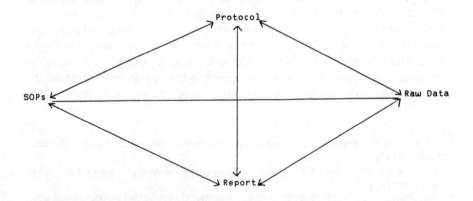

FIGURE 1. Key documents required to conduct an audit.

made, high in quality and properly priced can be easily marketed. The product of a toxicology laboratory is the final report and can conform to these same principles. The Quality Assurance professional's job is to assure:

- The study is being conducted according to the GLPs, sponsor approved protocol and the toxicology laboratory's SOPs;
- The sponsor receives a final report of high quality; and
- The cost of inspection does not dramatically increase the cost of the study.

SBA provides the Quality Assurance professionals with means to accomplish these principles.

Tables and appendices can be audited by three methods: 100% audit, *ad hoc*, and a sampling method based on the theory of probability, SBA. The method of inspecting all of the data points in a table or appendix diverts the responsibility for quality from the Study Director to the Quality Assurance Unit (QAU). Unfortunately, the QAU has no means of inserting quality into the study if the Study Director has not already done so. The result of 100% data point inspection is hard (unnecessary) work, high costs, and poor quality. The *ad hoc* method is not recommended, because it leads to uncalculated and unjustified risks. Furthermore, no criteria are given for either acceptance or rejection of the table or appendix being inspected. Two examples of *ad hoc* auditing are random row and column inspecting, or arbitrarily inspecting some percentage of the data points in a table or appendix.

SBA uses the theory of probability, although it has one disadvantage: some of the table or appendix's data points would not be inspected. However, the risks can be precisely calculated. The probability theory places the responsibility for study quality where it belongs, with the Study Director. This procedure can lead to less inspection work, lower costs and a high quality report.

Any form of probability has its associated risks. Basically, two types of risk exist:

- The toxicology laboratory's risk is the decision to reject a table or appendix when it should have been accepted.
- The sponsor's risk is the decision to accept a table or appendix when it should have been rejected.

PURPOSE

The purpose of the SBA system is to attain a table or an appendix acceptance rate at a level equal to or better than the acceptable quality limit (AQL). Furthermore, the designation or selection of an AQL does not imply that the Study Director or testing facility has the right to knowingly produce reports with errors.

DEFINITIONS

SBA system is a modification of British Standards 6000 and 6001, and MIL-STD 105D (the Standards), but before a detailed explanation of the specific

0.010	0.10	1.0	10	100
0.015	0.15	1.5	15	150
0.025	0.25	2.5	25	250
0.040	0.40	4.0	40	400
0.065	0.65	6.5	65	650
				1000

FIGURE 2. AQLs used by British Standards 6000, 6001, and MIL-STD 105D.

method can be discussed, definitions of key terms are required:

1. *Acceptable Quality Limit.* The acceptable quality limit (AQL) has already been mentioned above. The AQL is the target or desired average quality level, or to put it in other terms, the AQL is the lowest quality level that can be accepted as the table or appendix preparation average. The Standards state that the AQL is related to the quality required in the tables or appendices. Twenty-six specific AQLs are given and each is approximately one-and-one-half times as large as the previous one (See Figure 2). The average ratio between these values is 1.585 or the fifth root of ten. Both Standards use these 26 AQL values; if other values are desired, different tables must be constructed.

2. *Inspection Levels.* An inspection level is the relation between the number of data points in a table or appendix and the sample size selected for verification. Which level to choose is not clearly stated by the Standards, other than that if no previous experience exists, one should use General Inspection Level II (See Figure 3). The different inspection levels allow the Quality Assurance professional to increase or decrease the level of quality for specific inspection criteria without changing the AQL.

3. *Operating Characteristic Curve.* The graph used to display a particular sampling plan is known as the operating characteristic (OC) curve. It is the visual tracing of the probability theory for a specific sampling plan. The abscissa is the error rate and the ordinate is the probability of the table or appendix acceptance rate. The OC Curve shows the percentage of tables or appendices *expected* to be accepted, and not the percentage that will be accepted.

General Inspection Levels	Interpretation
I	Use when less discrimination or quality is needed to accomplish a specific inspection task.
II	Use when no previous experience exists.
III	Use when more discrimination or quality is needed to accomplish a specific inspection task.

FIGURE 3. Inspection levels.

Table/Appendix Size	Percentage of Data Points to Inspect
501 - 1200*	6.7 - 16.0
151 - 280**	28.6 - 53.0
	(11.4 - 21.2)**

SBA requires a sample size 80.
**SBA requires a sample size 32.

FIGURE 4. Sample size is constant at 80 data points.

4. *Sample Size.* Sample size or the number of the actual data points to be inspected is dependent on the table or appendix size. The reasons for this are:

- A correct random selection is more difficult to guarantee if the sample is too small a proportion of the table or appendix.
- Good tables or appendices become more likely to be accepted as the number of absolute data points increases, whereas bad tables or appendices conversely are more likely to be rejected.
- Large tables or appendices can afford a sample size that would be uneconomical for a small table or appendix (See Figure 4).

PROCEDURE

The conduct of an audit is more than reading the report, completing a GLP checklist and summarizing the findings. Each audit, whether it is a simple acute study or chronic/oncogenicity, requires advance planning. Hoover and Baldwin (1984) have explained their approach that advance planning is an essential ingredient in Team Auditing. (See Figure 5). SBA is involved either directly or indirectly with these four areas.

SBA requires the Quality Assurance professional to ask the following questions:

- What should the AQL be?
- What percentage of tables and appendices should be expected to be accepted?
- What inspection level is best for this study or phase?
- What error rates are we willing to accept?

The hardest decision to make is selecting the correct AQL. Essentially, this translates to how much error you are willing to accept. An AQL of 1.0 and an error rate of 1% states that approximately 95% of tables or appendices inspected

- Preparation
- Conduct of the Audit
- Summary
- Follow-up

FIGURE 5. Team Auditing.

Table Size	% Error Rate	0.65	AQL's 1.0	1.5
151 – 280	1		91	96
	2		81	88
	5		27	46
281 – 500	1		91	99
	2		81	92
	5		27	56
501 – 1,200	1	83	94	99
	2	54	80	92
	5	9	23	42
1,201 – 3,200	1	87	96	
	2	52	75	
	5	5	14	

FIGURE 6. Percentage of tables or appendices expected to be accepted (Approximate %).

are *expected* to be accepted. This information is taken directly from OC curve. Figure 6 displays the percentage of tables or appendices expected to be accepted by holding the AQL and percent error rate constant. As the table size increases the expected acceptance rate also increases. Figure 7 shows how the percent error changes when the AQL and the expected acceptance rate are held constant. These relations show that a 1% error rate and a 95% expected acceptance rate are the minimum criteria a Quality Assurance professional should use.

Table Size	0.65	AQL's 1.0	1.5
51 – 90	---	0.394	0.64
91 – 150	0.256	0.394	1.13
151 – 280	0.256	0.712	1.13
281 – 500	0.444	0.712	1.66
501 – 1,200	0.444	1.03	1.73
1,201 – 3,200	0.654	1.09	2.09
3,201 – 10,000	0.683	1.31	1.99
10,001 – 35,000	0.829	1.26	1.96
35,001 – 150,000	0.796	1.23	1.85

FIGURE 7. Error rate for 95% table or appendix expected acceptance rate.

The selection of the inspection level is now an easier task than what the Standards state, e.g., when no experience exists, use General Inspection II. Based on the auditing requirements for a particular study or the importance of placed specific data (e.g., urinalysis vs. neoplasms), the Quality Assurance professional may want more or less discrimination during the verification phase. A short review of the questions presented above is needed:

- What should the AQL be?

  Answer 1.0

- What error rate is acceptable?

  Answer 1%

- What percentage of tables and appendices should be expected to be accepted?

  Answer 95%

- What general inspection level should be selected?

  Answer   I. When less discrimination is satisfactory.

  II. When normal or average discrimination is acceptable.

  III. When more discrimination is required.

The best way to explain the SBA system is to conduct an actual table verification. Figure 8 is a condensation of the Standards and provides the Quality Assurance professional with necessary information to inspect a table or appendix. For example, a Body Weight table from a 90-day dog study has been selected for inspection. The procedure is:

1. *Count Data Points.* Count all the data points in the table. A specific method should be used to number the data points as they are counted, so those selected for inspection can be easily located. For example, count down each column and record the cumulative total. (See Figure 9). The total number of data points in this example is 112.

2. *Sample Size and Acceptance/Rejection Numbers.* Using Fig. 8, start in

Number of Data Points		Sample Size	Acceptance Number	Rejection Number
2 –	50	100% inspection	---	---
51 –	90	13	0	1
91 –	150	20	0	1
151 –	280	32	1	2
281 –	500	50	1	2
501 –	1,200	80	2	3
1,201 –	3,200	125	3	4
3,201 –	10,000	200	5	6
10,001 –	35,000	315	7	8
35,001 –	150,000	500	10	11

FIGURE 8. SBA sampling plan.

DOSE LEVEL (PPM)	MALES WEEKS ON TEST				
	0	1	2	. . . .	13
0	168.1	217.7	266.0	. . . .	475.2
10	166.4	220.2	267.8	. . . .	483.7
100	167.3	218.7	266.1	. . . .	469.3
1000	168.1	211.0	256.8	. . . .	450.9
FEMALES					
0	139.5	160.4	181.4	. . . .	270.5
10	140.8	165.0	184.2	. . . .	269.7
100	139.8	160.3	184.5	. . . .	269.6
1000	136.1	158.8	178.8	. . . .	261.9
Cumulative Totals	8	16	24	. . . .	112

FIGURE 9. Counting the data points and recording the cumulative totals by columns.

the left hand column labeled "Number of Data Points" and locate the row which contains the same number of data points as in the example (e.g., 112). To find the sample size, move one column to the right (e.g., 20). The sample size (20) is the number of points to be verified. Twenty data points out of a total of 112 will be inspected. The next two columns to the right are the acceptance and rejection numbers (e.g., 0 and 1, respectively). The acceptance number is the maximum number of errors that can occur without rejecting the table. The rejection number is the minimum number of errors needed to reject the table.

3. *Random Selection of Sample Data Points.* The inspection can begin once the table's data points are randomized and 20 have been selected. A number of methods can be used to randomize the data points. Figure 10 is an example of a SAS program that can randomize data points when specific information is given. Other methods of randomization can also be used, but will not be discussed at this time. Once the 20 data points out of 112 have been randomly selected, they should be highlighted for verification.

4. *Inspection.* The highlighted data points are now verified by comparing the reported value to the value found in the raw data. If an error is found, the corrected value is recorded on the table and a note is made to discuss this during the debriefing conference.

5. *Accepted or Rejected?* The table or appendix is accepted only if the number of errors found are equal to or less than the acceptance number. The table is rejected as soon as the number of errors is equal to the rejection number. Possible outcomes and procedures are:

   a. Table or appendix is accepted, no errors were found.

b. Table or appendix is accepted, but some errors were found. These errors are reported to the Study Director for verification and correction.

c. Table or appendix is rejected. Once the number of errors is equal to the rejection number, the inspection ceases. The Study Director is informed during the debriefing that a table or appendix has been rejected and these errors were found. Since a statistically based sampling system was used to evaluate the validity of the table or appendix, the Study Director must correct the errors found and retabulate the entire table or appendix because a high probability (95%) exists that other undiscovered errors are still present. Once the table or appendix has been corrected by the Study Director, it is resubmitted to Quality Assurance for reinspection. The SBA procedure is again initiated; however, one more step is added. Those errors reported by the first inspection are also verified at this time.

Figure 11 is a summary of the steps used to inspect a table or appendix.

DISCUSSION

The explanation presented above should provide a Quality Assurance professional with an understanding that he or she can streamline the auditing process and save time and money without sacrificing the quality required by management and the sponsor. However, proof is needed to substantiate that this system works. The Gulf Oil Corporation and the American Petroleum Institute's (API) Task Force on Quality Assurance (PS-47) began using SBA and Team Auditing

```
        Program

OPTION LS = 75;
PROC PLAN;
FACTORS BW = 20 of 112;

                                    SAS                                    1

                                    16:37 Tuesday, September 17, 1985

PROCEDURE PLAN.   RANDOM NUMBER SEED = 372705024

FACTOR       SELECT       LEVELS       RANDOMIZED?

------       ------       ------       -----------

BW              20          112           RANDOM

        BW

---+----+----+----+----+----+----+----+----+----+----+----+----+----+----+-
  5   19   49   87  ·77   44   56   69   50   72   63   95    8   73    3
 68   78   40   92   22
```

FIGURE 10. SAS randomization program and standard printout.

a. Select a table or appendix to be inspected.
b. Count the number of data points.
c. Based on the number data points counted, use the SBA Sampling Plan and determine:
   1. Sample Size
   2. Acceptance Number
   3. Rejection Number
d. Randomize the data points and select the specified sample size.
e. Compare the selected data points with the raw daa, and record any errors found.
f. Is the table or appendix accepted or rejected?
g. Report any errors found and tables or appendices rejected during debriefing conference.
h. Reinspect any rejected tables or appendices using the SBA system. Be sure to check the errors previously discovered.

FIGURE 11. Procedures to use SBA system.

in 1982 when the Chronic Inhalation Unleaded Gasoline Study was to be audited. The Task Force that was assembled to conduct this first Team Audit was composed of three member companies' toxicologists (two toxicologists who specialize in Quality Assurance) and API's expert in Toxicological Quality Assurance. The procedure presented in Figure 11 was used to perform the table and appendix verification. Each team member was required to prepare certain items prior to the audit. The actual audit took approximately 125 hours, but required 40 hours of preparation and 20 hours to summarize the audit results.

Figure 12 shows the results of the first audit conducted on the Chronic Inhalation Unleaded Gasoline Study and subsequent API audits on other studies. The 1982 audit (I) rejected 42% of the tables inspected. However, a year later, an 89% acceptance rate was achieved and clearly demonstrated the usefulness of SBA system. The improvement seen between the two audits shows the unwillingness of the testing facility to modify their report preparation process in an effort to produce a quality report. The audits conducted in 1984 and 1985 continue to show improvement. While table or appendix acceptance rate is approaching 95%, it has not yet been reached. This can be explained by reviewing Figure 13. Figure 13 shows that for tables or appendices which contain 500 or

| | | Percentage | |
Study	Audit Number	Rejected	Accepted
Chronic Inhalation	I (1982)	42	58
Unleaded Gasoline	II (1983)	11	89
Chronic Inhalation Petroleum Coke	I (1984)	9	91
Reproduction Toluene	I(1985)	9	91

FIGURE 12. Table and appendix acceptance rates from team audits.

Table Size	Percent
151 - 280	91
281 - 500	91
501 - 1,200	94
1,201 - 3,200	96

FIGURE 13. Percentage of tables and appendices expected to be accepted. (AQL = 1.0 and Error Rate = 1%)

fewer data points, assuming AQL of 1.0 and an error rate of 1%, the expected table or appendix acceptance rate is 91%. As the table or appendix size increases, so does the expected acceptance rate. This would appear to indicate that the majority of the report's tables or appendices contained less than 500 data points. However, to validate if this is a trend or an artifact, additional data from other audits would have to be evaluated.

Toxicology testing consists of many types of studies. Which ones can be evaluated by the SBA system? Figure 14 contains a list of studies that have been audited using SBA system. Furthermore, acute aquatic and genetic studies may lend themselves to the SBA system, but it will depend on how the report is presented. Acute mammalian studies are usually 100% inspected, because it is faster to conduct 100% audit than initiate the SBA process.

The Quality Assurance toxicologist can now add the statistically based auditing system to his or her standard report inspection procedure. This method establishes and quantifies the *risks* without sacrificing the quality. Management should be made aware of this system and informed about its time-saving and cost-saving features.

ACKNOWLEDGEMENTS

The author would like to thank the Gulf Oil Corporation for encouraging the development of streamlined quality assurance methods; API for recognizing the utility of Team Audits, and API's first Team Audit Group: Drs. Randy Roth and Judith Baldwin, and Ms. B. Kristin Hoover, who worked with the author. Finally I would like to thank Ms. Karen Huston, who typed the manuscript.

Subchronic	Teratology
Chronic Mammalian	Multi-Generation Reproduction
Oncogenicity	Fertility
Repeated Dose	

FIGURE 14. Types of studies that have been audited by the SBA system.

REFERENCES

BRITISH STANDARD 6000: 1972. (1972). Guide to the Use of BS 6001, Sampling Procedures and Tables for Inspection by Attributes. British Standard Institute, London.

BRITISH STANDARD 6001: 1972. (1972). Specification for Sampling Procedures and Tables for Inspection by Attributes. British Standard Institute, London.

HOOVER, B. K. and BALDWIN, J. K. (1984). Meeting the Quality Assurance Challenges of the 1980s. Team Auditing by Toxicologists and QA Professionals. J. American College Toxicology 3(2):129–140.

MIL-STD 105D. (1963). Sampling Procedures and Tables for Inspection by Attributes. Department of Defense, Washington, D.C.

SAS USER'S GUIDE: BASICS, 1982 Edition. (1982). SAS Institute, Inc.

SAS USER'S GUIDE: STATISTICS, 1982 Edition. (1982). SAS Institute, Inc.

SICONOLFI, R. M. and HOOVER, B. K. (1984). API's Approach to Quality Assurance. In: *Advances in Modern Environmental Toxicology* (M. A. Mehlman, C. P. Hemstreet, III, J. J. Thorpe, and N. K. Weaver). Chapter 20, pp. 271–279.

SICONOLFI, R. M., MARINO, D. J. and LAPLANTE, B. T. (1980). Quality Assurance in Toxicology—A Sponsor Perspective. 35th ASQC Midwest Conference Transactions—Tulsa, 1980, pp. 123–129.

WARD, C. O. and SICONOLFI, R. M. (1979). Quality Assurance in Industrial Toxicology. Quality Progress Vol. XII(8):34–36.

PANEL-AUDIENCE DIALOGUE
STUDY CONDUCT QUALITY

Chairperson:
Desmond L. H. Robinson
UK GLP Monitoring Unit
Department of Health and Social Security
London, England

Panel:
James P. Dux, Dexter S. Goldman, Richard M. Siconolfi,
Glenn S. Simon, Morrow B. Thompson

Desmond Robinson (Department of Health and Social Security, UK): If you look at your main program, you will see that there is a discussion period. Could we have some questions please?

Patricia Royal (Stauffer Chemical Company): We've heard a lot about the possibility of establishing criteria for acceptable data and perhaps for what is an acceptable study. We've heard Dexter Goldman say a few minutes ago that it's outside of the role of QA to make evaluations on the science of the toxicology studies, and yet, we also hear that the study director wants to hear all comments proposed and discovered by QA people doing inspections. If I have any question about the interpretation of the data, whether or not it's a statistically significant or a biologically relevant point, the study directors I work with want me to address the point in my audit report, so that they can respond to it. In this way, all questions are answered before that report leaves our office. I'd just like you to comment on that.

Dexter Goldman (EPA): Within your independent organization, you have certain ground rules for the relationship between the study director and the quality assurance unit. I'm more concerned with the regulatory inspection, or the actions of inspectors who are there to look at a study. My instructions to the inspectors are that, with a few exceptions, they are to stay away from the science of the study because that has already been decided between the laboratory and the sponsor. There are certain exceptions to that. I suggest if an inspector finds an exception which needs discussion, it is not a point to be discussed with the laboratory because they are following what they were told to do. Rather, it needs to be directed to the regulatory division to whom we report.

235

Royal: The problem involves, quite often, situations where the study director will say, "That's not your responsibility. Interpretation is not your realm. You are a number cruncher and that's all I want you to do." There are other study directors who want me to point out each finding to them, in writing. Then they respond to it so that there's a question and answer that has been documented. What I'm saying is that if we are getting to the point where we must establish criteria for acceptable data and reports, where are we going to draw the line as far as comments to be made by QA personnel on the interpretation of data?

Glenn Simon (Rhone-Poulenc): From my standpoint, I wouldn't object to having any questions raised. For example, is this particularly statistically significant point also biologically significant? Or, is this difference between means, which appears not to be statistically significant, biologically significant, anyway? If the answer is yes, then I'm very glad it was brought to my attention; if the answer is no, then, at least, I will have had it brought to my attention and the issue will have been laid to rest. So, from where I sit, I would much prefer to have the questions asked. Someone else suggested that those kinds of comments be put into a document separate from the strict GLP findings. For me, it wouldn't really make a difference. I think the comments need to be addressed either way. I don't think that it necessarily adversely affects the quality of the study if somebody asks a question about whether or not a relationship might have been overlooked, i.e., that a particular data point might be significantly different from controls. Therefore, I would like to hear about it.

Steve Harris (Consultants in Teratology): We have to continue amongst all of us this discussion concerning the QA specialists' input into toxicology studies. I really believe that there are a number of quality assurance specialists who are scientifically sounder than the study director who is monitoring the study. If they don't have the right to comment on the science of these studies, there is something wrong. We need to incorporate into our final reports an area in which that QA specialist can make some type of judgment. I don't know how you can consider a QA specialist a number cruncher. They have to be able to have some input, some place in our final reports, and EPA and/or FDA has to be able to accept that. We have to continue, through this type of meeting or small workshops, discussions concerning their input.

Simon: I agree with you.

John McCandless (Atlantic Richfield): We have third party QA audits done in our contract work. When the auditor audits a study, we request him to make GLP comments and reference the specific part of the regulation that his comment is applicable to, as well as making general comments concerning anything they see at that facility pertaining to the study. We're not specifically looking for interpretational, scientific judgment calls, but just more input into what's going on. We're not there; we contracted the work to these people; we trust them; we have another set of eyes there, and it's foolish not to take advantage of that.

Andrew S. Tegeris (Tegeris Laboratories, Inc.): Official government documents, both in this country and overseas, ask sometimes for half a loaf, which is a lot worse than no loaf at all. For instance, they'll ask for cholesterol assays which by themselves are totally meaningless. Either we should incorporate things like triglyceride and lipoprotein analyses or just get rid of the cholesterol. The same thing with electrolytes. Sodium, potassium, and chloride determinations are frequently listed as a requirement; yet, without carbon dioxide, any deviation in these electrolytes is meaningless. Even with carbon dioxide, you may have the same set of values in diametrically opposite clinical conditions. For instance, in primary respiratory alkalosis and compensatory metabolic acidosis, you also need the blood pH to interpret the data. I am making these points because we are talking about QA. Even if you recommend this to sponsors, some people want to do only that which is absolutely required by the regulations. I think this should be addressed and changed.

Morrow Thompson (NIEHS): I agree with you. We must be concerned about using appropriate tests for toxicology studies. I am particularly concerned about indicators of hepatocellular necrosis or function. From my standpoint, some tests that are used are not particularly helpful, but you see them used time and time again in toxicology studies. The enzyme asparate aminotransferase is not specific for hepatocellular necrosis. Some of the better enzymes that we should be using are sorbitol dehydrogenase, alanine aminotransferase, and even the serum concentration of bile acids. The same is true of the example you mentioned, lactate dehydrogenase. It is not specific for any particular system in the body. We need to be looking very carefully at the assays that we are using. Are they sensitive and are they specific for the particular system with which we are concerned?

McCandless: Dr. Thompson, you compared white blood cell counts from animals that were bled from the orbit with animals that had blood drawn from the right side of the heart. I realize there was a different anesthetic used, but did you open the chest and expose the heart on the animals that you eye bled? The trauma that would be introduced by the activity, even though the animals were anesthetized similarly, may affect blood parameters.

Thompson: No, I did not. However, there were also significant differences between samples collected from the heart and from the vena cava using the same anesthetics. Both of these procedures required surgical intervention and trauma. While your point is valid, I am not convinced the differences between the sites were related to sampling techniques.

Brian Short (CIIT): I have another question for Dr. Thompson. The toxic, fluorine-containing chemical, one of the three anesthetics used for the rats, has been shown to be nephrotoxic, especially to Fisher rats. It may be an idiosyncratic thing, but do you think that has any adverse consequence on clinical chemistry parameters?

Thompson: I have not done any studies myself. I am aware of reports that repeated use of methoxyflurane is nephrotoxic in the Fisher rat. For that reason, I would not recommend using it for studies that would require sequential bleeding in the rat. We will be recommending that carbon dioxide be used to anesthetize animals before blood collection in NTP studies.

Raj Chabra (NTP): I would like to clarify one thing about the design of NTP studies. We always include animals as concurrent controls, so we compare all of our data in treated animals with the controls.

Thompson: That is true, control animals are always included in NTP studies. I maintain, however, that this alone is not adequate. Using standardized, reproducible techniques and methods in a laboratory—between time points within a study and between different studies—is essential if comparable, reliable data are to be published. A laboratory should establish procedures that are used in all experiments regardless of the time (interim or terminal). With the establishment of a reliable data base, deviations from historic ranges, particularly in control animals, can be detected and appropriately investigated.

The NTP is in a unique situation. We have to assimilate data from more than a dozen separate laboratories. Because clinical pathology data are easily affected by sample collection, handling, and analysis, if we are to evaluate the quality of the data and to ultimately interpret the findings, standardization of techniques is imperative.

Kent Shillam (Huntingdon Research Center): Mr. Siconolfi has presented what is a tricky subject very well, indeed. I think even the uninitiated should be able to understand that here is a tool for QA which is a very valuable aid. We have been using a statistically based auditing method for perhaps eight years at Huntingdon. Initially, we started with sequential analysis, but we soon switched to the British standard 6000/6001. So we've had a lot of experience with this, and I would like to say that I agree wholeheartedly with your standards of being right 95 percent of the time. When you reject a report, and being confident when you accept a report, you are right 99 percent of the time. But what I do query is, in these days, is an A.Q.L. of 1.0 percent good enough? This is—don't forget the percentage error-rate that you consider is satisfactory as a process average. On a table in a report on a page, it is not uncommon for there to be 300 to 400 data points on a single page. Now, an A.Q.L., or an error rate, of 1.0 percent would mean with 300, 400 data points, there could be about six to eight errors on that page; and, yet, you are saying, "This is an acceptable level." I don't like it one little bit. If I saw a single page, and I accepted that report, and there are six to eight errors somewhere on that page, I don't think it is good enough. I don't think it is good enough for the laboratory; I don't think it is good enough for a regulatory authority to accept it as being a reasonable presentation of the findings of the study.

Now, in our instance, this 1.0 percent was an unofficial verbal statement given to us by the FDA, going back in 1977, as to what might be an acceptable error rate in the report. We thought we could do better than that, and we went for 0.4. At that time, we were using sequential analysis and 0.5 percent errors is what we thought was satisfactory. The nearest we could get was 0.4 in the tables. We've been using that for a number of years. I'm seriously now considering dropping to 0.25 percent errors, although it will probably increase the work of the quality assurance unit and time to audit a report. That is my thinking on it, Dr. Siconolfi. I don't know whether you care to comment on my suggestion that your 1 percent is not good enough.

Richard Siconolfi (Sherex): Well, I'm actually glad that you have information on using 0.4 and 0.25. As I've stated, 1.0 was the minimum, and I had to start some place, and that's where I started because it was easy to go through the tables and pull this information out. By all means, if you decrease the acceptable quality limit, you're going to increase the work in the quality assurance unit. Now, this is where you have to make a decision. Where do you balance out the increased work in QA against the quality report that you want to develop? That's something that you and management have to sit down and agree upon. I have no objection to going down as low as 0.1; I know of one facility that is using that A.Q.L., but they're all acceptable; it depends on what your criteria are in developing your own inspection procedures.

Judith Baldwin (Exxon): You introduced me to that method of auditing in 1982. I remember walking into a room filled with volumes of appendices and tables that we were supposed to inspect and get out in 125 hours. Do you happen to recall the number of data points? Do we still have some records of that, and do I recall that we found 20,000 additional data points the next year that hadn't even been presented to us? Yet, we were still able to do a pretty quick turnaround on a major study of great importance.

Siconolfi: If I remember correctly, I think the number of data points was approaching 100,000.

Baldwin: Not a bad return on the investment of time.

J. C. Bhandari (Dynamac): I think I do see the value of the system when the data are objective and quantifiable, such as body weight, organ weight, clinical pathology data, etc. Has this been applied to pathology data, particularly for carcinogenicity studies?

Siconolfi: We used all the data that were reported. For example, when we audited the unleaded gasoline inhalation study, we used this method for everything that was in tables or appendices; this included pathology data, clinical signs, and clinical chemistry data. Anything that's in a table can be audited using this method.

Bhandari: Again, talking about pathology, especially, because it's so subjective, you may have 10,000 data points or diagnoses, but only 50 of them may be valuable. Furthermore, perhaps only three tissues may be of real interest and must be investigated in detail. I fear that by using this method, you may take a sample which might not be truly representative of the significant findings and considerable time may be wasted going through a large amount of irrelevant data. There are many spontaneous, age-related findings (90% or more) in a carcinogenicity study and an experienced pathologist can review the distribution of lesions to easily select out and concentrate attention on the significant findings in a shorter period and more efficient manner.

Siconolfi: That's a very good question, and that would not come out in the presentation. One person on the audit team is assigned to verify 100 percent that the written report is validated line per line. So if there are significant tumors and they are in the report, one person's job is to read the report and make sure everything that the lab says in the report is, actually, in the data; so that is being looked at. One of the members of the inspection team was a pathologist at that time. We sat him down at a microscope and had him review some of the questionable tissues.

Andrew Waddell (Inveresk Research International): I, too, would like to join my colleagues in thanking Mr. Siconolfi for your excellent, evangelical presentation of this complicated matter. However, wherever there's an evangelist, there's usually a devil lurking in the background. Regrettably, this is the form he takes, because what concerns me about this approach is that we assume that every data point has an equal opportunity of being flawed. Now, all tables that I have audited are two-dimensional; they don't tend to be linear. So you have one variable, which may be the animal, and in the other direction, you may have different time points on which an observation has been made; or in clinical chemistry, for example, you may have different parameters that have been assayed. Now, my concern is that on occasions when I discover a mistake, it's because an error affects a complete group for some reason. For example, a miscalculation in the dilution factor in clinical chemistry. Without in some way structuring the points which are to be audited, there is the possibility that you could miss the completely flawed group. The second thing about this approach on which I'm not clear is, if you discover that you have errors in a table, but the total number of errors is small enough for you to accept the table, do you actually chase up the related points, either on that animal, or time, or do you stick very strictly to the previous allocated random number? The point is that if I have, for example, a creatine value that's wrong, I'll check some other ones to see whether, in fact, the error might be going through the group.

Siconolfi: To say that we use this procedure exactly and don't look at any of the adjacent data points would be a lie. For anybody who's done auditing with me, your eyes look at not only the column that you're on, but the adjacent columns as well. Although we didn't spell it out here, if we happen to find an error adjacent to one of the points highlighted, we count that as an error. With respect to your first question that had to do with a dilution factor miscalculation, it is possible to miss a whole row of animals. This is one of the disadvantages of the system; but we're relying on a correct random sample to find those errors, and 95 percent of the time it works. One way you can get around this disadvantage is by moving up to 99 percent. You can go back and retabulate the plan that I showed to have a 99 percent acceptance rate, but it's going to change your rejection/acceptance numbers. It might change your sample size as well.

Waddell: To continue in the theme of imp, if not devil, what concerns me is that while this makes it nice and clear cut, i.e., what we accept and reject, I personally would put a lot of store by the QA professional's judgment as to what is to be accepted and what should be changed. The statistical approach to auditing is very nice, very clear cut, and very clinical; but I think the element of professional judgment must still be in there, which this approach, to a certain extent, eliminates.

Siconolfi: Yes, I agree with you.

James Fernandez (International Minerals & Chemical Corporation): In your opinion, will not that 1 percent error lead to further errors? For example, where you have the body weights (rat 0, rat 1, rat 2, rat 3, there are ten, perhaps), and all of them fall into the range of 120 to 140 grams, but one type of error may be 910. That single, large error would be the one which offset the percent change, statistics, and a lot of things. Do you see why we ought to really go for less than 1 percent?

Siconolfi: Oh, I agree with you. To raise another point, the first team audit we did came up with something similar to that. One of the members was calculating mean body weight. He rejected the table of over 500 data points after seven data points were calculated. He just flat out rejected it. During a debriefing, we found that the lab was using the wrong formula for doing standard deviations. Once we corrected that, the rest of the table was fine. We got to the same result, but the statistical approach saved us time. Instead of inspecting all the data points, we highlighted because we had reached our rejection number. So, we recognize that you do have to have some flexibility when you're using this sytem.

David Ford (Life Science Research in England): Like my UK colleagues, we have experience with this system, since we have used it for more than a half a decade. We have found it a useful system, there's no doubt about it; but I think you have to realize its limitations. Some of those were suggested by Andrew Waddell. Another one is that it does allow some errors. I think you must be selective about its use. For example, if you are looking at a carcinogenicity study, one single tumor error might be absolutely pivotal to the study. So, for that reason, I think you have to look at the acceptability of what you're actually suggesting. For tumor tables, I would suggest that you have to check them all 100 percent, because you cannot brook one single error.

Another problem, and it's a practical one, is that you do have to use statistically-based auditing in a way that doesn't, in fact, cause you more work. If you try and use it, for example, on a pathology incidence table, we have found that it takes us longer to use a sampling scheme than it does to check one group or two groups, or something of that nature, because you are continually having to filter through all of the individual findings every time you check a point. I don't know if you have any comments on that.

Siconolfi: We haven't had that problem when we looked at histopathology at all. When we get the table set up the way the raw data from the pathologist were collected, we usually go right through without any problem.

Ford: I guess it is depends on how the pathologist presents his data.

Siconolfi: I'd have to look at it, or you have to tell them to use a different format to make your inspection easier.

Ford: Do you have any comments about the judgment that you use as to whether you should utilize the statistical approach or not?

Siconolfi: I would use this system any chance I got because it saves time, it saves money, and you can quantify the risks ahead of time.

Ford: Sure, I agree with that, but do you agree that there may be certain data in the report which are just too important to allow the possibility of any error?

Siconolfi: There's always that possibility. If you feel before a study starts that there might be a data category like that, then I would sit down with the contract lab and negotiate ahead of time that I wanted an A.Q.L. of 0.1 for this data set, or do a 100 percent audit. I'd rather see negotiations ahead of time on establishing the acceptable quality limit so that everybody up front knows what quality, especially what minimum quality requirements are expected.

Ford: I might just add that the way we have handled that is to write into our SOPs the acceptable quality limits and the type of check that we will use for each piece of data.

Carl Schultz (Cosar Inc.): What I don't believe was made clear by earlier comments is that the system's validity is based on the assumption that every data point that you are looking at is an independent variable, totally independent of the other variables in the table. Therefore, if you're checking, for instance, body weights, you would not include the average body weights with the individual body weights in that checking procedure.

Siconolfi: That's not true, because usually the tables are presented as a summary of all the means and standard deviations. Those derived data are handled by one inspection. The individual body weights collected during the study are presented in the appendix and are inspected separately following a separate plan.

Schultz: Okay if they're done separately, but sometimes they aren't. Sometimes you get the individual body weights with the average at the bottom of the page. That requires separate sampling and checking of those things. The other point I want to make is that this system is designed to uncover random errors. If within a given animal or a given measurement, there's a source of systematic error, you will not pick it up if you are only taking a random sample and a very small sample at that; for instance, if a balance is out of calibration. Your method is for picking up random errors, not systematic ones.

Siconolfi: Random or systematic errors, 95 percent of the time, will be picked up.

Schultz: The probability of picking them up is different.

Siconolfi: No, the probability is the same. It is 95 percent. We have seen audits work out that way. So, 5 percent of the time you're going to miss systematic as well as random errors, granted, but you're going to be missing that more often if you don't look at that particular row or column, as well.

Sharon Keener (Independent Consultant): In support of using this system, I think there are a couple of things you have to remember. Some of the systematic errors should be picked up during your in-life phase monitoring of the study and should be noted to make sure that they don't show up in a final report. In doing a retrospective audit, even on a study that has been monitored, I use the statistical method as a first tier approach to doing a final report inspection. As you're doing this, I don't think you can discount the inherent ability of QA people to be able to discern where problems lie in data. Once the first tier is finished, it is then necessary to go in and do a little more inspection and, like Carrie Whitmire said earlier, become somewhat of a detective.

Heinrich Fleischhauer (Schering A.G.): Not to repeat all these comments my colleagues already made, we found this step for randomizing and identifying the figures to be checked quite cumbersome. Furthermore, we found that most of the mistakes are clustered somewhere, and you have to follow your expertise to identify them. Speaking on behalf of the system, we have found one case where it's very applicable, and that is if you have raw data recorded by hand and then transferred to a computer system. Now we have a program that takes care of identifying the figures to be checked and sampling them. This is fine, because then you have complete documentation of those figures to be checked, and the work is very easily done. In this kind of system we gained the most from using a statistical approach to auditing.

Siconolfi: In a system like that, you'd always go back to the hand-recorded data to make sure they were inputted correctly. Then you would validate to make sure that your computer was operating correctly, the program software, the hardware, the output.

Ira Friedman (Pfizer): Rich, I don't know if you emphasized this, but the actual error rate, the actual number of errors in the report, is less than the A.Q.L. because you've corrected the errors that were found. So in the long run, you actually end up with a lower error rate in the report than your standard.

Siconolfi: That is correct.

Mary Ellen Cosenza (Revlon Health Care): We're looking into setting up this system and I have a couple of questions. When you get back a table that has been rejected, do you alter the A.Q.L. the next time you look at it, to make it tighter?

Siconolfi: I haven't normally, although I have heard of people tightening the A.Q.L. If you feel that there might be problems from a specific section within the lab, then your requirement of tightening that area is well founded. I would recommend that. I have not gone into tightening or relaxing the standard because I didn't want to cover too much information all at once. I just gave you the average acceptable.

Cosenza: I think, also, that a lot of people tend to tighten it for future inspections of that area. Say, if the errors increase, the next few reports might be tightened up a little bit.

Siconolfi: That's right. Normally, you would tighten it depending on what the standard dictates, but it's usually three or four more inspections. If they come out satisfactorily, then you can go back to the normal inspection rate. If an error occurs again, you can tighten it back up.

Cosenza: I have another question, which perhaps other people who use this system could help answer. How does the toxicologist accept the idea of getting back whole tables rejected without all the errors highlighted? Usually, we outline every error for them and I think they've kind of gotten dependent on us to find any errors. Now you're going to hand it back and say, "there are at least three errors; there may be more."

Siconolfi: Well, if we reject the table, I expect them to retabulate the whole thing. It's in our SOPs; management has signed it. I've heard a lot of grumblings from the toxicologists, but they usually found a way to do it.

Margaret Minosh (Northrop): If you're validating a large number of data points or a large number of tables, your auditors also risk making mistakes in their validation. Have you ever considered adding a second level of testing—of auditing the auditors?

Siconolfi: No, not really. Can you give me an example where you feel that the QA auditor would make a mistake in inspecting the table?

Minosh: I just know from having looked at tables myself, that as you go through a large series of numbers, you start seeing backwards, sort of. It's not a high probability, but if you were evaluating 1,000 or 2,000 points in a short period of time, it becomes more probable.

Siconolfi: The amount of data required to look at 2,000 data points at any one time would require a table of 1 million points. Most of the tables that we inspect are usually 1,200 points or less.

Minosh: Right, but you have an example on one of your slides where you accepted 40 tables and rejected 50, or something. So, you looked at 100 tables, and if you had 1,000 points—

Siconolfi: That was a team audit and we had four people looking at that. They only looked at one table at a time. I would guess that the average number of data points inspected for each table was 50, and they're not right in a line because they're randomly dispersed throughout the table. So, it requires the QA professional to look at that point that's supposed to be inspected, to find out where it is, to go to the raw data, to look at them, go back to the tables, compare that to what's in the raw data. Now, the only problem that would occur with what you said is, if we're doing means and you've got 50 animals, but you miss one, then there's going to be an error. So, if we miss it, that's a QA error. Now, when we come up with a different answer (we're generating a tape as we go along), we can check the tape against the raw data. If it's still an error, then we might input it again, because, you know, calculators occasionally make a mistake.

Minosh: Is that two separate people making that check, or is that the same person?

Siconolfi: No, that's just one person. Now, it has been known that on Thursday afternoon, when tempers are short, we will ask somebody else to run those numbers.

Minosh: Exactly.

Robinson: Okay, I think at that point we might usefully draw the discussion to a close.

Chapter VI
QUALITY OF PATHOLOGY

A MANAGER'S VIEW OF THE "MUSTS" IN A QUALITY NECROPSY

Hugh E. Black
Schering Corporation
Lafayette, New Jersey

ABSTRACT

The importance of the necropsy, one of the shortest phases in most toxicology studies, should not be underestimated. If done carefully and completely, the necropsy provides the means for tying together clinical observations with morphologic changes observed in tissues. By contrast, a careless necropsy jeopardizes the investment in time and resources in both the dosing and post-mortem phases of a study, and could even jeopardize persons currently being exposed to the test substance if significant changes are not recognized and reported. Ventilation, lighting and equipment must permit safe, comfortable working conditions with instruments and personnel available to complete any special techniques. Times set aside for the necropsy must be sufficient to allow proper tissue evaluation. Descriptions of findings by the pathologist must be complete, accurate and meaningful. Trained, experienced prosectors must collect tissues as required by protocol and trim them in a uniform manner following defined laboratory procedures. A system of accounting must be used to assure completeness of tissue collection. The system for recording observations must be a validated system that tracks lesions noted clinically through the necropsy on to histology and microscopy and must permit correlation of clinical, gross and microscopic findings. Upon completion of the necropsy, individual and tabular data must be available quickly for management action, should results indicate that action is required. Limited access to and appropriate approvals for editing must be in place with edit trails on all changes in data. A backup system for manual recording must be available in case of computer failure. The QA professional monitoring the necropsy must be capable of evaluating the quality and completeness of the tissue collection and be concerned with who is making the lesion observations and generating the descriptions.

1. Address correspondence to: Hugh E. Black, D.V.M., Ph.D., Schering Corporation, P.O. Box 32, Lafayette, NJ 07848.
2. Key words: clinical observation, morphologic changes, necropsy.
3. Abbreviation: QA, quality assurance.

BASIC PRINCIPLES

The necropsy is a short but important phase of a toxicity study. It represents the beginning of data generation in the postmortem phase of the study and is the link between the findings observed in the "in life" portion of the study and the findings observed when the tissues are reviewed microscopically. The necropsy process provides the opportunity to evaluate the organs for gross evidence of spontaneous disease, procedure-induced alterations and compound-induced lesions. Gross changes can be described as to their location, color and tinctorial characteristics, their extent and approximate age. An opinion may be rendered, based upon what is observed, as to the possible cause of death. Potential target organs of toxicity may be identified and, in some cases, sufficient evidence of toxicity or carcinogenicity may be gathered to pass to management an early warning to proceed cautiously or even to stop a clinical study.

A quality necropsy has some essential components: careful planning and preparation; adequate equipment; facilities that are well ventilated and well lighted; sufficient time to work carefully and thoroughly; trained, competent staff; data collection and tabulation procedures that complement rather than hinder the process; and appropriate supportive documentation. If these essential requirements are met, the product of the necropsy will be data of the highest possible quality.

PLANNING AND PREPARATION

Planning and preparation for a necropsy are essential to its success. In the allocation of personnel resources, managers often overlook the number of physical actions that must be completed in the preparative stage. In our laboratory, preparation for the necropsy actually begins at the time the study starts. The first step is the establishment of a numbered pathology notebook. This notebook is considered to contain raw data, is kept in a secured location and is eventually archived. By establishing this notebook at the beginning of the study, a location is established for holding all information generated manually, either from interim deaths or sacrifices as well as from the terminal necropsy (i.e., gross observations or organ weight data). Besides containing a copy of the protocol and all amendments, the notebook holds a list that identifies all participants in the necropsy, identifies their position and has samples of each person's signature and written initials. All paper generated during necropsy and associated with the study is held in the notebook as raw data. In one section the names of all individuals who enter manually collected data into the computer are listed and the date and data entered are identified. The final section of the notebook is an event log that is used to document events that, at some future date, may be needed to reconstruct the events around the particular study.

After establishing the notebook, the next step for the technicians is to carefully review the written protocol and compare the written protocol to the protocol on the computer. The purpose is to assure that all organs to be collected or weighed, etc., are accounted for on the computer, since the computer protocol will drive the system during its use at necropsy. The review of the protocol also forces the technicians to familiarize themselves with the type of study, the type and number of animals involved, the types of fixatives to prepare and any special procedures that will have to be carried out. This review also serves to remind the technicians of any difference in procedure that will be followed for interim deaths and sacrifices compared to the procedure for the terminal necropsy. After reviewing the electronic protocol, the technicians print sufficient labels for each animal to label all containers, capsules and other receptacles that will be required during the conduct of the necropsy. They also generate the manual data collection forms to assure that should the computer fail during the session, data collection will continue smoothly. Finally the fixatives and containers are brought to the necropsy room in sufficient quantities to meet the needs for the particular study.

Approximately one week prior to the initiation of the terminal necropsy, a pre-necropsy meeting is held, involving the pathologists, technicians and study director. A pre-necropsy meeting is an important part of the process for a quality scheduled necropsy, providing the forum for the final review of the protocol and affording the opportunity to identify all participants in the necropsy and define what will be their respective functions and responsibilities. Finally, the pre-necropsy meeting is the ideal setting for reviewing what has been observed in the "in-life" portion of the study. In addition, changes in clinical pathology data can be discussed and what has been observed during the necropsy of any dead or moribund animals can be described. By having a meeting prior to beginning the terminal sacrifice, the pathologist and necropsy team may have some indication of potential target organs of toxicity and will be aware of other findings that they might expect to see while terminating the study.

Three pieces of documentation are needed in the necropsy room prior to terminating a study: the protocol and any amendments, the clinical observations and the standard operating procedures. These documents represent essential information that must be readily available for the conduct of a necropsy on any study. The protocol defines the objectives and methods of the study and takes precedence over all other documents. As stated above, the written protocol must be checked against the protocol entered into the computer. Only if the written protocol and amendments are consulted and compared to the electronic protocol can costly and embarrassing errors be avoided, since once the necropsy starts, the electronic protocol is in control.

The latest clinical findings represent the second piece of important documentation that has to be available prior to necropsy for every animal, whether it is sacrificed moribund, found dead, or is to be sacrificed at the termination of the study. Because the necropsy links the in-life observations with the microscopic findings, a careful review of the clinical signs for each animal immediately prior to necropsy assures that unusual findings observed in the in-life portion of the study are identified and collected for future microscopic evaluation.

The third piece of documentation needed in the necropsy room is the standard operating procedures. There should be no doubt in anyone's mind how the necropsy is to be conducted but, should a question arise, the procedures must be immediately available for consultation.

THE NECROPSY PROCESS

An adequate amount of time is essential to completing a necropsy and gathering the available information. Because the necropsy procedures are repetitive but at the same time exacting, the necropsy becomes tiring. Technicians pressed to keep up a frantic pace throughout the workday are prone to making errors as they become tired. Mistakes made in tissue collection cannot be corrected once a carcass has been discarded. If the quality of the necropsy is poor, then time spent to plan and conduct the dosing phase, with all the attendant costs, followed by the time and cost required to prepare and read the tissues, are all in jeopardy. The few days and dollars saved by shortening the necropsy interval can become exceedingly expensive if the loss in quality causes the final report to be questioned, delayed or even rejected.

To conduct the necropsy efficiently and effectively and generate usable, meaningful data requires well-trained prosectors. Prosectors need to be proficient in their knowledge of the anatomy of the species they are prosecting, well-versed in the specific necropsy laboratory procedures, know how to handle and trim tissues to avoid artifacts and be capable of operating all equipment in the laboratory. At least some of the technicians should be trained in certain special techniques used for collecting and fixing tissues; i.e., if tissue is to be collected for ultrastructural study, the responsible technician must understand and be proficient in the tissue collection, preparation and fixation procedures that are required. Finally, it is counterproductive to expect that technicians can be moved in and out of an ongoing necropsy as they become available. A necropsy develops a rhythm. Certain actions depend upon previous actions and if someone new is introduced into the process or someone who has been involved is removed, it disrupts the flow of the process.

THE ROLE OF THE PATHOLOGIST

A pathologist must be in attendance at the necropsy, not on call, if the accuracy of the necropsy observations is to be assured. It can be argued otherwise, but it should be pointed out that all compound-induced changes are not as obvious as are tumors. Certainly there is a dollar savings if a pathologist is not in attendance, but the quality can suffer. Anyone who has spent time supervising a group of technicians and who has listened to the conversations around the table watched the individuals work as the day progresses and knows that the attention to detail is directly related to the size of the necropsy, the time allocated to complete the process and finally, the time of day.

The role of the pathologist is to supervise the necropsy process. He or she makes the determination on what is or is not abnormal, describes changes in accurate and meaningful terms and assures that the data generated by the necropsy are both complete and accurately reflect what was observed in the laboratory. The pathologist should attempt to determine the most likely cause of death for animals that died while on study. Because the gross changes noted at necropsy may be of a type and occur at a multiple of the human dose that indicates a potential hazard for humans receiving the compound, it is essential that these changes be recognized and reported immediately. By the same token, it is important that lesions that reflect intercurrent disease or changes caused by the dosing procedure not be confused with and be considered compound-induced changes.

TERMINOLOGY AND IDENTIFICATION

Finally, terminology is important. The individual documenting the changes observed must be aware of the significance of the terms being used. An extreme example would be the use of the term "tumor" to describe a subcutaneous swelling on the ventral abdomen of a female rat or a firm yellow focus in a lymph node. Although both lesions may in fact be tumors, there is an equal probability that they are not. It must be recognized that how the term "tumor" is perceived versus the term "swelling" or the description "firm, yellow focus," is significantly different. Similarly, if an increased incidence of masses or nodules is occurring in compound-dosed animals and by virtue of the character of the masses or nodules they are consistent with being neoplasms, it is essential that they be recognized at the time of the necropsy and collected.

A quality necropsy procedure must have a mechanism incorporated into it that makes it possible to identify and follow specific lesions from necropsy through histology to the microscopic review process. A relatively simple procedure is as follows: for each animal, sequentially number lesions after describing them, place each lesion in a capsule bearing its number, fix it, process it in the numbered capsule, number the block and slide with the same number, then record the microscopic observation against that lesion number. Such a process ties together the gross and microscopic description for a specific lesion.

The significant role of the representative from the quality assurance (QA) unit should not be overlooked in the necropsy process. To be a constructive adjunct to the necropsy, the individual must have a clear understanding of the necropsy process and be familiar with all the procedures. Similarly, the individual should be capable of reviewing the quality of collected tissues and should be able to randomly check fixed tissues from selected animals for completeness of the tissue collection. The QA monitor should pay particular attention to the thoroughness of the review of the carcass and individual organs for each animal as it is conducted by the pathologist. It is this review that is essential to the generation of all the information available at the necropsy table, and which cannot be sacrificed in order to speed the mechanical processes in the necropsy procedure.

DATA HANDLING AND COLLECTION

The purpose of automation of data handling at the necropsy is to provide a method for rapid tabulation of data and decrease the number of errors introduced by manually tabulating and typing results. Tabulated gross observations

253

should be available shortly after completion of the necropsy in a format that can be readily interpreted. The format of tabulated organ weight data also is important because of the volume of numbers generated. Ideally the data will be presented by organ as both absolute and relative values with both individual and mean values, will be statistically analyzed and will be accompanied by terminal body weight information.

Although the value of organ weight data is sometimes challenged, it can occasionally identify a pharmacologic effect of a compound that otherwise has no morphologic correlate, i.e., a compound-induced decrease in heart weight. For this reason, the collection of organ weight data requires consistency in procedures. All organs must be trimmed similarly and the weighing process must be consistent from animal to animal. The process must include steps that clearly identify the organs by animal number as they move from the necropsy table to the scale and back. Similarly, the process must move sufficiently quickly and include procedures that avoid drying of the tissues prior to their being sectioned and placed in fixative.

Since the collection of organ weight data requires gathering a voluminous amount of numerical information, the organ weighing system, if computerized, needs some essential features to minimize errors. It should always identify the animal being weighed, list all organs to be weighed, and accept and store weights of one or more organs from that animal. It should then be capable of moving to and accepting data from one or more additional animals before completing the set of weights from the first animal. The system should identify the organ that is on the scale and check its relative value against an internal control weight range for that organ by species and age; any weight outside that range should require a reweigh. A capability to add notes to flag selected organ weight data must be available. Flags provide a method for signaling the system to not include a weight in mean value calculations or any statistics. Finally, the system must require that the scales be properly calibrated as part of the start-up procedure to assure that the scales are accurate. The system should require recalibration at selected intervals.

With any electronic data collecting process, consideration must be given to an efficient method of manually recording data for later entry into the system, should there be a computer failure. Because necropsy data collection is an ongoing process that cannot stop because of a computer malfunction, manual recording forms for both gross observations and for organ weights must be available in the necropsy room at all times. Once used, these forms become original raw data and must be handled as such. In developing forms for manual data collection one must carefully consider the format to be used, since it is from these forms that the data will then be entered into the computer at a later date.

The value and completeness of the necropsy observations and the quality of the tissues collected are directly influenced by the condition of the carcass of the animal at the time it is evaluated. Very frequently there is the temptation for the study director to attempt to retain animals that clearly are not going to survive to the end of the experiment. Instead of being sacrificed these animals frequently die and, depending upon when they died, twelve or more hours may have lapsed before they are necropsied. The net effect is that significant autolytic changes have occurred which make microscopic evaluation of some tissues impossible. This problem tends to be more significant in rodent studies. Clearly, the gain to be had by sacrificing and evaluating moribund animals far outweighs the additional data to be gained if the animals survive another two or three days.

An established procedure for handling animals that die on study is essential to the quality of the postmortem data generated on these animals. To slow the autolytic process, a refrigerator must be available to hold the carcass until the necropsy. Dead animals must be placed in the refrigerator as soon as they are found. As a further step to improve quality of postmortem data in our facility, all studies are checked at least twice daily, once in the early morning and again in the mid-afternoon. Moribund or dead animals are then necropsied in the morning or late afternoon of that day. On weekends and holidays, moribund and dead animals are necropsied each morning. By using these procedures, the quality of the tissues and ultimately the quality of the postmortem data is maintained.

SUMMARY

In conclusion, the key to a quality necropsy is having qualified, dedicated people given adequate time to carry out a clearly defined process. The process must include all of the steps that are necessary to gather information completely and accurately. The data handling mechanism must complement the process and be capable of rapidly providing the data in a tabular format that facilities the review process and makes immediate action possible, should it be necessary.

IMPORTANCE OF UNCUT LESIONS
AND ANIMAL IDENTITY

Paul K. Hildebrandt
Pathco, Inc.
Research Triangle Park, North Carolina

ABSTRACT

Wet tissue examination has revealed that lesions can be missed at necropsy and at trimming. Also, animal identification in wet tissues can be difficult to verify in some studies. Missed lesions and unverifiable animals may impact considerably on the credibility of a study. Attention to detail by laboratory personnel can greatly reduce these discrepancies. The supervising pathologist should perform periodic in-house wet tissue audits to determine if discrepancies exist and to take appropriate action.

INTRODUCTION

Toxicological studies must be conducted in the most professional and accurate manner possible. The interpretation of experimental results can be no better than the raw data generated during the study. The Good Laboratory Practice (GLP) Act, with its quality assurance procedures, has had a positive impact on documenting raw data produced and provides an audit trail for such data.

There is an area in pathology when the laboratory can be in complete compliance with the GLP, yet errors can occur. If a lesion is missed at necropsy, no lesion is recorded and no paper trail is initiated for that lesion. An assessment of lesions missed at necropsy can only be determined when an examination (audit) of wet tissues is conducted. Wet tissue examination is not a requirement of GLPs. It has always been assumed that all lesions present at necropsy would be observed, identified and recorded. These lesions, in turn, would be trimmed, embedded and appropriate H&E slides prepared. The pathologist would examine the slides and make his/her histopathological diagnosis and evaluation. Gross-micro correlation would thus be possible, a paper trail would exist, and compliance with GLPs attained.

1. Address correspondence to: Paul K. Hildebrandt, D.V.M., Pathco, Inc., P.O. Box 12796, Research Triangle Park, NC 27709.
2. Key words: animal identity, lesions, necropsy, pathology, quality audit.
3. Abbreviations: GLP, Good Laboratory Practice Act; GLPs, Good Laboratory Practices.

Audits of wet tissues have revealed that lesions can be missed at necropsy. Some of these missed lesions have impacted considerably on the final interpretation of a study, actually reversing the original conclusion, while others have reduced the credibility of the studies to varying degrees.

In one study, 40 of 100 high dose rats (50 males and 50 females) had papillomas in the stomach which had not been observed at necropsy or at trimming (Fig. 1). This finding did not reverse the results of the study as a few papillomas had already been observed and diagnosed; however, the wet tissue examination changed the final statistics drastically.

In another study, liver lesions in control female mice were found which did, indeed, reverse the conclusion of the study. Hepatocellular tumors in female mice occurred at the following incidence: controls 3/50, low dose 6/50, and high dose 10/50. This particular compound was considered statistically significant as being carcinogenic for female mouse livers. During the slide/block match-up, it was found that one of the female mice with a hepatocellular tumor inadvertently had two slides prepared and one of these slides was present with the slides of another high dose animal which had no liver lesion described on the necropsy form or lesion in the wet tissue. The incidence of liver tumors was then: controls 3/50, low dose 6/50, and high dose 9/50. A wet tissue audit was performed and three additional lesions (hepatocellular tumors) were found in female control animals. The incidence of liver tumors was then: controls 6/50, low dose 6/50, and high dose 9/50. This incidence was not statistically significant and, thus, the original conclusion was reversed (Fig. 2).

Previously unobserved neoplasms such as papillomas of the tongue (Fig. 3), intestinal tumors (Fig. 4), fibromas of the foot (Fig. 5), and tumors of the kidney (Fig. 6) have been found during wet tissue audits. These findings can obviously impact on the credibility of any study in which such neoplasms have not been accounted for.

Animal identification in wet tissues is another area in which the credibility of a study can become suspect. When a container of wet tissue bears an animal number, it must contain the wet tissue from an animal that can be *identified as that animal*. Ear punches, toe clips, ear tags and tattoos are methods employed to number (identify) rodents. No method is 100% perfect; however, very good reliability can result from toe clips and ear punches (notches) if performed adequately. Ear punches and/or notches are usually located in one of the four quadrants of the ear, to designate a number preassigned for that quadrant. Several quadrants may be punched or notched to accommodate larger numbers and/or dose groups.

Problems that occur are punches that become torn and can resemble notches, and fight wounds (bites) to the ear which can resemble a notch or additional notches. Also, if notches/punches are not placed clearly in the appropriate quadrant, it can be confusing (debatable) as to which quadrant was intended to be punched/notched. A punch that is placed properly, well away from the margin and is subsequently torn, can usually be recognized as such. However, it

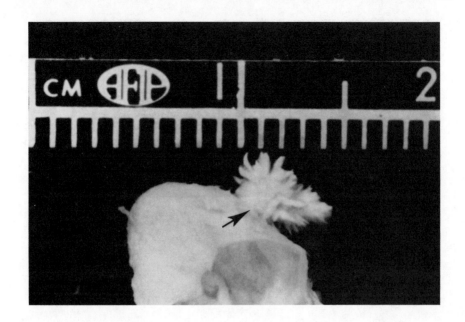

FIGURE 1. Example of one of 40 papillomas not seen at necropsy or trimming (rat).

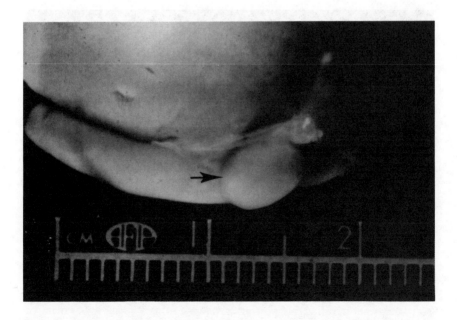

FIGURE 2. Example of liver tumor in mice not seen at necropsy or trimmed.

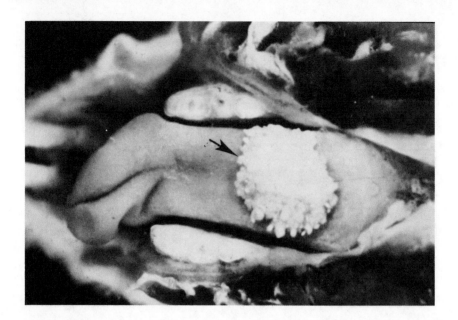

FIGURE 3. Papilloma on tongue. Mandible had been removed yet lesion not observed or trimmed.

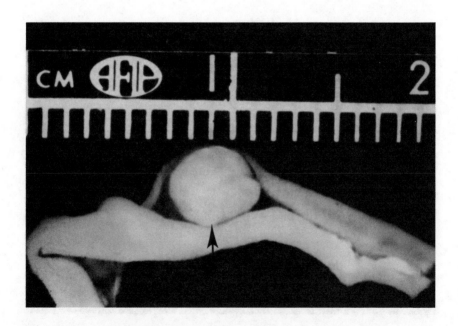

FIGURE 4. Intestinal tumor not recorded or trimmed.

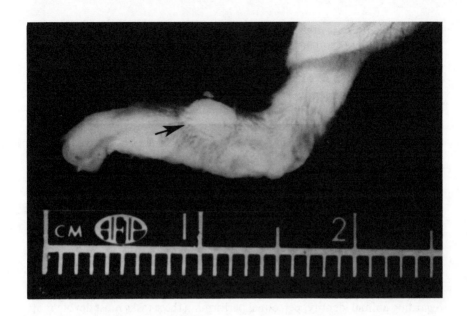

FIGURE 5. Lesion on foot (fibroma) not observed or trimmed.

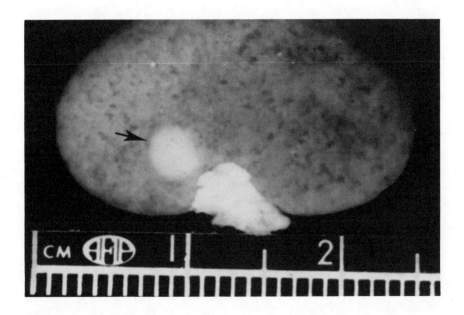

FIGURE 6. Tubular cell adenoma not observed at necropsy or at trimming.

can be very subjective if the punch was made near the margin and then torn. This can resemble a notch. If a notch was not placed well or is merely a small nick on the ear margin, it can resemble a healed bite wound.

Toe clips can also be somewhat confusing if the toe is not entirely clipped. Occasionally toes are bitten off by mice in the lower cage. This has been encountered when cages are stacked in inhalation chambers. However, mice seldom chew the entire toe; usually only the first phalanx is missing. During the toe clipping procedure, if the person clipping the toes does not clip a sufficient portion of the toe, confusion can later occur (subjectively).

When animals are numbered at the beginning of a study, the process should be done with patience and precision. If the numbering is performed adequately, most confusion at necropsy and time of wet tissue examination can be eliminated, or at least greatly reduced.

SUMMARY

To reduce the number of missed lesions at necropsy and reduce confusion regarding animal identity, personnel performing these tasks must devote more attention to detail. Necropsy personnel and the supervising pathologist must be aware of potential problem areas and adjust necropsy procedures to reduce the chance of error to a minimum. The laboratory pathologist should periodically perform a random sample wet tissue audit (approximately 10%), determine if errors exist and then take appropriate action.

NATIONAL TOXICOLOGY PROGRAM PATHOLOGY QUALITY ASSURANCE PROCEDURES

Jerry F. Hardisty
Experimental Pathology Laboratories, Inc.
Research Triangle Park, North Carolina

Gary A. Boorman
National Toxicology Program
National Institute of Environmental Health Sciences
Research Triangle Park, North Carolina

ABSTRACT

In a large scale toxicity and carcinogenicity testing program such as that conducted by the National Toxicology Program (NTP), rigid quality assurance (QA) procedures are necessary to verify and assure consistency and accuracy of the pathology data. The accuracy of the pathology evaluation is crucial to the outcome of toxicity and carcinogenicity testing and the conclusions to be drawn by the scientific community. The pathology data are often pivotal pieces of evidence used in the decision-making process that concerns the use of and human exposure to many economically important chemicals. It is essential that QA procedures be conducted so the scientific community and regulatory agencies utilizing these data are assured of the authenticity of the data used in decision making.

For studies sponsored by the NTP, a multistage QA program has been developed to monitor and audit studies to assure the quality of the pathology data. The data review proceeds in several stages of increasing detail which allows early detection and resolution of potential problems before the study review proceeds to the next stage. First, in a preliminary review, the quality of the pathology data is evaluated while pathology materials are at the testing

---

1. Address correspondence to: Jerry F. Hardisty, D.V.M., Experimental Pathology Laboratories, Inc., P.O. Box 12766, Research Triangle Park, NC 27709.

2. Key words: multistage quality assurance program; pathology evaluation; pathology working group.

3. GLP, Good Laboratory Practice; NCI, National Cancer Institute; NTP, National Toxicology Program; PWG, Pathology Working Group; QA, Quality Assurance; SOP, Standard Operating Procedure.

laboratory. Second, an assessment of the quality of the pathology materials (formalin fixed tissues, paraffin blocks and microscopic slides) is conducted. Third, an assessment of morphologic diagnoses is conducted by an independent pathologist who prepares a report documenting all discrepancies. This report and slides are reviewed by the NTP Pathology Working Group (PWG) to examine discrepancies and make recommendations for resolution by the study pathologist prior to production of a final pathology narrative and incidence tables.

INTRODUCTION

In a large scale toxicity and carcinogenicity testing program such as that conducted by the NTP, rigid QA procedures are necessary to verify and assure consistency and accuracy of the pathology data. The accuracy of the pathology evaluation is crucial to the outcome of toxicity and carcinogenicity testing and the conclusions to be drawn by the scientific community and society. The pathology data are often pivotal pieces of evidence used in the decision-making process that concerns the use of and human exposure to many economically important compounds and chemicals. Determination of toxicity and/or carcinogenicity is based upon a comparison of incidences, types and latency periods of lesions and tumors between control and treated animals. Even minor errors in tissue counts and incidence of lesions or variations in the nomenclature or sampling methods may distort the interpretations and result in misleading conclusions. It is essential that quality assurance procedures be conducted so that the scientific community and regulatory agencies that may utilize these data are assured of the authenticity of the data used in the decision-making process.

A quality assurance program for pathology was implemented by the National Cancer Institute's (NCI) Carcinogenesis Testing Program in 1977 to monitor and audit data resulting from two-year carcinogenesis bioassay studies which were being conducted at that time (Ward et al., 1978). In July 1981, the NCI Carcinogenesis Testing Program was transferred to the NTP. The procedures followed by the NCI for quality assurance were expanded by the NTP to include all subchronic toxicity studies and an intensified review of the chronic toxicity/ carcinogenicity studies to include pathology data from interim kills (Boorman et al., 1985).

A major responsibility of a study sponsor is the verification that the results of the toxicology or carcinogenicity test are supported by the raw data and that the conduct of the study is in compliance with the study protocol, laboratory Standard Operating Procedures (SOPs) and Good Laboratory Practices regulations (GLPs). This should be accomplished by periodic monitoring during the study and detailed assessment of the raw data and report upon completion. For studies sponsored at several testing laboratories by the NTP, a multistage quality assurance program has been developed to monitor and audit studies to determine if the quality of the pathology data is in conformance with GLPs and meets NTP standards. A multistage QA program allows early detection and resolution of potential problems. The review conducted by the NTP proceeds in

264

several stages of increasing detail. Problems or findings found during each stage are resolved before the study review proceeds to the next stage.

First, in a preliminary review, the quality of the pathology data is evaluated while the slides and tissues are still in the testing laboratory. Second, an assessment of the quality of the pathology materials (i.e., fixed tissues, paraffin blocks, microscopic slides) is conducted. Third, an assessment of the morphologic diagnoses is conducted by an independent pathologist who prepares a quality assessment report documenting all discrepancies. This report and slides are reviewed by a panel of pathologists experienced in toxicologic pathology to examine discrepancies which exist. This panel composes the NTP Pathology Working Group. The discrepancies are resolved by the study pathologist prior to the production of a final pathology narrative and tables. Each of these stages is described in more detail below.

PRELIMINARY PATHOLOGY DATA REVIEW

During the preliminary data review, the individual animal records and tabulated histopathologic diagnoses are examined for errors, inconsistencies and deviations from established NTP standards and guidelines. The individual animal records are reviewed to assure that the data have been entered correctly to eliminate entry of erroneous data into the computerized system used to tabulate the data (Linhart et al., 1974). The records are reviewed to verify that animal number, dose group, date and age of death, and disposition and condition codes are correct. The gross observations are reviewed and matched with histological diagnoses or descriptions to confirm that each group lesion has been considered. The morphologic diagnoses are reviewed to determine that only nomenclature acceptable to the computer software has been used and that each tissue with a microscopic lesion is recorded as examined microscopically. If satisfactory, then the data are tabulated by the computerized system for preparation of individual animal incidence tables and summary tables. If not, the individual animal records are returned to the laboratory for editing.

The tabulated data are examined by the study pathologist, who makes necessary changes or corrections and prepares a draft pathology narrative which describes the lesions, summarizes the data and makes conclusions on the study results. The corrected tables and narrative summary are evaluated by the NTP prior to a review of the morphologic diagnoses from an examination of the slides. Past experience with pathology data from NTP studies has indicated that the quality of some aspects of the data can be ascertained by simply examining the pathology tables and reviewing the pathologist's interpretive summary of the results. During this review, deviations from historical control data, duplications and inappropriate use of topographies and morphologies and tissues with low tissue accountability, when compared to NTP Guidelines (see Table 1), are identified. Studies which may be compromised either due to early deaths because of gavage errors or other causes unrelated to the compound, due to advanced autolysis or cannibalization, or due to animals not being available for histology for a variety of reasons may also be discovered at this time. If this

TABLE 1
Tissue Accountability in Subchronic and Chronic Studies

Organ Guidelines	Rat			Mouse		
	Good %	Fair %	Poor %	Good %	Fair %	Poor %
Gross Lesions	100	<100	<100	100	<100	<100
Lymph Node	≥ 96	92-95.9	< 92	≥ 94	88-93.9	< 88
Salivary Gland	≥ 98	96-97.9	< 96	≥ 96	92-95.9	< 92
Bone with Marrow	≥ 98	96-97.9	< 96	≥ 96	92-95.9	< 92
Thyroid	≥ 98	94-97.9	< 94	≥ 96	92-95.9	< 92
Parathyroid	≥ 80	60-79.9	< 60	≥ 70	50-69.9	< 50
Stomach	≥ 96	92-95.9	< 92	≥ 96	92-95.9	< 92
Duodenum	≥ 94	88-93.9	< 88	≥ 94	88-93.9	< 88
Jejunum	≥ 94	88-93.9	< 88	≥ 94	88-93.9	< 88
Ileum	≥ 94	88-93.9	< 88	≥ 94	88-93.9	< 88
Cecum	≥ 94	88-93.9	< 88	≥ 94	88-93.9	< 88
Colon	≥ 94	88-93.9	< 88	≥ 94	88-93.9	< 88
Rectum	≥ 94	88-93.9	< 88	≥ 94	88-93.9	< 88
Liver	≥ 98	96-97.9	< 96	≥ 98	96-97.9	< 96
Gall Bladder	NA	NA	NA	≥ 92	84-91.9	< 84
Testes/Ovaries	≥ 98	96-97.9	< 96	≥ 96	92-95.9	< 92
Epididymis/Seminal Vesicles	≥ 96	92-95.9	< 92	≥ 94	88-93.9	< 88
Prostate	≥ 96	92-95.9	< 92	≥ 94	88-93.9	< 88
Uterus	≥ 96	92-95.9	< 92	≥ 96	92-95.9	< 92
Preputial/Clitoral Gland	≥ 96	92-95.9	< 92	NA	NA	NA
Lung	≥ 98	96-97.9	< 96	≥ 98	96-97.9	< 96
Nasal Cavity	≥ 98	96-97.9	< 96	≥ 98	96-97.9	< 96
Larnyx	≥ 96	92-95.9	< 92	≥ 94	88-93.9	< 88
Trachea	≥ 96	92-95.9	< 92	≥ 94	88-93.9	< 88
Esophagus	≥ 96	92-95.9	< 92	≥ 94	88-93.9	< 88
Heart	≥ 98	96-97.9	< 96	≥ 98	96-97.9	< 96
Thymus Chronic	≥ 80	60-79.9	< 60	≥ 70	50-69.9	< 50
Subchronic	≥ 98	96-97.9	< 96	≥ 96	92-95.9	< 92
Pancreas	≥ 96	92-95.9	< 92	≥ 94	88-93.9	< 88
Spleen	≥ 98	96-97.9	< 96	≥ 96	92-95.9	< 92
Kidney	≥ 98	96-97.9	< 96	≥ 98	96-97.9	< 96
Urinary Bladder	≥ 96	92-95.9	< 92	≥ 96	92-95.9	< 92
Adrenal	≥ 98	96-97.9	< 96	≥ 96	92-95.9	< 92
Pituitary	≥ 96	92-95.9	< 92	≥ 92	84-91.9	< 84
Skin	≥ 98	96-97.9	< 96	≥ 98	96-97.9	< 96
Brain	≥ 98	96-97.9	< 96	≥ 98	96-97.9	< 96

NA - Not applicable

review is conducted while the slides and tissues are still at the testing laboratory, the study pathologist can more easily and quickly address questions raised during this review.

The tables are examined for inconsistent nomenclature used for diagnosis. This may involve inconsistencies in either topographical or morphological nomenclature. An example of a possible inconsistency in topography would be to have some diagnoses of *Uterus - Cystic Hyperplasia* and *Uterus, Endometrium - Cystic Hyperplasia*. The study pathologist must verify that these should both appear under one topography. An example of possible morphologic inconsistencies would be *Thyroid - Adenoma*; and *Follicular Cell Adenoma*. The study pathologist should review the cases where adenoma was diagnosed to properly classify the cell of origin. During this preliminary review, the pathology tables are examined for tumor incidence rates in controls that are unusually low or high when compared with historical rates (Haseman et al., 1984) and all negative and positive trends that may be treatment-related. The pathologist's narrative that accompanies these tables is studied to ensure that treatment-related trends and variations in control incidence rates are discussed. Deficiencies found during the preliminary review of the data are returned to the study pathologist for problem resolution before an evaluation of the diagnoses is conducted from an examination of the slides.

During this preliminary pathology data review, target organs are identified which will be examined during the study's QA review. Target tissues are identified by review of the pathology summary tables and consist of organs and tissues with lesions that are apparently related to compound exposure. Both positive and negative trends in the data are considered in the selection of target organs to be reviewed. Additionally, tissues and organs with reported incidences of lesions which vary with respect to historical control incidences may also be selected for review.

PATHOLOGY MATERIALS REVIEW

The purpose of an audit of the pathology materials is to confirm the authenticity of the data given in the NTP technical report. The pathology materials (i.e., individual animal records, fixed tissue, paraffin blocks, microscopic slides) are inventoried upon receipt. The slides are examined macroscopically for the quality of the histotechnique. This includes a macroscopic examination of each slide to evaluate for labeling, tissue and coverglass placement, air bubbles, and cracked coverslips or broken slides. During this evaluation, the slide identification penciled on the frosted end of the slide is compared with the printed slide label. Labels are also checked to see that changes are initialed and dated to meet GLP standards. A microscopic evaluation of the quality of the histotechnique is conducted by a histology technician on selected slides for such aspects as section thickness, knife marks, processing artifacts, holes and stain intensity that affect slide quality. The paraffin blocks are arranged next to the slides for a random sampling of animals in each group to confirm that slide labels match block labels, number and distribution of tissues in a particular slide match the block and that all blocks have been sectioned with corresponding sections on microscopic slides. Blocks are also examined for proper resealing to assure good preservation of tissues during storage. This slide to block match-up is routinely done for all slides and blocks from a random sample of control and treated animals. If any discrepancies are found, slides and blocks are returned to the testing laboratory for resolution of the problems noted.

After inventory of the bags containing fixed tissues, a random sample from each dose group is examined to assure that the label is appropriate to confirm the animal's identity from tissues (ears punched, notched or tagged or toes clipped) and to correlate the bag label identification with the individual animal identification. Wet tissues from these randomly chosen animals are reviewed by a pathologist for lesions that may not have been trimmed. Additional bags are opened when the clinical history suggests a possible mix-up in animals and in all cases where a gross lesion noted at necropsy was not described microscopically to assure that gross lesions have been trimmed for evaluation. In studies where gross lesions are found that were not trimmed or tissue identity suggests possible animal mix-ups, additional bags may be opened and examined until the extent of the problem is determined.

PATHOLOGY DIAGNOSTIC QUALITY ASSESSMENT

The Toxicity and Carcinogenesis Testing Program managed by the NTP involves many pathologists of diverse backgrounds from several laboratories throughout the country. A quality assessment program has been established to review the accuracy of the study pathologist's diagnoses. This program utilizes a unit of independent pathologists, with extensive experience with lesions in the strains of rodents used, to assess the histopathologic diagnoses. Disagreements in diagnosis and other inconsistencies in the data are examined by a panel of toxicologic pathologists who make recommendations for resolution.

The reviewing pathologist examines microscopically all tissues determined to be target organs during the preliminary data review, all neoplasms diagnosed in the study, and all tissues from 10% of the animals selected randomly from each experimental group. This microscopic review may also include all tissues with tumor incidences which are unusually low or high in the control groups. The reviewing pathologist's diagnoses are compared with the study pathologist's diagnoses and all disagreements are noted. At the same time, a technician prepares an inventory of the tissues on the slides for each animal. The quality assessment unit prepares a report of all discrepancies in tissue counts and diagnoses and an accompanying set of slides containing all target tissues and slides with noted discrepancies to be reviewed by the NTP Pathology Working Group.

The NTP PWG consists of a chairperson and a group of pathologists experienced in the lesions in question and knowledgeable about rodent pathology. The chairperson reviews the report and set of slides prepared by the quality assessment unit. Representative slides of the treatment-related lesions in target tissues and discrepancies noted in the quality assessment report are reviewed by the entire group. When there is a difference of opinion between the study pathologist and the PWG, recommendations are made to the study pathologist for reexamination. After the study pathologist reviews the slides in question, a final pathology table is generated and a final pathology narrative is prepared by the study pathologist. At this point the pathology is considered complete, and the drafting of the NTP technical report proceeds.

SUMMARY

We have focused on quality assurance in pathology utilizing extensive quality assessment procedures conducted by the NTP. Although not discussed, the NTP also conducts extensive audits of all aspects of the study, including toxicology, chemistry, health and safety and animal care. A summary of findings of the audits is included in the final technical report. Toxicology studies are expensive and time-consuming. Further, they are often pivotal pieces of evidence used in the decision-making process concerning the use of and human exposure to many economically important compounds and chemicals. Agencies that utilize these data should have quality assessment procedures to verify that the laboratory pathology quality control and assurance procedures are adequate and to confirm the authenticity of the data.

REFERENCES

BOORMAN, G. A., MONTGOMERY, C. A., HARDISTY, J. F., EUSTIS, S. L., WOLFE, M. J. and McCONNELL, E. E. (1985). Quality assurance in pathology for rodent toxicology and carcinogenicity tests. In: Handbook of Carcinogenesis Testing, H. Milman and J. Weisburger, eds. Noyes Publications, Parkridge, NJ.

HASEMAN, J. K., HUFF, J. A. and BOORMAN, G.A. (1984). Use of historical control data in carcinogenicity studies. Toxicol. Pathol. 12:126–135.

LINHART, M. S., COOPER, J. A., MARTIN, R. L., PAGE, N. P. and PETERS, J. A. (1974). Carcinogenesis bioassay data system. Comp. Biomed. Res. 7:230–248.

WARD, J. M., GOODMAN, D. G., GRIESEMER, R. A., HARDISTY, J. F., SCHUELER, R. L., SQUIRE, R. A. and STRANDBERG, J. D. (1978). Quality assurance of pathology in rodent carcinogenesis tests. J. Environ. Pathol. Toxicol. 2:371–378.

THE PATHOLOGY WORKING GROUP AS A MEANS FOR ASSURING PATHOLOGY QUALITY IN TOXICOLOGICAL STUDIES

Gary A. Boorman and Scot L. Eustis
Chemical Pathology Branch, National Toxicology Program
National Institute of Environmental Health Sciences
Research Triangle Park, North Carolina

ABSTRACT

Both quantitative and qualitative data need to be considered in determining whether the pathology portion of a rodent toxicity and carcinogenicity study is valid. Such a complex study often takes three to four years to complete and includes necropsies of hundreds of rodents and preparation of thousands of histological slides. The quantitative pathology data include animal identification, identification of paraffin blocks and histological slides, abnormalities described clinically or at necropsy, number and amount of tissues included for histopathologic evaluation and computer data entry and tabulation. These quantitative pathology data can be audited to determine whether problems exist that would affect the validity of the study. The histopathologic diagnoses represent the qualitative data that are equally important in study quality. These diagnoses represent an opinion by a pathologist about the nature and significance of each lesion. Most chemically induced effects are represented by a spectrum of lesions that may or may not appear similar to what occurs spontaneously. An individual pathologist's skill depends on background and training, familiarity with naturally occurring and chemically induced lesions and success in keeping current with the latest scientific knowledge. Since morphologic diagnoses are not simply right or wrong, special quality assurance procedures are needed to validate the qualitative pathology data.

1. Address correspondence to: Dr. Gary A. Boorman, Chemical Pathology Branch, National Toxicology Program, N.I.E.H.S., Research Triangle Park, NC 27709.

2. Key words: pathology quality assurance, rodent pathology, toxicological pathology.

3. Abbreviations: EPA, Environmental Protection Agency; FDA, Food and Drug Administration; GLPs, Good Laboratory Practices; NCI, National Cancer Institute; NTP, National Toxicology Program; PWG, Pathology Working Group; QA, Quality Assurance.

The National Toxicology Program (NTP) has two levels of review for morphologic diagnoses. First, a Quality Assurance (QA) pathologist reviews the diagnosis for all tumors, all tissues with a chemical effect and all tissues from 10% of the animals selected at random. A panel of pathologists serving on a Pathology Working Group (PWG) reviews discrepancies and induced lesions without knowledge of treatment group or prior diagnostic opinions. Each pathologist records his/her diagnosis separately. Each diagnosis is discussed and an attempt is made to arrive at a consensus. If the separate diagnoses represent agreement that is different from that of the original diagnosis, the study pathologist is requested to update the diagnosis. In cases of split decisions, the original diagnosis usually remains unchanged. The PWG members also discuss the nature of the lesions, suggest further studies that might provide useful information, or note factors that might affect the strength of the conclusions. The study pathologist, having evaluated the entire study, often provides insight and answers questions during the PWG discussions. The PWG procedure helps assure that the pathology diagnoses and interpretations for NTP reports meet current standards for rodent toxicology and carcinogenicity studies.

INTRODUCTION

The quality of toxicity and carcinogenicity studies has improved in recent years, due partly to increased genetic definition and monitoring of test animals, better laboratory animal management, improved chemistry procedures and improved quality of pathology data. Improved pathology data quality for National Toxicology Program studies is facilitated by quality assurance procedures that were initially implemented by the Carcinogenesis Testing Program of the National Cancer Institute (NCI) (Ward et al., 1978; Boorman et al., 1985) and by the establishment of uniform standards through Good Laboratory Practices (GLPs) mandated by the Food and Drug Administration (FDA) and Environmental Protection Agency (EPA).

Pathology data usually provide the endpoint for decisions concerning the potential hazard of a test article. Since these decisions may have significant economic and human health impact, it is important that the data be as accurate as possible and reflect current knowledge of laboratory animal pathology. Quality pathology data begin with careful study design and require frequent, detailed monitoring during the in-life portion of the study. Steps to assure pathology data quality during these phases have been described by Boorman et al. (1985).

At the completion of the study, when the study pathologist submits the pathology data and an interpretive narrative summary, the sponsoring agency should take several steps to validate that the data are consistent, accurate and complete. It is necessary to understand that pathology data have both quantitative and qualitative aspects that require different types of validation procedures. Quantitative data can be accurately measured and precisely validated. Such data include animal identification, number of lesions seen grossly, number of tissues examined, identifying numbers on histological slides, paraffin blocks

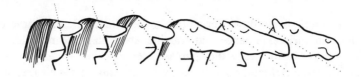

"Morphologic Evidence" (drawing by Siné)

(From Marcel Bessis' *Blood Smears Reinterpreted*,
Springer-Verlag NY, 1977)

FIGURE 1. A sequence of morphological appearances implies a transition but does not prove a relationship. Training and experience are needed for accurate extrapolation from morphology to the biological nature of a lesion.

and other factual data pertaining to pathology. On the other hand, the histopathological diagnoses are qualitative data that are less easily validated since they represent a judgment on the nature and expected biological behavior of a specific lesion. However, the biological behavior for a given lesion cannot always be precisely determined, since collection and fixation of the tissue for pathologic examination usually prevents further study of that lesion. The purpose of this paper is to present procedures that the NTP has implemented to assure quality of both quantitative and qualitative pathology data.

QUANTITATIVE PATHOLOGY DATA REVIEW

The quantitative data review is an important step at the end of the study that can be largely done by data clerks and histology technicians under the supervision of a pathologist thoroughly familiar with toxicity studies and GLPs. The raw data, including histological slides, paraffin blocks and formalin-fixed tissues, are carefully examined to verify that all are properly identified and correctly labeled. It should be possible to follow a lesion described clinically through necropsy, tissue trimming, slide preparation and histopathologic examination. All abnormalities described grossly must have an appropriate correlating microscopic diagnosis.

QUALITATIVE PATHOLOGY DATA REVIEW

The histopathologic diagnosis that a pathologist renders depends on the microscopic appearance of the tissue examined and how closely the lesion in question matches his/her mental perception of a lesion. The accuracy of this judgment is based on the totality of the individual's training and experience. For example, C-cell tumors are diagnosed in the rat thyroid gland based on the pathologist's knowledge of ultrastructural studies that have demonstrated secretory granules in these cells and the knowledge that antibodies for calcitonin will bind to these granules. Not all C-cell tumors are morphologically identical, and if a pathologist is experienced, he/she will also recognize rare spindle cell variants of this tumor, in which the C-cells are elongated instead of round.

Another example is a mouse uterine tumor for which different pathologists, depending on their experience and training, may diagnose reticulum cells, Schwann cells or histocytes as the neoplastic cell type.

In addition to interpretation of the cell type, a pathologist is also required to make a decision concerning the biological behavior of the specific lesion. This decision is not always possible to verify since further studies, such as transplantation or analysis for genetic alteration, are usually not done. This decision is very important, however, as it may determine the exposure hazard of the test article for the species being tested. From these results some judgment is often made concerning potential hazard to man. If a pathologist's opinion is that a proliferative lesion will regress when the stimulus (chemical) is removed, the lesion may be classified as hyperplasia. Proliferative lesions that are felt to represent slow autonomous growth but with minimal likelihood of invasion or metastasis are classified as benign tumors while lesions that grow rapidly, spread quickly and kill the animals are considered malignant tumors. The latter have the most ominous implication for risk assessment in humans. Since chemicals that cause cancer in humans frequently cause cancer in animals and often in the same organ or tissue (Wilbourn et al., 1984), this implication is not unfounded. If a pathologist cannot always verify the biological behavior of a specific lesion, how can he/she make these qualitative decisions accurately? Again, this depends on the knowledge, experience and training of the individual pathologist.

In the mouse, primary hepatocellular neoplasms with a trabecular pattern quite frequently metastasize to the lung, providing clear evidence of their malignancy. A pathologist will usually diagnose a small hepatocellular neoplasm as a carcinoma if it has a trabecular pattern, even if it is restricted to the liver. Training and experience help a pathologist to distinguish a true trabecular pattern carcinoma from a vascular tumor that might appear trabecular. There is abundant literature on rodent tumors to assist the pathologist in making these qualitative decisions. How can the scientific community be assured that the pathology diagnoses are as accurate as possible and reflect current knowledge about rodent lesions? In the NTP, this is done in two steps. First the histopathologic diagnoses are reviewed by a second pathologist. Then a panel of pathologists with experience in related lesions independently makes its decision about the biological nature of the lesions. The degree of agreement among the panel members provides an indication of the degree of certainty about the nature of the lesion in question.

In the first step a QA pathologist reviews all tumors diagnosed in the study, all tissues in which a chemical effect is expected, and all tissues from 10% of the animals selected at random. A report with the QA pathologist's diagnoses for all tumors and all target tissues plus the corresponding slides is submitted to the NTP. A PWG chairperson reviews selected slides and the report and prepares a series of slides for the PWG to review in a blind fashion. Representative lesions found in the study, as well as any significant lesions for which the study and QA pathologists had a difference of opinion, are reviewed by the PWG.

The type of lesions in question determines the composition of the PWG that will review the slides. If there are proliferative lesions of the nasal cavity, then the panel of pathologists will include scientists with experience in nasal cavity lesions and inhalation studies. The group will include members from academia, industry and government, each bringing his/her own experience and perspective. For controversial studies, eight to ten pathologists often constitute a PWG. Each pathologist records his/her diagnosis for each slide; after a series has been reviewed, the panel is polled and the lesions discussed. For unanimous or nearly unanimous decisions the study pathologist is requested to change the original diagnosis, if different, to reflect the consensus PWG opinion. For split decisions the study pathologist's diagnosis usually remains unchanged, but it is apparent that the nature of the lesion is less certain. The degree of certainty is considered in the final judgment concerning the study results. Often there is near unanimity with the study pathologist's and QA pathologist's diagnoses by the PWG. This validation, coupled with the QA of the quantitative aspects of the pathology, provides the best assurance that the pathology data are accurate, precise and state of the art.

CONCLUSIONS

It is crucial that the pathology data from rodent toxicology and carcinogenicity studies be validated for both their quantitative and qualitative aspects. Qualitative aspects can best be judged by an independent panel of experienced pathologists using a PWG format. This procedure has been highly successful for the NTP and has helped assure that the pathology aspects of the study are accurate and state of the art. It also quickly identifies controversial pathology findings so these may be considered before making conclusions or designing additional studies. PWG participation by study pathologists also serves as a useful educational experience. It helps NTP pathologists identify recurring diagnostic issues and gives study pathologists an opportunity to compare their opinions with those of their peers. In toxicologic pathology continuing education and peer review help maintain quality.

REFERENCES

BESSIS, M. (1977). Blood smears reinterpreted (trans. by George Brecher). Springer-Verlag, New York, New York.
BOORMAN, G. A., MONTGOMERY, C. A., Jr., EUSTIS, S. L., WOLFE, M. J., McCONNELL, E. E. AND HARDISTY, J. F. (1985). Quality assurance in pathology for rodent carcinogenicity studies. In: *Handbook of Carcinogen Testing* (H. A. Milman and E. K. Weisburger, eds.), pp. 345–357. Noyes Publications, Park Ridge, New Jersey.
WARD, J. M., GOODMAN, D. G., GRIESMER, R. A., HARDISTY, J. F., SCHNELER, R. L., SQUIRE, R. A. AND STRANDBERG, J. D. (1978). Quality assurance of pathology in rodent carcinogensis tests. J. Environ. Pathol. Toxicol. 2:371–378.
WILBOURN, J. D., HAROUN, L., VAINO, H. AND MONTESANO, R. (1984). Identification of chemicals carcinogenic to man. Toxicol. Pathol. 12:397–339.

GOOD LABORATORY PRACTICE AND THE TOXICOLOGY DATA MANAGEMENT SYSTEM

Charles A. Montgomery, Jr.
National Toxicology Program
National Institute of Environmental Health Sciences
Research Triangle Park, North Carolina

ABSTRACT

In the National Toxicology Program (NTP), histopathology data are collected and tracked through a computer system, the Toxicology Data Management System (TDMS). Histopathology data may be collected by use of paper, voice dictation or direct entry into the computer. The advantages and disadvantages of each will be discussed. Pathology quality is maintained through the use of a standardized pathology nomenclature. TDMS data are validated by the computer and the contract laboratory's quality assurance (QA) program. Individual animal pathology reports allow the pathologist to make a correlation between gross and microscopic pathologic lesions. Group summary data are available for neoplastic and nonneoplastic disease. Tracking of data will be discussed from the microslide to the final report.

INTRODUCTION

The NTP uses a multifunctionally designed computer system, named the Toxicology Data Management System, to collect both in-life and pathology data. TDMS is composed of two primary parts. The Experimental Information System (EIS) is responsible for in-life data collection, including body weights, clinical signs and dosing information. The Post Experimental Information System (PEIS) is responsible for both gross and microscopic pathology. The PEIS portion will be discussed in this paper.

1. Address correspondence to: Charles A. Montgomery, Jr., D.V.M., National Toxicology Program, N.I.E.H.S., P. O. Box 12233, Research Triangle Park, NC 27709.
2. Key words: data management, histopathology data, pathology nomenclature.
3. Abbreviations: CPB, Chemical Pathology Branch; EIS, Experimental Information System; IANR, Individual Animal Necropsy Record; NCL, No Corresponding Lesion; NST, No Section Taken; NTP, National Toxicology Program; OP, Original Pathologist; PCT, Pathology Code Table; PEIS, Post Experimental Information System; PWG, Pathology Working Group; QA, Quality Assurance; TDMS, Toxicology Data Management System.

The Individual Animal Necropsy Record (IANR) is the backbone of PEIS. The top of the document contains header information giving the name of the chemical, the weeks on experiment, dose, route of administration and individual animal identification data inclusive of species, sex, strain and histology number. The disposition of the carcass is recorded at the time of necropsy, e.g., moribund sacrifice, scheduled sacrifice, natural death. The condition of the carcass is also given, e.g., fresh, partially cannibalized. Several blocks on the form allow for tissue accountability and the status of each tissue required by the experimental protocol. This format allows the pathologist to trace a tissue from the time of necropsy through trimming and microscopic pathologic evaluation. A code is used to give the organ status, e.g., a - normal; b - lesion present; c - missing tissue; d - tissue present; not examined. There is also a column to record required organ weights.

This form contains space to describe at necropsy the types of lesions observed (inclusive of anatomic site), the morphologic diagnosis, and the quantity, shape, color and consistency of the indicated lesion. There is space to record the degree of severity and a method to document whether a photograph was taken of the gross lesion at the time of necropsy. Pathologists can use the PEIS IANR to trace a gross lesion through the interpretive stages and, finally, through to the point at which gross/microscopic correlations are required. All gross lesions are listed in numerical order. The pathologist can then use a plus sign to designate whether gross/microscopic correlations exist. If the lesion were such that it could not be embedded and a slide made, e.g., fluid in the thoracic cavity, the correct designation would be, "no section taken" (NST). If there were no corresponding microscopic lesion for the gross description, then the block on the IANR would be filled out with "no corresponding lesion" (NCL). The form includes signature blocks for the necropsy prosector, pathologist, trimmer and data clerk, if applicable. There are also blocks for notes and information on cause of death.

SYSTEM STANDARDIZATION

The PEIS uses a standardized nomenclature for gross and microscopic pathology which is referred to as the Pathology Code Table (PCT). The nomenclature was designed by members of the pathology staff at the National Center for Toxicological Research and the National Institute of Environmental Health Sciences in 1981. It has evolved over the last four years, and the fourth edition of the PCT was issued in November of 1985.

The PCT utilizes three types of terms. Topographies are the anatomic sites. The system is set up on a hierarchical scheme starting with the anatomic system, the organs within that system, and then the sites within those organs. The second type of term is the morphologic diagnosis. Qualifiers include items such as grade of severity of a lesion, specific types of degenerations, pigments, inflammations or types of cellular infiltrates. The PCT was designed to eliminate lump terms such as "toxic hepatitis" or "toxic nephrosis." These terms could have many interpretations depending upon the pathologist who read the slide. The NTP prefers the use of base terms (Figure 1). In this example, "toxic nephrosis" could be described as having the four component parts listed.

278

FIGURE 1
Histopathologic Diagnosis

Not preferred	• Toxic Nephrosis
Preferred	• Degeneration, focal, mild, renal tubule, kidney
	• Regeneration, focal, minimal, renal tubule, kidney
	• Karyomegaly, mild, renal tubule, kidney
	• Pigment, mild, kidney

DATA COLLECTION AND VALIDATION

The microslide is the raw data for the purpose of pathology computerization for the NTP. The data may be collected in one of three ways. The pathologist may elect to enter the data directly into a microprocessor. This is the preferred way for the NTP, and it allows the pathologist the capability of reviewing individual organ or individual animal data as they are entered directly. If the pathologist wishes, an individual animal histopathology record form can be used and a data clerk may enter the data into a microprocessor from the paper document. The pathologist may also dictate findings on tape and ask a data clerk to transcribe data directly into a microprocessor. The latter two methods require a second person to validate the data.

Once the data have been validated by a second data clerk or the original pathologist, histopathology work sheets or tapes can be discarded or erased. The microprocessor floppy disks are backed up daily and group data are transmitted to the main frame computer by telecommunication once a week. The pathologist or data clerk can obtain several different kinds of reports directly from the microprocessor for checking the accuracy of data. Once the data have been telecommunicated to the mainframe computer, a number of mainframe reports are available to the laboratory or the pathologist. Examples of mainframe reports are shown in Figure 2. One of the histopathology reports contains every piece of information the pathologist entered into the microprocessor for a given animal, inclusive of notes and "trace gross lesion" information. Individual and summary tables on neoplastic and nonneoplastic lesions are available, as are statistical analyses of primary tumor and survival data. A slide/block inventory is also available, which is useful when the laboratory transports material to the NTP Archives.

A schematic representation of NTP data flow is shown in Figure 3. Once the Original Pathologist (OP) completes the histopathologic interpretation and the

FIGURE 2
Examples of TDMS Reports Available from Mainframe Computer

- Individual animal histopathology
- Neoplastic diagnoses by anatomic site
- Non-neoplastic diagnoses by anatomic site
- Statistical analysis of primary tumors
- Statistical analysis of survival data
- Slide/block inventory

NTP PATHOLOGY DATAFLOW

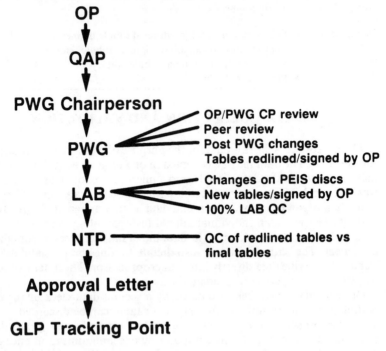

FIGURE 3. NTP Pathology Dataflow.

data have been checked by the laboratory quality assurance program, they are shipped to the NTP quality assessment pathology contract laboratory in Research Triangle Park, North Carolina. The pathology data undergo a rigorous review process. The QA report on the chemical study, along with the original pathology report, is shipped to the NTP, where members of the Chemical Pathology Branch (CPB) assign the study to a Pathology Working Group (PWG) chairperson.

The PWG chairperson reviews all aspects of the study, including toxicologic parameters, clinical medicine correlations and clinical pathology data. The chairperson reviews all diagnoses in which there is a discrepancy between the original pathologist's and the QA pathologist's diagnosis, as well as all neoplasms and target organs with chemically induced lesions. In addition, all microslides from a 10% random sample of each dose group are examined for missed diagnoses. A date for a pathology working group is set and Ad Hoc members identified to peer review the data. One day before the PWG is convened, the original pathologist on the study comes to the NTP and reviews slides with the PWG chairperson. The majority of discrepancies or differences of opinion are resolved on that day. The PWG reviews slides of chemically related lesions and any unresolved discrepancies during the peer review.

After the PWG, the individual changes are made on an individual histopathology table, initialed by the original pathologist and each individual page of the report signed by the original pathologist. A copy of this document is held at

NTP. The original is returned to the laboratory where data clerks make the individual changes on the PEIS floppy disk. New tables are then generated and 100% of the changes are quality assured by the laboratory. The reports are then signed by the original pathologist and forwarded to NTP for final review. NTP performs an additional 100% quality assessment, comparing the original tables with marked changes against the final tables. An additional 10% of the data are also checked to make sure that inadvertent changes were not made at the time of data entry. If at this point the data are approved by the NTP, the Chief of the Chemical Pathology Branch writes an approval letter and the GLP tracking points begin. If changes have to be made to the data after this point, a "reason for correction" form must be filled out and approved by the Chief, CPB, NTP or a designee.

CONDUCT OF THE PATHOLOGY AUDIT

Lucas H. Brennecke
Pathology Associates, Inc.
Ijamsville, Maryland

ABSTRACT

Pathology audits should evaluate one or all of the areas of raw data, tissue specimens, and final tables/reports. Raw data evaluation includes individual animal gross necropsy findings and microscopic diagnoses, and the preliminary pathology tables (if used) on which any changes are made. Tissue specimens include slides, paraffin blocks, and fixed wet tissue. Slides and wet tissue must be reviewed to resolve gross-microscopic correlation discrepancies found during the raw data evaluation. Wet tissues are examined for possible missed gross lesions and identification discrepancies. Slides and blocks must be examined for labeling and matching errors. A representative number of diagnoses should be compared with results presented in the report.

INTRODUCTION

The pathology audit is an important process in validating one of the final steps in biomedical research and has the express purpose of determining the adequacy of the necropsy and histopathological evaluations, identifying problems which could influence the interpretation of the study, and assuring that the raw data support those results found in the study report. Comprehensive or partial pathology audits may be undertaken at any step of the research process from necropsy of the animals to retrospective audits of final reports, depending upon the goals of the audit, expected shortcomings, and the immediacy of the information desired. Prior to beginning an audit, the auditor should familiarize himself with all requirements, guidelines, and conditions under which the study

1. Address correspondence to: Lucas H. Brennecke, D.V.M., Pathology Associates, Inc., 10075 Tyler Place, Hyatt Park II, Ijamsville, MD 21754.
2. Key words: audit, pathology, raw data, wet tissue.
3. Abbreviations: NTP, National Toxicology Program; PWG, Pathology Working Group; QA, Quality Assessment.

was conducted as well as with the findings of the study. If additional review programs were used, these reports should also be read. In the case of NTP studies, this includes the quality assessment (QA) report and the report of the Pathology Working Group (PWG). If such review programs are not used, then it may be desirable to incorporate a QA of slides looking specifically at target organs and neoplasms in all organs as well as an evaluation of tissue accountability.

PROCEDURES

Several particularly important checks are made to determine the validity, thoroughness, and completeness of the pathology. These audit checks can be broadly categorized as falling in the areas of raw data, tissue specimens, and final tables/reports.

Raw data include forms on which gross necropsy and microscopic findings are recorded as well as preliminary tables ("red-line tables") on which the pathologist may make corrections. The necropsy form is a particularly important document, in that it pinpoints those important areas (lesions) from which many of the microscopic diagnoses are made and ultimately reported in the final report. However, it is also the document on which the identification of the live animal appears. Data entry is, therefore, an important aspect of the audit. It is desirable to have a trained data technician check both the gross and microscopic entries for completeness and correctness to include changes (initialed and dated).

An important initial check by the pathologist is for gross versus microscopic correlation discrepancies. For each significant necropsy observation there must be a corresponding microscopic observation and/or diagnosis. The most common error is failure to address the lesion in any way. However, particular attention must be paid to insure that the microscopic diagnoses which are present actually correlate with the gross observations. In many cases, the auditor need not address every gross observation. Indeed, many of these do not fall in the category of "lesion" at all. Color changes are often in the eyes of the prosector, and it usually does not take long to see a pattern of "pet lesions" for a given prosector. Although all gross lesions are important, the pathology auditor may only want to concentrate on target organs and potential neoplastic lesions in all organs. While checking the gross and microscopic findings, the pathologist should also pay particular attention to the cause of death (disposition) of the animal. This is particularly important in gavage studies where tabulation of causes of death may be significant. While many deaths may have been recorded as natural deaths, gross and/or microscopic findings may indicate that the death was gavage-associated. During the review of raw data, all or a random sample of diagnoses should be compared to the tabulated data appearing in the final pathology tables and/or the final report.

In order to resolve discrepancies in gross versus microscopic correlation, appropriate slides should be reviewed. If there is not already a system of QA on slides and pathology reports and/or a peer review board, it may be desirable to do a random check on neoplasms and/or target organs. While reviewing the slides for lesions, the pathologist may simultaneously evaluate the tissues for proper histotechnique to include adequacy and accountability of tissues for histopathologic evaluation.

The final audit check to be made by the pathology auditor is on the wet tissue. Checking the wet tissues serves three important functions, identification of animals, evaluation of necropsy/trimming by checking for possible missed gross lesions, and resolution of gross/microscopic correlation discrepancies. When checking the wet tissue, attention must be paid to areas often overlooked by prosectors, such as stomach and urinary bladder mucosa, liver nodules and small skin lesions on the carcass. Necropsy and microscopic reports should be nearby to verify that lesions found were reported.

Animal identification verification is a simple, yet very important aspect of the wet tissue check. Nothing can invalidate or cast serious doubt on the validity of a study as easily as failure to properly identify the animals or properly label the wet tissue containers. The identification of the animal should be carefully compared to the necropsy form as well as the wet tissue container. If identification discrepancies are discovered, every attempt should be made to resolve them by looking at other wet tissues with which the identity may be confused.

While the pathologist is checking data and slides, a histotechnician can be making a slide/block evaluation. Discrepancies such as missing slides and/or blocks, mislabeled or unlabeled slides or blocks or slide/block mismatches should be noted, as should blocks which were not cut full-face, or which have been cut away. In addition, problems which may affect the long-term storage of slides and blocks, such as improper coverslipping or exposed drying tissue in blocks, can be pointed out.

SUMMARY

The pathology audit is a very important step in the technical evaluation of biomedical studies. Not only are the thoroughness and completeness of gross and microscopic evaluations determined, but the adequacy of documentation and the validity of the final report are closely scrutinized.

REFERENCE

NATIONAL TOXICOLOGY PROGRAM. (1984). SOP No. 1. Pathology Data Audit for Chronic Toxicologic Studies.

PANEL-AUDIENCE DIALOGUE
QUALITY OF PATHOLOGY

Chairperson:
Scot L. Eustis
Toxicology Research and Testing Program
National Institute of Environmental Health Sciences
Research Triangle Park, North Carolina

Panel:
Hugh E. Black, Gary A. Boorman, Lucas H. Brennecke,
Jerry F. Hardisty, Paul K. Hildebrandt, Charles A. Montgomery, Jr.

Dexter Goldman (EPA): Lucas Brennecke and Charles Montgomery have briefly alluded to raw data and audit trails and have discussed the NTP system. Not all of us have the luxury of pathology review and re-review. EPA, as a regulatory agency, has a different view of the definition of pathology raw data and audit trails. EPA considers that pathology raw data start with the original signed micropathology interpretation sheets or with the disk entry at the time it is made permanent on the disk by the pathologist before proceeding to the next case. Under this set of definitions, no change may be made in the pathologist's interpretation at any time without full compliance with GLPs. The pathologist may revisit the case as often as he/she wishes, but any change made in the diagnosis must be fully validated at all times.

Scot Eustis (NIEHS/NTP): The NTP system is really not much different from that described for EPA. The final pathology tables containing all of the individual animal histopathology data are signed off by the pathologist that these are the final diagnoses. Any changes made thereafter must be documented by a paper trail.

Goldman: We are in complete agreement with the sign-off by the pathologist. However, in EPA the data trail starts *before* the final pathology tables. EPA wants to know why the diagnosis was changed at all points along the system.

Andrew Tegeris (Tegeris Laboratories): Who actually enters the gross pathology comments in the necropsy room—the pathologist or the technician?

287

Hugh Black (Schering Co.): At Schering, the pathologist gives verbal directions to the individual operating the computer terminal. The pathologist can watch the overhead monitor to assure the correct entry is made into the computer. No technician is allowed to enter any pathology data into the system, even on weekends and holidays.

Tegeris: On weekends at our laboratory, we have a trained technician who is on call to do necropsies and enters his/her comments on a paper record. On Monday, the pathologist reviews the technician's comments and verifies them by reviewing the wet, fixed tissues. The pathologist may than accept or cancel the technician's record. The pathologist enters the gross necropsy findings into the computer (as verified from the wet tissues) and the Individual Animal Data Record sheet prepared by the technician is thrown away.

Black: In my opinion, you threw away the raw data. The only thing the pathologist can do in that situation is assure that what goes into the computer is, in his best estimate, a correct description of what the technician wrote down. The only time you really have raw data, as far as gross necropsy is concerned, is when you have the animal on the table before you, because that is where you have your information. If the technician misses lesions or incorrectly describes lesions, there is no way Monday morning you are going to be aware of that.

Tegeris: The pathologist looks at the fixed tissues on Monday and correlates that with what he sees in the fixed tissues and compares that with the technician's paper entry prior to entry into the computer. After that, the pathologist throws away the technician's record.

Black (Schering Co.): I would still say that the raw data are that original description of what was observed at the necropsy table by the technician.

Doug Bristol (NIEHS/NTP): Hugh Black indicated that prior to trimming, it would be helpful if quality assurance sat down with the trimmers. Please discuss where quality assurance can fit in with the entire pathology evaluation process.

Gary Boorman (NIEHS/NTP): It is very helpful to have a quality assurance person sit down with the histotechnologist at the time of trimming tissues and go through those tissues with the technician to assure that: a) all tissues are accounted for, b) the tissues are properly trimmed and, c) all lesions identified at necropsy are, in fact, in the container of tissues. At NTP, we have QA people who have worked in the histology laboratory, so they are competent in this type of review. This review gives the manager some assurance that the individuals who are prosecting are carefully collecting and placing all of these tissues in their proper place. During the large necropsy, there is a minimum amount of time to complete the process and people tend to become tired and may become somewhat careless. By participation of QA, there is assurance that the necropsy is carried out according to the protocol.

Bristol: Does this approach require the QA person to have expertise in pathology? If this is not possible, how can they achieve what you are describing?

Boorman: I think you can, because you have a technician who is used to doing this type of work sitting right beside you. You can simply ask them "here are the tissues and the tissue list, let us go through them and identify them and check them off."

Zachary Wong (Chevron): In your description of the Pathology Working Group, Gary (Boorman), individual tissues with equivocal lesions are looked at by the group and the individual members of the group write down their diagnosis prior to group decision. What is the disposition of these individual diagnoses and how is the group review of information handled in the final report? The review of materials by one or more pathologists is not uncommon. In our group, we have only one other pathologist, and the final decision is usually made by the study pathologist.

Boorman: This is a good question and we have given it some thought. We do not record the individual pathologist's diagnosis. Generally, we keep track of the votes and if it is unanimous there is nothing said about a specific set of lesions. If there is a split vote, this will sometimes be included in the Technical Report discussion. For example, "in the high dose animals, there was a series of lesions where there was difference of opinion as to whether it was a benign tumor, or malignant tumor or ...." We do not record the specific diagnosis per pathologist. It is used more as an advisory in our overall deliberation.

Eustis: If there is a consensus in disagreement with the study pathologist, he is asked to reconsider his diagnosis to reflect the PWG review. In most cases, he does so, and that becomes the final diagnosis. If the study pathologist disagrees on many cases where there is a clear consensus by the panel that he is incorrect, the original pathologist is still allowed to retain his diagnosis. However, NTP retains the right to print their own results in the Technical Report and make their interpretation based on the results of the PWG.

Boorman: We have on occasion published a Technical Report where we have two tables—the study pathologist's and the PWG's interpretation. When it reflects importantly on the overall conclusions, we would go with the PWG response which is what we make the call on, but we would still have the study pathologist's opinion in a separate table.

Chapter VII
INTERNATIONAL REGULATORY
ASPECTS OF QUALITY

DEDICATION – CHAPTER VII

The conference committee wishes to dedicate Chapter VII, "International Regulatory Aspects of Quality," to the memory of the late Dr. Desmond L. H. Robinson. Dr. Robinson's death in December 1985 was a great personal and professional loss to those who knew him and to those who will never have the pleasure. The members of the conference committee will always remember him as a true gentleman and fellow professional with a wry wit who was "hard but fair."

INTERNATIONAL REGULATORY ASPECTS OF QUALITY

Dexter S. Goldman
Laboratory Data Integrity Program, Office of Compliance Monitoring
U.S. Environmental Protection Agency
Washington, DC

CHAIRPERSON'S REMARKS

The Office of Pesticides and Toxic Substances (OPTS) of the U.S. Environmental Protection Agency (EPA) actively promotes the establishment of formal agreements between EPA's Good Laboratory Practice (GLP) authority, the Office of Compliance Monitoring (OCM), and GLP authorities in other member countries of the Organization for Economic Cooperation and Development (OECD). The purposes of such agreements are (1) to most efficiently utilize limited professional and financial resources, (2) to provide for acceptance of toxicity testing data by the regulatory authorities of one country when the testing was properly conducted and monitored in another country and (3) to the extent possible, to encourage equivalence in the training of inspectors and in the procedures followed in inspecting laboratories and auditing data.

The principal difficulties in achieving these goals include (1) the multiplicity of GLP authorities in some member countries, (2) the lack of final GLP compliance legislation in some member countries, (3) the reluctance of some member countries to have inspectors from another country join an inspection of a facility under their jurisdiction and (4) the sheer magnitude of the problem of testing volume being done on an international basis. It is not uncommon for required short-term toxicity testing to be done in one country and required long-term toxicity/oncogenicity testing to be done in a second or even a third country.

Another problem, real or not depending on many factors, is this: should we continue to define chemicals by legislation into pharmaceutical, agricultural and industrial? Should there be multiple authorities controlling categorized chemicals? In other words, to paraphrase Gertrude Stein, a chemical is a chemical is a chemical. This is, however, a political and not a scientific question and must be answered in political terms.

Sometimes language is a barrier, not to the testing, but to the understanding of the intent of the legislation. What is, for example, certification or accreditation of a laboratory? What is the value of repeated audits of an ongoing study versus a full audit of the final report against all of the original data?

Sometimes social and cultural backgrounds and standards have an effect on the appearance of procedures. What, for example, is the value of a stable professional testing staff in a laboratory in one country versus a mobile professional testing staff in another country? Does this have any relationship at all to the level of professionalism at either laboratory; is this a critical measure of professionalism? Usually the attitudes on this question depend on the country that asks the question, but is the question legitimate in the first place?

The EPA feels that the interests of all regulatory parties are best served by actively promoting those processes and procedures that will enhance the free interchange between participating countries of data properly generated, monitored and audited. To that end we have exchanged information on processes and procedures with the relevant GLP authorities in other countries. We have promoted the exchange of inspection teams between the EPA and interested OECD member countries and feel that the short-term future includes the establishment of bilateral or multilateral agreements on these matters. Of course, the Food and Drug Administration (FDA) has been working toward these goals for some time and the EPA has an active working relationship with the FDA which takes advantage of the FDA's experience in these matters.

In the discussion this morning by our distinguished guests from other OECD countries we will hear varied points of view and about varied degrees of progress in many areas of concern. I think it proper, however, to bear in mind that the variability reflects different approaches, not different goals. I have had the pleasure of discussions with several of our panelists and with my distinguished colleague from the FDA, Dr. Lepore, on these processes, procedures and goals and I am looking forward to rapid progress in these areas.

INTERNATIONAL MEMORANDA OF UNDERSTANDING ON GLPS

Paul D. Lepore
Office of Regulatory Affairs
Food and Drug Administration
Rockville, Maryland

ABSTRACT

The Food and Drug Administration (FDA) has the policy that the Good Laboratory Practice Regulations (GLPs) apply to all safety studies regardless of country or origin. Accordingly, FDA may refuse to accept, for regulatory purposes, any study conducted in a laboratory that refuses inspection or that is not operating in compliance with the GLPs. To facilitate policy implementation, FDA encourages bilateral GLP understandings with foreign governments. Phase I memoranda of understanding (MOUs) are executed to permit a period of time for each participating country to develop compatible GLP programs and harmonious working relationships. FDA has entered into Phase I MOUs with authorities in Canada, Sweden and Japan. Negotiations are in progress with the United Kingdom and Italy. Phase II MOUs afford reciprocal recognition to each country's GLP programs and permit the mutual acceptance for regulatory decision-making of safety studies conducted in the participating countries. FDA has entered into a Phase II MOU with Switzerland and is currently in negotiations with France and Japan.

INTRODUCTION

The publication of proposed rules for Good Laboratory Practice in 1976 represented a dramatic step for the FDA. For the first time in history the Agency was compelled to ensure the adequacy of product safety evaluation by developing specific procedures for toxicology data collection and documentation. It is not surprising that the proposal of these regulations sparked consider-

1. Address correspondence to: Paul D. Lepore, Ph.D., Office of Regulatory Affairs, Food and Drug Administration, 5600 Fishers Lane, Rockville, MD 20857.
2. Key words: data acceptability, foreign studies, Good Laboratory Practice, memoranda of understanding, monitoring program.
3. Abbreviations: EPA, Environmental Protection Agency; FDA, Food and Drug Administration; GLP, Good Laboratory Practice; MOU, Memorandum of Understanding; OECD, Organization for Economic Cooperation and Development.

able national and international activity. This paper will consider international activities in regard to the GLPs with emphasis on work done by the Organization for Economic Cooperation and Development (OECD). FDA's efforts in the international arena will also be discussed.

BACKGROUND

In 1979, the OECD established an expert group chaired by the United States to harmonize GLP requirements and laboratory monitoring programs among member countries. At the initial meeting of the expert group, two objectives were established. First and foremost, the group was to develop a set of principles of Good Laboratory Practice that constituted internationally agreed upon standards. Secondly, the group was to develop a plan for the implementation of the OECD GLPs which would promote the international acceptance of the resulting test data.

The first task was completed in 1980, and the draft GLP guidelines were accepted by the OECD Council with the recommendation that they be provisionally implemented in the OECD member countries. In order to implement these GLP guidelines, it was suggested that governments should first designate or establish a national authority to monitor compliance with the principles of GLP. Normally, the national authority would be a governmental body, but if a third party were designated, it was recommended that it be under the supervision of the government. The scope of the guideline was recommended to include the testing of all regulated chemicals such as industrial chemicals, pharmaceuticals, and pesticides. It was further advocated that OECD principles of GLP be incorporated into laws, regulations, codes of practice, or recommendations depending on the legal and/or administrative practices existing within a country. Compliance to GLPs was to be monitored by on-site laboratory inspections and data audits which would be patterned after the OECD guidelines for national inspections and study audits. The national authority should use properly trained inspectors to conduct inspections. These inspectors should be technically competent to assess the compliance status of the laboratories and scientifically familiar with the test procedures. The expert group urged that the product of the inspection be a written inspection report which would be the confidential property of the national authority. The report would be evaluated to determine the areas of noncompliance and the national authority would then take whatever follow-up actions were necessary to assure that adequate correction was taken by the laboratory.

FDA's ACTION

These recommendations were accepted by the OECD governing council in 1981 and they guide FDA's actions on the acceptability of international test data. These efforts are important since there is no question that foreign toxicology laboratories do submit a considerable amount of data to the Agency. Data derived from New Drug Applications sent to the National Center for Drugs and Biologics in 1981 showed that 48% of the studies submitted were foreign studies. These data also showed that foreign laboratories conducted 54% of the studies submitted. Both categories were substantially increased since 1976, when similar figures were gathered.

In view of this extensive international activity, it is not surprising that FDA has adopted the policy that the GLPs apply to all safety studies regardless of country of origin. FDA will not accept, for regulatory purposes, any study that has been conducted in a laboratory that has refused inspection by the Agency. The basis of this policy is the belief that a single standard should apply to all work submitted to the Agency. FDA instituted a foreign laboratory inspection program in 1977 in order to implement this policy. FDA carries an inventory of some 150 foreign toxicology laboratories, over 70 of which have been inspected. The criteria for inspection include the need to audit the data of a critical study as well as inspection of those laboratories that frequently submit data to the FDA. To date, laboratories have been inspected in West Germany, France, Belgium, Italy, Japan, the United Kingdom, Canada, Sweden, Switzerland, Australia and the Netherlands. Results of these inspections have been quite favorable, as it is apparent that foreign laboratories have been assiduous in adoption and implementation of GLP regulations.

MEMORANDA OF UNDERSTANDING

Throughout the past eight years, FDA has also been engaged in bilateral agreements with parallel agencies in foreign governments. The purpose of these agreements is to afford mutual recognition to each country's GLP program and to permit the mutual acceptance for regulatory decision-making of safety studies conducted in either participating country. FDA embarked on a two-tiered program whereby a Phase I agreement provides for a period of time during which each country can develop compatible GLP regulations. Phase II of this program affords reciprocal recognition to both countries' programs and provides for the mutual acceptance of safety studies conducted in the participating countries.

Phase I programs should include the development of acceptable principles of Good Laboratory Practice as well as effective inspection programs and compliance strategies. During this time, joint inspections by both national authorities are conducted and assistance is provided to reduce any program difficulties. Administrative program information such as inspection reports or inventories is traded between countries.

Near the end of a Phase I agreement period, each country conducts a formal assessment of the respective toxicology laboratory monitoring programs using the implementation criteria developed by the OECD. If the assessment results in a determination of the equivalency of the respective programs, negotiations are initiated on the Phase II agreement. Reciprocal recognition would be given to the programs of each country, providing for the mutual acceptance of data from studies conducted in both countries.

Phase I agreements have been executed with Canada, Japan and Sweden and negotiations are presently underway with the United Kingdom and Italy. Discussions with the United Kingdom have included the Environmental Protection Agency (EPA) for the first time and an attempt will be made to include the concerns of both EPA and FDA in one agreement. A Phase II agreement is in place with Switzerland while negotiations continue with Japan and France. Other Phase I and Phase II agreements may occur in the future.

GOOD LABORATORY PRACTICE REGULATIONS AND THEIR IMPACT ON STUDIES CONDUCTED IN FRANCE

Remi Glomot
Centre International de Toxicologie
Miserey, France

ABSTRACT

Since December 22, 1978, the publication date of the final set of rules by the Food and Drug Administration (FDA), French authorities began to become involved in the application of Good Laboratory Practices (GLPs). Nevertheless, no official statement was made on the subject until May 31, 1983, when the French Ministry of Health published a legal text on GLP for pharmaceuticals and set up a national inspection system. Other approaches were taken in the chemical and agrochemical fields, but none has yet drawn an official response. The past and present status of GLP in France is described.

INTRODUCTION

Since 1976, with the FDA's publication of proposed guidelines on GLP, and later, in 1978, with the final version of such guidelines, the French authorities and private companies of my country have become involved in GLP. Although they had the impression that these regulations were essentially the consequences of local problems and that during many decades, studies were conducted throughout the world in a proper way without any official GLP rules, the French private firms considered it necessary to cooperate in setting up national guidelines. However, the authorities did not undertake any official action at that time.

May I remind you that the FDA started its first set of inspections in foreign countries, including a few French laboratories, in late 1979 and early 1980. May I also remind you that during a meeting in Sweden in 1978, the representatives of the Organization for Economic Cooperation and Development (OECD)

1. Address correspondence to: Dr. Remi Glomot, Centre International de Toxicologie, Miserey Cedex, France.

2. Key words: inspection system, pharmaceuticals, regulation.

3. Abbreviations: AMM, Autorisation de Mise sur le Marche; EEC, European Economic Community; FDA, U.S. Food and Drug Administration; GLP, Good Laboratory Practice; ILAC, International Laboratory Accreditation Conference; OECD, Organization for Economic Cooperation and Development; RNE, Reseau National d'Essais.

member countries stated that one of the priorities of this international organization was defining GLP principles. Several experts acted for France in the Expert Committee and took part for more than two years in various meetings in the U.S. and in some European countries.

In order to be in compliance with the scope of the OECD, it was necessary for member countries to have a GLP inspectorate. The French authorities made some proposals in that field in 1980. The different ministries concerned, including Industry, Health, Agriculture, Environment, Education and Labor, as well as public and private organizations, met together to harmonize their approach to the problem. During the meeting the French Ministry of Health proposed a single inspection team under its own responsibility, as they already had an inspectorate working on both GLP inspections and inspections of retail pharmacies.

But until the government changed in 1981, no other action was undertaken to incorporate the OECD principles of GLP into national guidelines. At the end of 1981 the Syndicat de l'Industrie Pharmaceutique, the pharmaceutical organization that is the equivalent of the PMA in the U.S., pointed out the urgent need to establish GLP guidelines. A combined government/industry and academic task force prepared a draft document which defined GLP for the toxicological testing of pharmaceuticals. The task force worked mainly on two documents, the FDA and OECD guidelines.

THE INSTRUCTION OF 1983

After a final agreement by the Ministry of Health, an Instruction to inspectors was published as an official statement on May 31, 1983. This Instruction is not legally binding on pharmaceutical firms, and concerns only the inspectors who visit the laboratories. This was done to preserve a quick modification of the procedure if required. In the case of noncompliance, any study carried out in a laboratory would not be considered in support of the Autorisation de Mise sur le Marche (AMM), equivalent to an NDA or product license, until all corrective actions have been taken and the facility again complies with GLP standards. This information about the GLP status of a country can be brought to the attention of authorities in other countries.

Inspectors belong to the Direction de la Pharmacie et du Médicament, which is a division of the Ministère des Affaires Sociales et de la Solidarité Nationale—Secretariat d'Etat charge de la Sante. They are all graduates in pharmacy and their responsibility is to inspect private, cooperative and hospital pharmacies as well as manufacturing units for GLP compliance. For the most part, they are regionally based. Some of them, five at the present time, completed supplementary training on GLP at the National School of Health. Two of these have spent two weeks in the U.S., mainly at the NCTR, and have participated as observers of an FDA inspection of a U.S. laboratory. They also took a course at a summer school organized by a non-profit organization, the Fondation de l'Industrie Pharmaceutique pour la Recherche, in which representatives of the NCTR, FDA and officials from other countries participated.

Furthermore, it was felt that a compliance manual was required. The working party met again to draw up a draft for the inspectorate to comment on the manner in which the inspections must be carried out. This document was mainly derived from the FDA manual, and the final version was published on September 3, 1984, after agreement by the Ministry of Health, as an Instruction to the inspectors.

So far as I know, six inspections have already been conducted in France, two of them in conjunction with FDA inspectors, and two with Japanese inspectors belonging to the Ministry of Health and Welfare. Reciprocal agreements on the mutual recognition of the validity of inspections are under discussion with FDA, Japan and Canada, but I have no precise knowledge on the stage of the agreement reached to date.

Quite recently this year, the pharmaceutical companies operating in France and requiring an inspection have been asked to notify the Ministry of Health. During a first phase, the inspections will be done on a voluntary basis. Gradually they will be transformed into a more international comprehensive system, similar to that operating in the U.S., with inspections conducted both on a periodic basis and in response to specific product issues. Furthermore, the dossier presented by any laboratory to support the registration of a drug must include a statement in compliance with French GLP and signed by the Study Director and Quality Assurance Unit (QAU) management. If the dossier is prepared by a French expert, he has to sign it, taking the responsibility that all the work has been done according to GLPs. In order to meet the actual demand for inspection, 12 inspectors have been trained in France this year; probably 5 or 6 of them will be selected as GLP inspectors.

Apart from the pharmaceutical field, France is also considering the application of GLP principles to other fields, such as chemicals, agrochemicals and veterinary drugs. In our country, chemicals are subject to a law published on July 12, 1977. In order to be in compliance with this law, every new chemical, prior to being launched on the market, must be tested for adverse effects on man and his environment.

After the publication of the OECD guidelines, the chemical companies gradually followed the guidelines of this international organization regarding methodologies and GLP. This was done on a voluntary basis in order to fulfill one of the basic conditions for export production.

THE RESEAU NATIONAL d'ESSAIS

Until now, no official action has been undertaken to control the chemicals for GLP purposes according to a system comparable with that of pharmaceuticals. However, a system for accrediting the testing laboratories, called the Reseau National d'Essais (RNE), was set up in 1978. This non-profit organization is governed by the law of 1901, which organizes the test function in France, in order to establish a multidisciplinary coordinated group of testing laboratories at a national level and on a federative basis. When the RNE was founded, the authorities expressed the wish that "a better coordination of testing activities be undertaken at the national level, and that every effort be made to make the quality of testing services carried out in France known and appreciated abroad."

The RNE was set up both in the context of international talks and the mutual recognition of test results held in conjunction with the first meeting of the International Laboratory Accreditation Conference (ILAC) in Copenhagen, in the light of GATT action to draw up a standards code and within the framework of the United Nations Economic Commission for Europe with respect to laboratory accreditation.

All of the economic partners concerned with the test function were consulted, including the Technical Ministerial Department, professional organizations, public and private laboratories. A Board of Directors was nominated with the participation of public and private laboratories and professional organizations. The French government has a representative in the organization with the right of veto.

The RNE is characterized by:
- the purely voluntary mode of participation of each member, since the Reseau possesses no regulatory action;
- its accessibility, since all laboratories may resort to it on the unique condition of proving their competence;
- its representation of all technical fields.

One of the RNE's committees is devoted to controlling chemical laboratory testing facilities, including toxicological laboratories. After an inspection phase, some of these laboratories have already been accredited.

In another area, I would like to remind you that France is a member state of the European Economic Community (EEC), and, as such, must apply the directives voted by the Commission Council. Accordingly, France is affected by the proposal published in the EEC official paper of August 29, 1985 under the reference 85/C 219/05. In the first proposed article, it is mentioned that to perform the test mentioned by the EEC directive 67/548, "the member states must take the appropriate measures in order that the laboratories apply the GLP principles specified in the annex No. 2 of the OECD Council decision concerning the mutual acceptance of data for the evaluation of chemical products."

In the field of agrochemicals and veterinary drugs, some actions have recently been undertaken in France. Most importantly, under the leadership of the Ministry of Agriculture and more precisely of the Quality Directorate, a meeting will be organized with all of the public and private bodies concerned. A task force will probably be set up to propose a text of GLP guidelines and establish an inspection system which could have a connection with the pharmacy inspectors. To date, the majority of agrochemical companies doing research in France voluntarily follow the OECD and EPA guidelines, both in their methodologies and adherence to GLP. This voluntary compliance is not surprising when we consider that the four main research firms in that field are also pharmaceutical companies. This is also true of the veterinary drug companies, although to a lesser extent.

302

CONCLUSION

Finally, what is the impact of such regulations or guidelines on studies conducted in France? Generally speaking, study quality has been improved during the last few years. This is no doubt the opinion commonly expressed by members of the national committee for AMM. As in other countries, the most difficult thing was probably the establishment of a GLP spirit. To accomplish that, many meetings were organized to explain to laboratory personnel what the GLPs were and how to handle them. The second step was to convince people that they should follow GLP not only to achieve compliance but also to perform better scientific work.

Today, the great majority of French pharmaceutical companies work under GLP conditions for pharmaceutical testing. Nearly all of them have a QAU. Their GLP managers meet together regularly, and more than twenty attend national meetings. They also have an annual meeting with their colleagues from other European countries to exchange their experiences on this subject.

The same level of quality has also been noted in the main agrochemical and veterinary drug companies, although as I mentioned previously, the voluntary application of GLP must be controlled by inspections. We are all hoping that this will be done in the near future.

Reciprocal agreements on the mutual recognition of inspection for pharmaceuticals are now underway with the FDA, Japan and Canada. We hope that these agreements will reach the final or the operating levels soon.

GOOD LABORATORY PRACTICE AND ITS IMPACT ON STUDIES CONDUCTED IN GERMANY

Hartmut Uehleke
Federal German Health Office
Bundesgesundheitsamt
Berlin, Federal Republic of Germany

ABSTRACT

Pitfalls and public argumentation about sometimes doubtful and unclear circumstances in the conduct and documentation of safety studies in toxicology culminated some ten years ago. Nonuniform acceptance of toxicological studies in and between different countries produced additional arguments. Consequently, the draft "Nonclinical Laboratory Studies, Good Laboratory Practice Regulations" of the FDA (Fed. Reg. *41*, Nov. 19, 1976) revived the "1967 Guideline of Dangerous Substances" of the European Economic Community. In 1978, the cabinet of the Federal Republic of Germany (FRG) decided to incorporate aspects of GLP into the draft of a new and unified law on dangerous substances (later Chemikaliengesetz). However, the term "Quality Assurance" was much less used and considered in the FRG and in Europe. The ECETOC (European Chemical Industry Ecology and Toxicology Center) document of March 15, 1979 expressed the opinion that specialized QA groups must not be installed in addition to the responsible investigators. Various groups had to be convinced that GLP is not the official "cookbook" for perfect toxicology. Some legal authorization for supervision and inspection of the conduct of animal experiments did exist in the FRG.

Other activities started at the OECD in Paris, more pronouncements about international cooperation, leveling of trade obstacles, improving international exchange and acceptance of scientific documents, less duplication of animal experiments, and similar aspects. What has been accomplished? GLP and QA

1. Address correspondence to: Dr. Hartmut Uehleke, Bundesgesundheitsamt, Department of Toxicology, Thielallee 88, D-1000 Berlin 33, Federal Republic of Germany.

2. Key words: Good Laboratory Practice, mutual acceptance of data, regulatory agencies.

3. Abbreviations: ECETOC, European Chemical Industry Ecology and Toxicology Center; EEC, European Economic Community; EPA, Environmental Protection Agency; FDA, Food and Drug Administration; FRG, Federal Republic of Germany; GLP, Good Laboratory Practice; NIH, National Institutes of Health; OECD, Organization for Economic Cooperation and Development.

may not directly interfere with pitfalls and opportunities in toxicology, or more generally, in experimental medicine. However, better planning and conduct, standard (minimal) operation procedures and other factors have also improved documentation, acceptance of protocols, interdisciplinary and international cooperation. With the GLP guidelines, the majority of protocols appeared clearer, in a better layout, with more comprehensible condensation and evaluation. Retention of materials and specimens gave a fair chance to answer the critical doubts and questions of scientific organizations, and of various agencies.

INTRODUCTION

There were many starting points for Good Laboratory Practice (GLP) and quality assurance activities in Germany. Dubious experimental toxicology studies and pitfalls in their conduct caused controversy and public concern. Many instances of ambiguous results, doubtful statistical significance and varying evaluations of animal carcinogenicity studies all contributed to the need for stricter planning and conduct of animal experiments.

For practical reasons, the major pharmaceutical houses and chemical companies in Germany (and in central Europe), either approached or adopted the current rules, protocols and standards of conduct observed by the United States Food and Drug Administration (FDA). However, questions of governmental surveillance and control of study conduct were not identical in Europe and the United States. In Europe, individuals connected with universities and learned societies in the fields of pharmacology, toxicology, pathology, medicinal biochemistry and biostatistics raised strong objections to test plans and protocols that were too rigid and imposed by official rules and laws.

Nevertheless, since 1975, scientific organizations and government agencies have been cognizant of the importance of study requirements such as the quality of laboratory animals, diet and environment in developing reliable and reproducible toxicology data. Tight official rules and standardized protocols have also been beneficial to industrial corporations, and it is generally less expensive and faster to fulfill strict ("cookbook") working procedures in toxicology and pathology. It should be stressed that the procedures used by competent people to ensure the quality and reliability of studies were not greatly altered by mere prescriptions (WHO, 1978; Paget and Thomson, 1979).

In many private and industrial laboratories and in certain agencies, the mere routines and skills necessary to organize and condense raw data from sometimes thousands of pages and data entries in various disciplines have greatly improved. By its nature, science must place more emphasis on insight and understanding of modes of action in toxicologic safety investigations. Indeed, it is more conducive to proper health protection to know the mechanism(s) of action of any chemical instead of evaluating samples of "perfect" protocols.

Contract laboratories and companies must pay high prices for errors, bad planning, human negligence, defective organization and poor understanding of the scientific disciplines. All of these factors have contributed to a common approach among the various interests.

306

In the European Economic Community (EEC) and in the Federal Republic of Germany (FRG), the proposed draft of FDA's "Nonclinical Laboratory Studies: Good Laboratory Practice Regulations" revived the EEC Commission document, "1967 Guideline on Dangerous Substances" (FDA, 1978a). After the official GLP rules appeared in the United States in 1978, the cabinet of the German government decided to incorporate aspects of GLP into a draft of a new and unified "Law on Dangerous Substances" (later "Chemikaliengesetz"— Chemical Act) (FDA, 1978b). Additional activities began at the Organization for Economic Cooperation and Development (OECD) in Paris, which advocated international cooperation, leveling of trade obstacles, international exchange and mutual acceptance of scientific materials with more uniform protocols (OECD, 1979). The EEC Commission and the U.S. Environmental Protection Agency (EPA) also reached some provisional conclusions regarding GLP (U.S. EPA, 1979; EEC Commission and U.S. EPA, 1980; Paget, 1979).

The term "quality assurance" was used less frequently in the FRG and in parts of Europe. The document issued in March 1979 by the European Chemical Industry Ecology and Toxicology Center (ECETOC) at Brussels expressed the opinion that specialized quality assurance groups must not be installed in addition to the responsible investigators (ECETOC, 1979). At that stage, various groups in foreign ministries, agencies and the press had to be educated and convinced that GLP was not an official "cookbook" for faultless toxicology. This point bears repeating: GLP is no substitute for education, qualifications, experience, peer review and state of the art techniques in toxicology and related specialties. The rules, guidelines and explanation for GLP were laid down in the 1982 document of the OECD (OECD, 1981; 1982) and are valid for the FRG.

PREVIOUS REGULATORY MEASURES IN GERMANY

The background for any possible control of animal experimentation and the production of biologic data in the U.S. and the FRG were neither identical nor comparable. The existing Animal Welfare Law (Tierschutzgesetz) and the activities of the German Society for the Study of Experimental Animals had achieved many agreements and rules, including some for supervision. The National Institute of Health (NIH) "Guidelines for the Care and Use of Laboratory Animals" are a counterpart to these agreements (Moreland, 1978).

Therefore, any legal rights for inspection and control of animal facilities were never such a necessary issue for GLP development in Central Europe. In the FRG, any establishment for animal breeding and/or experimentation must receive permission from the local government district (Regierungsbezirk) staffed with competent veterinarians and a Chief Medical Officer. Additional permission is also necessary from Factory Inspection (Gewerbeaufsicht). The final authority is the Department of the Interior of the corresponding Federal Country (11, with Berlin). This obvious distribution of central power is also valid for supervision and execution of legal aspects in the areas of food and drugs. Of course, legislative power remains with the Federal Ministries, the Bundestag and the Bundesrat.

Those local authorities have the right to supervise, inspect and control. Every animal used for any experiment which may involve pain must appear on appropriate protocols. Bulk reports are sufficient for nutritional investigations, animals sacrificed for isolated organs or for the preparation of isolated cells, cell cultures and subcellular particles. Approval for the conduct of animal experimentation is given only for a specified institution (e.g., an industrial laboratory) in connection with competent and certified individuals. With this background in mind, it may be easier for an American to understand that the idea of any foreign inspector's being empowered to control animal facilities and protocols could produce objections and even horror among chemical companies.

The trilateral agreement among the United States, Canada and the United Kingdom for mutual exchange, inspections and audits for drug applications compelled the OECD member states to more open positions. Some progress and official agreements between the U.S. and the FRG have been achieved with respect to GLP and therapeutic agents. FDA's intimidation of European Drug Companies to approve only data from laboratories accepting U.S. inspection and audits finally opened the doors of the big multinational German chemical companies. It is hard to describe the feeling of top people in industrial science and management within large, reputable enterprises when the non-academic U.S. inspector appears with bundles of lists to fulfill his national duty. The same is true when the decision is made to perform at least some research at a United States subsidiary (in the "glasshouse").

The official notice in the *Bundesanzeiger* on German Drug Law specified the competent authorities, agencies and individual experts responsible for executing the law (Bundesanzeiger, 1982). Subsequent administrative regulations of August 25, 1983 concerning the implementation of the Drug Law determined the purpose, authorization, inspection, sampling, conduct of clinical trials, supervision and legal cooperation of authorities with respect to GLP. These administrative regulations became effective on January 1, 1984 and empowered the cited authorities to perform inspections and study audits in accordance with the OECD guidelines for national GLP inspections.

In 1985, negotiations concerning GLP inspections and audits for the mutual acceptance of data on chemicals were in progress, and the OECD is presently attempting to remove the remaining obstacles so that an agreement can be reached. Open questions of legal competency, legal jurisdiction and other judicial aspects still exist with respect to local supervision by any foreign inspector. The OECD and EEC adopted a "Decision on the Mutual Acceptance of Data" which states that "data generated in the testing of chemicals in an OECD member country in accordance with OECD test guidelines and OECD principles of GLP shall be accepted in other member countries for purposes of assessment or other uses relating to the protection of man and the environment" (OECD, 1981; 1982). The right of any recipient country to be an observer (not the inspector) at a corresponding national audit has been laid down in these documents. At the present time, however, these agreements are limited to chemicals.

Another point should be mentioned. The classic German laws on weights and measures (Eichgesetz) offered some additional legal means to supervise laboratories. The classification and use of very pure chemicals (*pro analysi*) was born in Central Europe and has contributed to reliable results. In such fields as medicine, chemistry, pharmacy, physics, biology and biostatistics, the tradition of semi-academic careers and professions with apprenticeships involving technicians and laboratory assistants guarantee that personnel meet certain standards. The proper handling of animals by certified and educated "Biologie-laboranten" (biology assistants) was beneficial and rewarding.

CONCLUSION

What has been resolved and what remains open in relation to GLP and quality assurance? The struggle and public pressure to reach perfection and to quantitate nearly any possible risk during life have urged many people to demand more and more animal experimentation. In cases of doubtful statistical significance involving alteration of biologic parameters by a chemical, the public and the agencies are inclined to ask for large numbers of animals. Bigger dosage groups and additional doses may be required. This is not a primary aspect of GLP. Nevertheless, we may forget the truth that statistics are frequently comparable to a lantern in a dark harbor serving more to halt a drunken seaman than to enlighten the public.

Without a doubt, GLP has increased the costs for toxicology studies through sophisticated animal facilities, more hygienic supervision, defined inbred animal strains, strict diet and fodder control, animal handling by trained, certified persons, and large organizations and supervisory groups. As a consequence, there is a trend in Central Europe for expensive animal research establishments to move to other countries with lower manpower costs. However, this trend reveals little experience in managing long-term animal studies. Scientists, for well known reasons, have always objected to strict rules for the conduct of toxicologic investigations. "Do it according to the best available knowledge and to the presently accepted scientific standards." That was the good answer of a reputed British Scientific Committee to a letter inquiring exactly the "required special investigations expected for this compound ...." "Less formalism, more brain" was the very sound opinion of our British colleagues 10 years ago.

GLP and quality assurance should not interfere and should not be misused for trade regulations or as a trade weapon. Otherwise, they develop into a boomerang for international cooperation of the scientific disciplines. Today, the heart of the scientific toxicologist is really warmed when he or she reads a fine and translucent protocol. This is a positive outcome of all of the GLP and quality assurance activities. One can hope that in the future a proper balance may exist between public and political "necessities" and the development of a free scientific community delivering new methods and new insights. Remember that in the past 30 years it is mainly the unexpected and the unknown that have produced the more significant events in the field of toxicology.

REFERENCES

BUNDESANZEIGER. (1982). Bekanntmachung der fur den Vollzug des Arzneimittel-gesetzes zustandigen Behorden, Stellen und Sachverstandigen. 34th Year, No. 234a, Dez. 16, Bonn.

ECETOC. (1979). European Chemical Industry Ecology Centre, Monograph No. 1, Brussels.

EEC COMMISSION and U.S. EPA. (1980). Quality Assurance of Toxicological Data. Proc. of the Colloquium Luxembourg, Dec. 11–13, Luxembourg.

MORELAND, A. F. (1978). Guide for the Care and Use of Laboratory Animals. DHEW Publ. No. (NIH) 78–23. U.S. Dept. of Health and Human Services, NIH, Bethesda, MD.

OECD. (1979). Principles of Good Laboratory Practice (GLP). OECD Document 79.17, Paris.

OECD. (1981). OECD Guidelines for Testing of Chemicals, and Continuing Series. Paris.

OECD. (1982). Good Laboratory Practice in the Testing of Chemicals, Paris.

PAGET, G. E., ed. (1979). Good Laboratory Practice, MTP Press, Lancaster.

PAGET, G. E. and THOMSON, R. (1979). Standard Operating Procedures in Toxicology, MTP Press, Lancaster.

U.S. EPA. (1979). Good Laboratory Practice Standards for Health Effects. U.S. Fed. Reg. **44**(91):27334–27376.

U.S. FDA. (1978a). Non-Clinical Laboratory Studies, Good Laboratory Practice Regulations. U.S. Fed. Reg. **41**(225):51206–51226, Proposed Regs.

U.S. FDA. (1978b). Non-Clinical Laboratory Studies, Good Laboratory Practice Regulations. U.S. Fed. Reg. **43**(247):59986–60020, Final Rule.

WHO. (1978). Principles and Methods for Evaluating Toxicity of Chemicals, Part I. Environm. Health Criteria 6, WHO, Geneva.

GLP REGULATORY ASPECTS OF THE MINISTRY OF AGRICULTURE, FORESTRY AND FISHERIES IN JAPAN

Kazuo Okutomi
Agricultural Chemicals Inspection Station
Ministry of Agriculture, Forestry and Fisheries
Kodaira, Tokyo, Japan

ABSTRACT

There are four different Good Laboratory Practice (GLP) systems for the respective regulatory authorities in Japan. The GLP system for agricultural chemicals will be described here. New GLP guidelines were implemented on October 1, 1984 after four-and-a-half years' consideration by the Ministry of Agriculture, Forestry and Fisheries (MAFF). MAFF GLPs are compatible with other GLPs such as those of the U.S. Environmental Protection Agency (EPA) and the Organization for Economic Cooperation and Development (OECD). Actual GLP operation is carried out by Agricultural Chemicals Inspection Station (ACIS) inspectors. They have already filed more than 30 petitions for confirmation. This petition system, unique to MAFF in Japan, facilitates the GLP inspection, as MAFF can inspect the testing facilities for agricultural chemicals on a timely basis. MAFF is now trying to make some bilateral arrangements for GLP to facilitate the mutual acceptance of data.

INTRODUCTION

In Japan there are now four GLP systems in operation that have been established by four different ministries. The first three have been established according to the distinction of regulatory authorities for industrial sectors, and include the Ministry of Health and Social Welfare for pharmaceuticals, the MAFF for agricultural chemicals, and the Ministry of International Trade and Industry for industrial chemicals. The fourth GLP system has been established by the Ministry of Labor for workers' safety. In this paper, the GLP system for agricultural chemicals will be described.

1. Address correspondence to: Kazuo Okutomi, Agricultural Chemicals Inspection Station, Ministry of Agriculture, Forestry and Fisheries, 2-772, Suzuki-cho, Kodaira, Tokyo, Japan.
2. Key words: bilateral arrangements, GLP systems, regulatory authorities.
3. Abbreviations: ACIS, Agricultural Chemicals Inspection Station; EPA, U.S. Environmental Protection Agency; GLP, Good Laboratory Practice; MAFF, Ministry of Agriculture, Forestry and Fisheries; OECD, Organization for Economic Cooperation and Development.

ESTABLISHMENT OF THE GLP SYSTEM

In the agricultural chemical field, GLP guidelines were published on August 10, 1984 by the Director General of Agricultural Production, Bureau of MAFF. These regulations became effective on October 1, 1984. Until the publication of GLPs for Agricultural Chemicals, MAFF carefully studied the concept and every detail of GLPs and planned the schedule for introduction. The study was begun in 1980 and included a survey of the management and practice of toxicological testing facilities in Japan.

OPERATION OF GLPs

Although MAFF GLPs are substantially the same as and compatible with other GLPs, we have some specific features for operating the system effectively. One main feature is a "self-claiming system." Before the actual test data submission is made to the regulatory agency, the test facility must submit a petition to the ACIS of MAFF for confirmation as a suitable test facility. This facilitates the regulatory agency's planning of the inspection schedule and conduct of a proper inspection. We now have about 30 petitions in our file and, according to our schedule, these laboratories have been inspected or will be inspected in the near future, at least once every three years. We have a data audit system, so in cases where a test facility has passed the facility inspection, data audits will be done if necessary.

These inspections are conducted by MAFF GLP inspectors mainly from ACIS, within which an organization for dealing with GLP inspections was established in 1983. If data are found to be unsatisfactory by these inspections, they cannot be used for the application of agricultural chemical registration and the test facility that carried out the study for compiling the data is not recognized as a testing facility in compliance with GLP. In such a case, the test facility must submit a petition for confirmation after the necessary improvement. The facility will then be inspected and must prove its conformity to conduct toxicological testing for application of agricultural chemical registration.

I would briefly like to introduce the practice of inspection for confirmation of quality and integrity of toxicological data.

1. Manner of Inspection
   A. The inspection shall be conducted with sufficient care not to cast excessive burdens on the person seeking confirmation.
   B. For the inspection, care shall be taken not to interfere in the private affairs of the Applicant or his employees.
   C. The inspection shall be conducted during the normal business hours of the Applicant except in unavoidable cases.
   D. The inspection shall be conducted in the presence of the Applicant or his representatives.
   E. The inspections shall always maintain dignity as a person who conducts fair and strict inspection and strive to gain complete confidence in the inspection.

2. Execution of Inspection

The review shall consist of inspection by documents and an inspector's visit to the testing facility. Both types of inspections shall be conducted as follows.

A. Inspection by Documents. The inspection by documents shall be conducted on the matters pertaining to overall operation and control of the testing facility, the condition and maintenance of testing equipment, testing capability of the test facility, and other items that can be inspected by documents.

B. The inspection by site visit shall be conducted on the following items: confirmation of arrangement of the protocol, standard operating procedure and final report; confirmation of custody of raw data, specimens, etc.; confirmation of the facilities and working conditions; confirmation of activities of the quality assurance unit; examination and verification of the raw data, specimens and final report of the toxicological studies prepared by the testing facility.

Other necessary items. In addition, the testing facility shall submit test substances, specimens, raw data, personnel records of researchers and other documents and materials when considered necessary for further inspection.

3. Preparation of Reports

On completion of the inspection, the Inspector shall draft a report and submit the draft to the Chief Inspector. The Chief Inspector shall call a meeting to check the test facility for conformity to the GLP. The Chief Inspector shall prepare a report based on the results of the study in the meeting and submit it to the Director General of the Agricultural Production Bureau. The Chief Inspector may have the Applicant give full explanation when such explanation is considered necessary. The Director General will notify those who have submitted a petition for confirmation of the result of the inspection.

INTERNATIONAL ASPECTS

As I mentioned previously, MAFF GLPs were finalized considering not only the harmonization with other GLPs in Japan, such as those of the Ministry of Health and Social Welfare for pharmaceuticals, but also with other GLPs such as those of EPA and OECD. Because of the international nature of agricultural chemicals, which are commonly used on a worldwide basis, toxicological data are usually submitted to a foreign authority in addition to that of the country of origin. In this context, international harmonization of GLPs is necessary for the smooth development of agricultural chemicals indispensable for agricultural production.

Toxicological data are now frequently used for obtaining registrations in countries other than the country of origin. Although regulatory authorities must check the credibility of data, there was no internationally accepted rule before the idea of GLP was introduced. In Japan, we formerly adopted the rule that, in principle, toxicological testing data must be generated by the authoritative test facilities in Japan for assuring data credibility. In this new stage for GLPs, in order to facilitate the mutual acceptance of toxicological testing data, each country which has adopted GLPs must develop and practice a proper operational schedule.

If the GLP system is operated successfully in many countries, data exchange will be far easier than before. We are now trying to make bilateral arrangements for GLPs in order to facilitate the mutual acceptance of toxicological testing data. For the time being, we believe that bilateral arrangements are the most successful way for achieving mutual acceptance. We believe that achievement of international harmonization in this area is genuinely important, and we will do our best to achieve this goal.

GOOD LABORATORY PRACTICE AND ITS IMPACT ON STUDIES CONDUCTED IN THE UNITED KINGDOM

D. L. H. Robinson
UK GLP Monitoring Unit
Department of Health and Social Security
London, England

ABSTRACT

Monitoring of facilities for compliance with the Organization for Economic Cooperation and Development principles of Good Laboratory Practice began in 1982. Initially, monitoring was concerned only with laboratories generating toxicological data for industrial chemicals. More recently, monitoring has been extended to pharmaceuticals, agrochemicals and cosmetics. Responsibility for all monitoring now rests with one regulatory authority.

The changes and progress which have been made on the home and the international fronts will be described and discussed. A detailed account of the present position and planned developments for the future will be given.

INTRODUCTION

When we consider the probable impact of Good Laboratory Practice (GLP) implementation in any country, it is necessary to take account of a number of factors. Among them, the following are of major importance:

- The preexisting situation with regard to control of the various laboratory procedures;
- The existing legislation concerning the submission of preclinical data;
- The extent to which GLP principles have already been voluntarily implemented;

---

1. Dr. Robinson died in December 1985. Address correspondence to: Dr. Derek Jennings, UK GLP Monitoring Unit, Department of Health and Social Security, Elephant and Castle, London SE1 6TE, England.

2. Key words: implementation, monitoring, voluntary implementation.

3. Abbreviations: DHSS, Department of Health and Social Security; EEC, European Economic Community; FDA, U.S. Food and Drug Administration; GLP, Good Laboratory Practice; OECD, Office of Economic Cooperation and Development; QA, Quality Assurance; QAU, Quality Assurance Unit; SOPs, Standard Operating Procedures.

315

- The GLP monitoring unit requirements needed to achieve compliance;
- The benefits which are expected to be gained, particularly concerning an enhanced quality of toxicity studies.

In the United Kingdom, monitoring of toxicology facilities by UK government staff has only been recently introduced, first to comply with a European Economic Community (EEC) directive for industrial chemicals and then in response to Japanese requirements concerning pharmaceuticals. Some facilities, however, had implemented GLP principles some years before this, but for those who had not and particularly for those requiring compliance statements for foreign regulatory authorities, rapid and sometimes radical reorganization was necessary. In many instances this involved changes in systems, procedures, staff responsibilities, attitudes, habits and even structural alterations to buildings.

But even when such a reorganization is made in complete accordance with national regulations or OECD guidelines, such a change only shows that when the facility was inspected, all recommendations had been implemented to demonstrate that the facility was complying with GLP principles at the time of inspection. Because inspections involve a completed study review, many studies will have been conducted before GLP principles were implemented. Even when GLP implementation occurred at a relatively late stage, many completed studies evoked little criticism when they were reviewed.

The U.S. Food and Drug Administration (FDA) conducted a pilot inspection program during the two years before GLP regulations were finalized. In 1977 they visited two UK facilities and conducted inspections and audits. In one instance no action was indicated; in the other, voluntary action was indicated. However, no adverse comments were made about the quality of the toxicology data. In 1977, apart from making arrangements for written observations to be collected and stored, there had been no attempt by UK facilities to introduce probable GLP requirements. Thus, although the various requirements itemized in GLP guidelines and regulations had not been met, the UK toxicological studies reviewed appeared to be perfectly satisfactory.

THE PRE-GLP IMPLEMENTATION SITUATION IN THE UK WITH REGARD TO LABORATORY PROCEDURES

Animals. Although the nature of the preclinical data which must be generated in support of a new chemical submission has steadily increased in diversity and complexity over the last two decades, the focal point in any toxicology study is still the direct toxicity tests carried out upon animals. In the UK, wide-ranging control over the use of animals for all types of experimentation has been in force since the introduction of the Cruelty to Animals Act in 1876. In order to accomplish the main objective of not allowing the laboratory worker to conduct experiments which are calculated to cause pain to living vertebrate animals, the Act made many requirements which are analogous, appropriate to and sometimes even more stringent than those contained in GLP guidelines and regulations.

The Home Office accepts applications for carrying out experiments on living vertebrates only from suitably qualified applicants. Applications must be supported by two presidents of learned societies; if authorized, experiments are only to be carried out at registered premises to monitor a variety of activities, many of which clearly cover GLP requirements:

- Inspection to ensure that appropriate and specific environmental conditions are being maintained in animal rooms to assure the healthy state of the animals.
- Inspection to ensure adequate caging and housing for the different animal species.
- Examination of records in the animal house:
  1. The name of the license for any experiment;
  2. Identification of each experiment;
  3. Identification of each animal used.
- Examination of records in the laboratory:
  1. Records of experiments done by each licensee;
  2. Records of the number and type of animals used in tests;
  3. Details of the nature of the experiments.

Obviously, the record keeping demanded of a licensee automatically requires personnel to maintain detailed records of the studies for which the animals were used.

Staff Training. In response to demands from establishments engaged in all types of scientific work, a wide range of training courses and qualifications for staff at all levels have evolved over the last 40 years. All branches of industry have organized introductory courses and in-house training. In addition, they have encouraged staff to pursue external training, obtain qualifications and, even when this has involved day release, have adopted a generous, almost philanthropic, attitude toward staff education. Thus, apart from school leavers, unqualified staff are not and have not for many years been employed to work on toxicology studies.

EXISTING LEGISLATION AFFECTING SUBMITTING OF PRELIMINARY DATA

The control of animal experimentation and the extensive training received by toxicology facility personnel did much to lessen the impact of GLP implementation in the UK. But before 1975, records of all work on animals were regarded fairly widely as the personal property of the licensee, as indeed were most of the data recorded in laboratory notebooks. Therefore, there was some difficulty in retrieving raw data, because personnel often discarded these data after reports or publications had been issued. The need to store raw data had never been established.

Although raw data for some old studies are not available, many studies conducted after 1960 would probably have survived study audit because regulatory demands over the last 25 years for new pharmaceuticals and veterinary products necessitated the development of efficient data recording systems in toxicology laboratories; most of these data were kept. Most of the data generated to support submissions to the voluntary Pesticides Safety Precautions Scheme have also been kept. However, secure archive facilities with storage and retrieval systems were much later developments, as were many of the systems and facilities required to be introduced before GLP compliance could be achieved.

VOLUNTARY IMPLEMENTATION OF GLP PRINCIPLES

At present, the only mandatory requirement in the UK for generating toxicology data in compliance with Office of Economic Cooperation and Development (OECD) Guidelines involves industrial chemicals marketed in quantities greater than one ton. However, since the publication of FDA regulations in 1978, UK firms aware of the possibility that the FDA would conduct an audit on their submissions which would also involve a facility inspection began to implement GLP principles.

The Quality Assurance Unit (QAU) is the point of contact between the GLP inspectorate and a toxicology facility. Implementation of GLP principles without Quality Assurance (QA) staff is inconceivable. Thus, QA staff were appointed to UK toxicology facilities at an early stage. These QA staff members tackled their tasks efficiently and enthusiastically and soon organized a QA Group which gave authoritative advice and assistance and attracted membership from most of the sites that generated toxicological data.

In the absence of UK GLP regulations, it was the QA personnel who have had the task of convincing facility management that although the serious problems experienced by the FDA have not been observed in the UK, the efficiency of toxicology facilities and the integrity and international acceptability of toxicology data would be enhanced if GLPs were implemented.

Many FDA requirements caused major difficulties during these early days. One such problem was that a study director should be responsible for the overall conduct of a toxicology study. The word "director" has a different connotation in the UK from that in the U.S. Traditionally, UK directors are members of the Board of Management and in toxicology laboratories are responsible for the studies. Some time elapsed before the status of a study director was fixed at its correct level, well below that of a company director.

Between the introduction of FDA regulations in 1978 and the commencement of UK GLP monitoring, most UK sites generating toxicology data progressed toward full GLP compliance under the guidance of their QA personnel. By 1982 all contract houses and many in-house facilities were known to be working in compliance with GLP principles. However, the major spur for all UK facilities to effect full GLP compliance and for the UK government to extend GLP monitoring to facilities generating toxicology data on pharmaceuticals, and then on agrochemicals, was the Japanese regulatory requirements. In October 1984 the UK DHSS (Department of Health and Social Security) GLP Monitoring Unit became responsible for all GLP monitoring in the UK. The Unit was appropriately located in the DHSS Division concerned with Toxicology and Environmental Protection. At the present time, all contract houses in the UK and about half of the in-house facilities have been inspected by UK GLP Monitoring Units.

REQUIREMENTS OF THE GLP MONITORING UNIT
FOR COMPLIANCE

A major advantage of beginning GLP monitoring at a relatively late stage is that one can benefit from the experience of other regulatory authorities. But there are also disadvantages. Regulatory authorities who have introduced GLP regulations since 1981 have based them on OECD Guidelines. The problem for the UK and other countries currently preparing inspector's manuals, advisory documents on GLP requirements and GLP regulations is that of ensuring that an inspected facility meets the varied requirements of these regulatory authorities. Another complication is that some regulatory authorities have not nominated GLP inspectors but use scientists from government establishments. Inherent in this system is the great risk of inconsistent interpretation of requirements. In order to introduce as consistent an approach to GLP monitoring as possible, UK inspectors are nominated scientists with toxicological and regulatory experience. To cope with inspections and study audits in contract houses, industry and academic laboratories, a team of up to three inspectors will be necessary.

During the course of an inspection, all deviations are noted and the QA manager informed. Many deviations are small and can be corrected before the end of the inspection. Nevertheless, all deviations are recorded in a further statement which is given to management and discussed at a formal exit interview. If the statement is agreed to, management is required to give written confirmation of its acceptance. Although no major deviations have yet been observed, management must correct all deviations and inform us in writing of how the corrections were made before we are prepared to issue a compliance statement. We also reserve the right to reinspect before agreeing that compliance has been achieved. Should routine study audits be required, the inspectorate can cope, but where the science of a study is in question, we would ask an appropriate specialist from another government department to join the team. Inspectors, specialists and administrative staff of the unit are, therefore, all government employees and are subject to the Official Secrets Act.

THE BENEFITS OF GLP

As far as the majority of toxicological sites are concerned, it is difficult to determine the extent to which GLP implementation has improved data quality. However, GLP does give all concerned—bench worker, QA manager, facility management and regulatory authority—assurance that the study has been conducted according to an accepted set of guidelines. Most importantly, the various systems ensure that all personnel concerned with a toxicology study are aware of their duties and responsibilities. Of paramount importance is the protocol, which demands careful planning to indicate clearly to all operatives the details of the study, specifications of the various animals and materials to be used and the observations to be made. Second in importance are the Standard Operating Procedures (SOPs), many of which were communicated verbally until recently. The writing of SOPs has involved tremendous thought and effort, but has obvious advantages.

Validation of results by study supervisors and study directors ensures ongoing surveillance of the work, while inspection of critical phases by QA personnel completes the in-house monitoring of a study to ensure that all possible care has been taken.

In conclusion, it is clear that in some areas, such as with regard to control of animal use, experimentation and husbandry, the required changes have not necessarily been great. In other areas, enormous effort has had to be deployed. Even at sites of modest proportions, the cost has been considerable. The ultimate benefit to industry is, of course, international acceptance of the way in which the data for a submission have been generated. But it would be completely wrong to assume that compliance with GLP principles implies complete acceptance of the integrity of the work, because the inspector, although experienced in toxicology, is not employed to judge the science. The scientific evaluation is done by the regulatory authorities, and any queries raised are investigated by specialists at study audits.

Although many of the benefits of GLP are intangible, scientists who once deeply resented inspection of their work now take pride in demonstrating their ability to carry out their studies in compliance with the requirements of GLP guidelines.

PANEL-AUDIENCE DIALOGUE INTERNATIONAL REGULATORY ASPECTS OF QUALITY

Chairperson:
Dexter S. Goldman
Laboratory Data Integrity Program, Office of Compliance Monitoring
U.S. Environmental Protection Agency
Washington, D.C.

Panel:
Remi Glomot, Paul D. Lepore, Kazuo Okutomi,
Desmond Robinson, Hartmut Uehleke

Zachery Wong (Chevron): I would like to ask Mr. Okutomi to comment on the status of bilateral agreements for Good Laboratory Practice between the Ministry of Agriculture, Forestry and Fisheries in Japan and other foreign countries.

Kazuo Okutomi (MAFF): At this moment, there are no bilateral arrangements between Japan and foreign countries.

Desmond Robinson (Department of Health and Social Security, UK): We will be signing a bilateral agreement with Japan as soon as the Japanese have time, as they are very busy. The Japanese MAFF is in contact with quite a number of OECD signatories with a view to making bilateral agreements.

Dexter Goldman (EPA): I would like to add that EPA recently submitted a draft of an agreement to MAFF with respect to harmonization of GLP regulations, inspections, inspection methodologies, and so on, with a view to obtaining a signed bilateral agreement. I would expect that this will be completed in the next few months.

Pat Royal (Stauffer Chemical Co.): There has been some discussion over the last few years about the possibility of laboratory accreditation for licensing as a result of GLP inspections. Has any further movement been made in this area in either the United States or in Europe?

Robinson: We would not touch accreditation with a right long barge pole.

Goldman: That takes care of the U.S. and the U.K.

Remi Glomot (CIT, France): We have a data and laboratory auditing system for pharmaceuticals, but we do not have one for chemicals.

Hartmut Uehleke (German Government): That's true in our country. Accreditation is required for any laboratory performing animal experiments, but not in compliance with GLP. It's just a very general license that is given to the establishment only in conjunction with individual people. It is competent people who are important; you can't separate this.

Goldman: So your accreditation is for facilities conducting animal work. It would be like our AAALAS or AALAC programs.

Uehleke: Yes, similar.

Steelman (McNeil Pharmaceuticals): Dr. Goldman's introductory remarks discussed joint venture agreements in which studies are conducted in several countries on the same test material. The proliferation of co-marketing agreements means that today's toxicologists are dealing with data from sometimes two, three, or even four different countries on the same compound. If I understood you correctly, the quality of those data varies from unsatisfactory to outstanding. Assuming that we are dealing with the submission of data that span this range of quality, I understood that you had a problem with a rat study done in one country and a mouse study done in another country.

Goldman: I would say that you are taking something out of context that I did not mean in that respect. First, I didn't comment on quality of studies, I commented on quantity of studies. My comment on a rat study being done in one country and a mouse study being done in another country was simply a matter of surprise to me from my background. It had nothing to do, whatever, with the corporate decision to do that or the quality of the study that results. My background was more with the NTP where we would expect the rat and mouse study to be done at the same facility, but we have all seen variants on this theme that had nothing to do with quality.

Kent Shillam (Huntingdon Research Laboratories, U.K.): Mr. Okutomi mentioned that so far the Japanese MAFF has received 30 petitions for confirmation. Could we know what proportion of these are from overseas companies? What might be the total number of petitions anticipated? Has the Japanese MAFF got a new building on the drawing board to accommodate the volume of information that we are having to submit to them?

Okutomi: We have received about 30 of these documents, and among them, about 25 are from Japan. The remainder would be from several other countries. We have no idea how to anticipate how many petitions we will get from other countries.

Robinson: Mr. Okutomi works at the testing station and not for the headquarters of MAFF. The sort of question that Kent put to him would be difficult for him to answer. When I was in Japan and quizzed the people, I can tell you that foreign countries put in an enormous amount of paper. The average Japanese submission was much smaller. Perhaps the Japanese have a capacity to put things down more concisely.

Terry Bromley (Wellcome Foundation, U.K.): At a meeting in Cambridge, England earlier this year, it became clear that there was a growing leaning towards the first data entry being the start of the data trail that would lead ultimately to the final signed pathology report. Is that situation changing?

Goldman: Not from the chairman's point of view.

Paul Lepore (FDA): Not from my point of view either. For six years, FDA has interpreted raw data collected by the pathologist to be the final, signed and dated report. We see no need to change this particular definition, because it has been successful. It is based on the GLP provision for raw data that says that raw data are number one. It is a note, document or record that represents the original observation. There is also the proviso that raw data are necessary for the reconstruction of a study. This includes slides which have been discussed before. The NTP scenario is somewhat problematic, because it is difficult for a Pathology Working Group not to affect the raw data. It depends on how they work. The original pathologist—the first reader of the slide—writes the final report. The Pathology Working Group can influence the original pathologist to change his mind and thereby change the final report. If the Pathology Working Group has an alternative interpretation of the data, then that becomes a separate piece of raw data that must accompany the report of the original pathologist. I don't know how much NTP deals with that, but that is the way it must be. The original pathologist can reconsider the diagnosis and modify the report, or there can be a formal report amendment such as what the Pathology Working Group would do if they had a different diagnosis. In summary, we interpret the raw data definition to mean that information required to reconstruct the study. Interim conclusions that sharpen as the experiment continues are not considered to be raw data. We do not consider this scenario to be different from the responsibility of each data collector in a study to verify the data collection observation. The person who takes in-life measurements may change his mind hundreds of times before he records an observation on paper. The data collector is the first point of verification and that person must testify, certify and so designate by proper documentation that a finding is accurate. We feel that the pathologist must have the same kind of freedom to make a decision.

Bromley: I understood from talking to you at Cambridge that the FDA had some regrets in making a decision in the first place and that the agency could see some merit in having data prior to that report.

Lepore: Yes. At that time I was concerned that some of the revisions in the pathological findings were being made absent from the proper data trail by subsequent pathological readings.

Glomot: Even if the pathology is not being done by a working group, it is impossible for the pathologist to have in mind several hundred slides in the early stages of the diagnostic process. His opinion will vary during the course of this review and I agree with Paul Lepore when he said that the final, signed report constitutes the raw data.

Charles Montgomery (NIEHS/NTP): I would like to clarify one point that Paul Lepore made about the Pathology Working Group. At the NTP, the original pathologist is held responsible for his diagnosis. In a court of law, that is the diagnosis that stands. The Pathology Working Group is not a judge and jury; it is scientific peer review. If at the end of the meeting of the Pathology Working Group there is a significant difference of opinion that would alter the interpretation of the study, a separate document would be added to the report by the Pathology Working Group. This group does not alter the original pathologist's thinking—it is a second opinion. To my knowledge there have only been two cases in which this happened in all of the studies that we have done. For the most part, the Pathology Working Group functions to clean up the data. It keeps the original pathologist from saying "chronic inflammation" one time and "cellular infiltration, lymphocytic" in another case when it is really the same lesion. That is what all of this QA business is about and I agree with Paul Lepore that the tracking point is now where it should be. To back it up to any other point would be devastating.

Goldman: EPA does not have the broad experience that FDA has had or the levels of quality assurance that the NTP has for pathology. Therefore, we take the view that the audit trail starts at an earlier point in the procedure. Whether we ultimately retain that view depends on how the results come in.

William Farland (EPA): I would like to make a comment on some international aspects that have not been discussed relative to testing guidelines. We have a U.S. ad hoc group of OECD test guidelines centered in our office of EPA. We have representatives from a number of different constituencies on that group. You can either contact me or one of the following representatives: Dorothy Canter, NTP; Tom Schellanberger, Tegeris Laboratories for National Association of Life Science Industries; Robert Moolenaar, Dow; and Ellen Silbergeld from the Environmental Defense Fund. Let us know if any of these people or I can act as conduits of information for status reports or provide you with documents to comment on guidelines related to the OECD testing program.

Chapter VIII
JOINT CONFERENCE SUMMATION

CONFERENCE SUMMATION: INDUSTRIAL VIEW

Robert W. Naismith
Pharmakon Research International, Inc.
Waverly, Pennsylvania

During the three days of the conference we have shared our perspectives and widened our horizons about the importance of managing the conduct of toxicology studies, and ensuring the quality of the data that are derived from those studies. A very clear message of the conference was the recognition for the need and value of quality assurance, and of the increasing role quality assurance must play in the acceptability of the data from toxicology studies.

The conference was unique in its joint sponsorship by, and the cooperation of, several trade associations, the National Toxicology Program and the National Institute of Environmental Health Sciences. Another milestone in the history of toxicology and in the new science of quality assurance was that government and industrial scientists, management and quality assurance personnel participated as partners. We have exchanged important concepts and strategies to improve the quality of toxicology studies, beginning a dialogue which needs to continue for the successful realization of this partnership. A successful quality assurance program requires commitment from management, sound judgement from the scientific team and diligence from the quality assurance professional.

In his opening remarks for the conference, Dr. David Rall, Director of the National Institute of Environmental Health Sciences, emphasized the impact on society and the importance of decisions made from data derived from toxicology studies. He also reminded us of the ongoing need to continue to improve these tools used in the decision making process. Dr. Frank Press, President of the National Academy of Sciences, also summarized the importance of these and brought to our attention the fact that there are currently twenty-five laws and six agencies that regulate or rely upon the data from toxicology studies. He cautioned us of the need to ensure the quality and scientific validity of the experiments used to comply with these laws.

Dr. Robert Scala examined the concept of quality and reminded us that it requires an individual, professional diligence from each of us. Quality is an ongoing task for everyone, and maintaining this quality requires a constant

1. Address correspondence to: Dr. Robert W. Naismith, Pharmakon Research International, Inc., P.O. Box 313, Waverly, PA 18471.
2. Key words: cooperation, partnership, quality.
3. Abbreviations: FDA, U.S. Food and Drug Administration; GLP, Good Laboratory Practice.

renewal of commitment by the working scientist. Quality must be a pervasive attitude, beginning with management and infectious among the entire staff.

Dr. Sidney Green discussed the history and background leading to the implementation of Good Laboratory Practice (GLP) regulations within the Food and Drug Administration (FDA), and the problems associated with their implementation. The openness and candor of Dr. Green's description of the difficulties uncovered through internal inspections within the agency set the stage for frank discussion during the conference. There is no question that a mature cooperative attitude towards GLPs has emerged from the FDA. The FDA has been flexible and responsive, and continually reexamines the impact of these regulations on the conduct of toxicology studies.

Presentations by management personnel support the idea they are committed to quality. Dr. Richard Steelman reiterated the corporate policy of Johnson & Johnson, which recognizes "good quality is good business." His description of the process that assures the quality of every activity leading to a final product, and how it involved all management and the workforce, was very enlightening.

Dr. Jerry Smith emphasized that Good Laboratory Practices are not necessarily Good Toxicology Practices. He reminded us that industry must not only sponsor and conduct toxicology studies of the highest quality, but must also sponsor and conduct full, complete toxicological evaluation programs of the highest quality. In support of that theme, Dr. Judith Baldwin reminded us that quality is a process and this process should not stop when quality assurance completes an audit. Management needs to react not only to the summary findings of quality assurance, but also to the process.

Much of the conference dealt with the importance of the protocol, the facility, animal quality, environmental factors, necropsy procedures, pathology, and test article characterization. Ira Friedman described the ways in which the protocol is an essential tool for management, the study director, the quality assurance unit and the regulatory authorities, and how a well-written protocol and a complete data file bolster the confidence, credibility and reliability of the study. The suggestion that quality assurance people be responsible for putting the protocol, once written by the study director, into a computer may prevent questions about whether quality assurance is an integral and informed part of the process.

As the quality assurance process continues to mature, we as professionals have to decide what is right, what is wrong, what is proper, what is improper. One of my grave concerns was amplified by the very frank assessment of Attorney James Phelps. He explained that in today's legal climate "we have to keep records to disprove fraud." I feel that open discussions in meetings like this will help to prevent that attitude from becoming pervasive in our field. The relationships and the professional dignity by which we interact must be carefully guarded. It is essential that we encourage a climate of trust and integrity. We have to be certain what information is necessary and what we are capable of properly evaluating during a laboratory inspection. Also, we must be cautious, recognizing where expertise ends and presumption begins.

A discussion of the toxicologist's expectations of quality assurance and how the toxicologist can utilize the expertise of quality assurance was presented by Dr. Glenn Simon. He recognized the different skills required of a study director and reiterated the need for cooperation between the study director and quality assurance personnel. The role of the study director as the arbitrator of data acceptance, from a scientific standpoint rather than in a functional audit performed by quality assurance, was also emphasized. It is therefore important that we recognize these two roles as separate, and be sensitive to the different concerns each has in the conduct of any study.

The need for developing new methodologies to deal with the problems of quality assurance was emphasized by Richard Siconolfi's presentation on statistical approaches to study auditing. Prior to the suggestion of statistical approaches for study audits, the validation of toxicology reports was limited to auditing every data point or performing it in an *ad hoc* fashion. The development of formal methods for data auditing is particularly apparent in studies in which large data bases develop, such as in reproductive or chronic bioassays.

Speakers representing regulatory agencies outside the United States ably presented international concerns about quality assurance. Scientists must be cognizant of the appropriate international regulations, especially when submitting data to foreign countries. International cooperation and bilateral understandings of GLPs need to be forged to facilitate the international acceptance of toxicology data. Quality does not know national boundaries. It continues to be an international concern, regardless of country of origin, that Good Laboratory Practices be employed in the conduct of toxicology studies.

Another recurring theme throughout the conference was the array of skills and depth of knowledge required of quality assurance personnel. Frank Press referred to the new technologies and the remarkable opportunities these new technologies are going to present, namely, the impact of biotechnology on toxicology and quality assurance. It is worth mentioning that in our laboratory we are already using a mammalian cell with an inserted bacterial gene to make decisions about a chemical's ability to cause mutations. Use of this genetically modified mammalian cell line assists us in making safety decisions. Quality assurance must be prepared to handle such novel technologies. These problems are not coming; they are here and will increase in scope as we expand the use of the new tools now available.

Several speakers spoke continually about the problems associated with toxicology experiments conducted at academic institutions. Many universities generate toxicology data, and reports of these experiments find themselves in the safety arena. Scientists often use the lay press to report that chemicals cause cancer, are teratogenic or mutagenic, or have other toxic effects. There is a need for academic scientists who generate data which greatly impact on safety decisions, risk assessment and society's concerns to support their experiments and conclusions with complete data. Because of the potential emotional and financial consequences of these experiments, we need to bring academic scientists into this partnership. To do this we are going to have to rely on quality assurance. Inadequate results in press releases on new cancer cures, carcinogenic substances or other hazards are unfair to the public.

A timely suggestion about how to deal with these issues occurred during the question period following Frank Press's presentation. To assist the public in interpreting new scientific advances, a TV program similar to "Wall Street Week In Review," entitled "Science Week In Review" and aired on the Public Broadcasting System, is worthy of serious consideration. The science of toxicology needs the public's understanding. It is a science of high visibility and what better way to reach the public than through television?

Several questions were asked about whether quality assurance was only intended to be "number crunching." Has the science exceeded its intended purpose? That view is archaic and has no place in modern regulatory science. Quality assurance has, and is going to continue to ask questions, and this is the very essence of science. As an illustration, over the past ten years uncertainty has been expressed about the genetic stability of several mouse strains. It is certainly appropriate for quality assurance to ask questions about genetic stability and the importance of monitoring it. Such questions have been overlooked by many scientists. However, if deemed to be germane, it is up to the scientist to design experiments that answer these questions.

Finally, I feel it appropriate to summarize many issues from this conference which still need to be addressed and require action:

1. Quality assurance is a partnership and this partnership needs assistance. We need to support the quality and integrity of our science through quality assurance. This assurance must include career opportunities and rewards commensurate with its value.

2. It is appropriate that the topic of this meeting be reexamined in a similar fashion within the next several years to monitor the impact of quality assurance.

3. At this critical point, due to its embryonic nature, quality assurance as a discipline needs to be nurtured. It will need assistance from leaders in the field, including the organizers of this conference. Quality assurance must also be addressed by the professional societies. Do not be overly possessive and restrict such activities to the Society of Quality Assurance. It is important that the Society of Toxicology and the American College of Toxicology include continuing education programs which emphasize quality assurance in their professional meeting schedules.

4. It is essential that many of the suggestions and ideas raised during this conference be implemented. I ask the organizing committee to carefully consider these suggestions and comments. This industry has been, is, and will be committed to study Good Laboratory Practices. Training courses are urgently needed to allow young professionals to function in quality assurance positions. These courses could be offered in the form of one- or two-day symposia or in conjunction with the professional societies. We have heard an appeal from the World Health Organization at this meeting that the need for training courses transcends national boundaries. They have offered to assist in planning this effort. We have also heard a university, the Centers for Disease Control and the National Toxicology Program offer their services. Suggestions that we consider certifying

people for quality assurance may be premature, but formal courses offering continuing education credits should be available to quality assurance personnel. This effort needs the support of both industry and government. I believe industry and government are prepared to support it.

5. It also may be necessary, after hearing many questions, to begin to define the type of person qualified to serve as a quality assurance professional. The proceedings of this conference certainly have shed light on the multi-faceted skills necessary to function in a quality assurance position. Dexter Goldman very aptly asked during the conference, "why was this person selected?" If he were to ask us this same question on an individual basis during an inspection, the tone of the question and the importance of its answer would take on a different perspective.

6. Management, both in government and industry, must be reminded of the need to examine quality assurance findings. We cannot afford to repeat mistakes. Quality assurance is a management tool, and it should allow us to do things right the first time.

In conclusion, we have spent three days focusing on the interactions between management, the scientist and quality assurance in order to improve standards of quality in the conduct of toxicology studies. As the gate-keepers of this field, our continued demand for such scientific integrity will have enormous benefit for both the science and the society we serve.

CONFERENCE SUMMATION: GOVERNMENT VIEW

Bernard A. Schwetz
Systemic Toxicology Branch, Toxicology Research & Testing Program
National Institute of Environmental Health Sciences
Research Triangle Park, North Carolina

Since the implementation of Good Laboratory Practices (GLPs) in 1978, quality assurance has matured significantly as a critical part of toxicology. As with other scientific areas, this process of maturation is associated with growing pains. One sign of maturity is the concern expressed at this conference for the identity and responsibility of the quality assurance program. This concern is reflected in uncertainty about who the quality assurance person should be, what training he or she should have, and how we might provide additional training in quality assurance.

Another clear evidence of quality assurance's maturation is the ability of the Food and Drug Administration (FDA), through Dr. Sidney Green's talk, to share the learning process experienced by the Agency during their early involvement with quality assurance in their own laboratories. The problems encountered and the resolution of those problems were openly discussed on the basis of the learning experience. Another significant sign of the maturing of quality assurance is the recent formation of the Society of Quality Assurance. The formalization of this society from the Quality Assurance Roundtable is a major step in bringing together people of more backgrounds, including representatives from academia and government, in the growth of quality assurance efforts.

Numerous speakers at the conference highlighted management's role in quality assurance. Dr. Richard Steelman mentioned that management is cause, while all else is effect, a concept that was considered to be as true in quality assurance as in any other area of laboratory management. Dr. McConnell referred to the "top-down" method of management used by the National Toxicology Program. This management style also applied to quality assurance. Clearly, management was considered to be the driving force for implementing quality assurance. In my opinion, one concern over this allocation of responsibility is the fact that management responds to problems on a priority basis. Unless the audit process reveals significant problems, it is easy for quality

---

1. Address correspondence to: Dr. Bernard A. Schwetz, Systemic Toxicology Branch, Toxicology Research and Testing Program, N.I.E.H.S., P.O. Box 12233, Research Triangle Park, NC 27709.

2. Key words: Good Laboratory Practices, management, monitoring, quality assurance.

3. Abbreviations: FDA, Food and Drug Administration; GLPs, Good Laboratory Practices.

assurance to become a low priority. The commitment to GLPs is highly vulnerable to apathy. In the future, a significant challenge to toxicologists and quality assurance people will be to maintain the commitment to quality assurance and GLPs at the level needed for ensuring the quality of toxicology studies achieved during the past few years.

Many speakers throughout the conference mentioned the cost and cost effectiveness of quality assurance in toxicology. Dr. Robert Scala spoke of the rationale for doing work right the first time, a good management practice that is a logical means of managing toxicological work. However, as most of us have seen in real-world laboratory operation, we seldom have enough money to do the work properly, but we always have enough to do it over. Good management practices would determine that if work is done right the first time, we could spend less money, resources and career time of toxicologists in repeating studies.

A considerable part of the conference focused on the source of problems or uncertainties in conducting toxicology studies, including preparation of protocols, standard operating procedures, the nature of the facility itself, animal health, environment, pathology procedures and test article characterization problems. It is unclear whether these factors were given visibility because they are the highest priority concerns for quality within our toxicology studies, or whether they are areas in which sufficient progress has been made that we have the experience to talk about them. These items have received considerable attention during the evolution of Good Laboratory Practices, and the need for continued discussion should be balanced against their actual priority. Perhaps their prominence relates to the need to continue educating new people coming into toxicology and quality assurance about these important issues.

The conference brought out clearly the vacillation between the responsibility of toxicologists versus that of quality assurance personnel, an emphasis which is consistent with the need for clarifying the identity of quality assurance personnel. Perhaps it is not surprising that quality assurance monitors are concerned about their identity, since many of them have been "borrowed" from other disciplines in toxicology laboratories, such as chemistry, pathology or animal care. It is natural for such individuals to assume responsibility for the quality of work as well as the nature of the science in toxicology studies. But this vacillation between being a toxicologist and being a quality assurance monitor has caused considerable stress in the evolution of quality assurance. It seems most appropriate that people involved in quality assurance monitoring should assume highest priority responsibility for the quality assurance aspects of the auditing and monitoring and, as permitted, comment on the quality of the science after data quality has been monitored. As the interface between quality assurance and other areas of toxicology becomes better defined, it is very likely that the relationship between toxicological responsibility and quality assurance responsibility will become better defined.

Data quality in toxicology studies is independent of the type of study and discipline, the regulator involved with the ultimate use of the data and the data's nation of origin or place of intended use. While this conference focused primarily on carcinogenesis studies, quality assurance efforts are clearly important in all types of toxicological studies, and the same principles of quality are applicable. While quality assurance and GLPs were associated most strongly with the Food and Drug Administration during the early years of implementing their guidelines, data quality certainly is not limited to the FDA. The same principles of quality assurance apply to data intended for all uses, not just for one or two regulatory agencies.

Likewise, the quality of data is independent of its nation of origin or nation of intended use. Quality is important for all types of data and uses, not just for selected situations. Data quality and the attitude of scientists are closely interrelated. Through the years, some people's attitudes and work habits were such that GLPs were inherent in their activities, even before the GLPs were implemented. Other people have great difficulty working in a manner consistent with GLPs because of their work habits and attitudes, regardless of the presence of strict guidance from GLPs. Work habits that are consistent with high quality are truly a function of personal attitudes, which are influenced by the presence of guidelines for study conduct. Dr. Sidney Green referred to scientists as being independent and assuming that matters of GLP were someone else's responsibilities. Such attitudes were part of the early problems within the FDA's laboratories as well as at other facilities.

The conference considered the topic of ethics only tangentially. Intuition suggests that ethics are important in the field of quality assurance, but perhaps no more so than in any other area of science. It is interesting to learn that the newly formed Society of Quality Assurance incorporated a code of ethics into its original constitution and bylaws and to note that the Society of Toxicology has recently approved a code of ethics for all of its members.

A frequent question asked during the conference was how we should be teaching quality assurance. One possibility was through the use of short courses given over several days using an intense program that would cover all aspects of quality assurance and GLPs. The involvement of the university as a teaching center and the question of auditing university courses was also discussed. Since many university research laboratories have not adopted GLPs, it is difficult to expect university departments to teach GLPs in their toxicology courses. Many universities are, however, including some course work on quality assurance and GLPs, and today's graduate students as a group have a much greater awareness of the implications of GLPs in their own work than their predecessors. In addition to short courses and university-taught efforts, the government and perhaps the World Health Organization should play a role in teaching quality assurance principles and practices. Additional conferences prepared jointly by government and industry might be an important way of continuing the evolution of quality assurance and providing teaching opportunities. The potential role of the government toxicology laboratories in the future teaching of quality assurance needs to be investigated.

One of the more complex issues to surface during the conference was the consideration of minimum criteria for accepting or rejecting data and studies. Mr. Siconolfi provided information on an elegant approach, based on statistical considerations, for auditing data. While not necessarily totally acceptable to everyone, such an approach does serve as a reference point for future activities in auditing data. Dr. Steinberg commented that the criteria for data acceptance are based on experience. While this is certainly true and logical, it does not provide for consistency between organizations or scientists in making decisions about the acceptability of data. Dr. Smith clearly identified the difference between good laboratory practices and good toxicological practices. This is not to say that GLPs are unimportant; on the contrary, they can enhance the quality of data but are not a remedy for inadequate toxicological practices. It was recommended that rather than identifying minimum criteria for acceptance or rejection, typical cases sufficient for rejection of data might be identified as reference points.

There was general agreement throughout the conference that a greater awareness of quality control and quality assurance has made our data, and therefore our decisions, more reliable. Better quality data have narrowed the confidence limits around our predictions as toxicologists.

Future considerations in the area of quality assurance include the questions of training additional people, criteria for acceptance or rejection of data, audit of university-conducted studies, and audit of new types of data, such as those associated with biotechnology. As quality assurance continues to evolve, perhaps through the assistance of the Society of Quality Assurance, the highest priority issues and needs should be identified to permit a concentration of effort on these high-priority needs rather than continuing to work diffusely on many different aspects. How these needs can be related to future conferences should be considered. Perhaps future meetings should focus on more specific topics rather than the broad scope of topics addressed here. The Society of Quality Assurance should collaborate with the Society of Toxicology and the American College of Toxicology to assure interface with these other groups of toxicologists to whom quality assurance must continue to be a high priority.

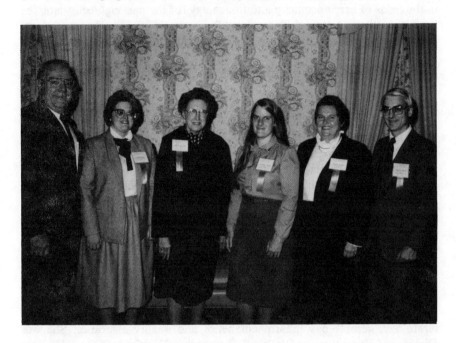

From left to right: Arthur F. Uelner, Monsanto; B. Kristin Hoover, ARCO Chemical Company; Carrie E. Whitmire, NTP/NIEHS; Christine L. Davies, NTP/NIEHS; Judith K. Baldwin, Exxon Corporation; and Douglas W. Bristol, NTP/NIEHS.

ARTHUR F. UELNER received his B.S. degree in chemistry from the University of Iowa. He has had more than thirty years' experience in quality control and quality assurance with the Monsanto Company in all aspects of multi-product manufacturing and large industrial laboratory operation. Currently he is Manager of Quality Assurance in the corporation's Department of Medicine and Environmental Health.

B. KRISTIN HOOVER received a B.S. degree in biology from Ball State University and an M.A. in environmental biology from Hood College. She was instrumental in the development of a quality assurance program for the American Petroleum Institute and is widely published in the field. Ms. Hoover is currently a senior toxicologist for ARCO Chemical Company, a division of Atlantic Richfield Company.

CARRIE E. WHITMIRE received her B.A. from the University of Texas and an M.A. and a Ph.D. from the University of Kansas. She has had forty years' experience in biological research with three major pharmaceutical corporations, in government laboratories and on contracts with the National Cancer Institute and The Council for Tobacco Research, U.S.A. She has been working in the fields of carcinogenicity and toxicology for the past eighteen years, the last six with the National Toxicology Program (NTP). She has over forty publications in the field of viral and chemical carcinogenicity. During the past four years, one of her primary responsibilities has been the Quality Assurance and Good Laboratory Practices program for NTP.

CHRISTINE L. DAVIES received a B.S. in chemistry from New Mexico Tech and has done graduate studies in biochemistry at New Mexico Tech and North Carolina State University. She has conducted research at the International Center for Environmental Safety and in the Laboratory of Reproductive and Developmental Toxicology at the National Institute of Environmental Health Sciences. Chris has coauthored several papers on the action of estrogens in the mouse reproductive tract. With the National Toxicology Program she has participated in monitoring all aspects of the chemistry performed for toxicity/carcinogenicity studies and has played an active role in performing retrospective quality assurance audits of completed studies.

JUDITH K. BALDWIN holds an M.A. from Trenton State College and received her B.S. and Ph.D. from Rutgers University. During her more than twenty years of experience in toxicology, she has published in the fields of teratology, gerontology, pharmacokinetics and quality assurance. She was Director of Toxicology at Wallace Laboratories (Division of Carter-Wallace Inc.) prior to assuming her present position as Senior Staff Scientist in the Research and Environmental Health Division of Exxon Corporation.

DOUGLAS W. BRISTOL received a B.S. in biology from St. John Fisher College and a Ph.D. in chemistry from Syracuse University. Doug has held positions in academia (University of Utah, Instructor; North Dakota State University, Assistant/Associate Professor of Biochemistry and Head, Residue Research Laboratory), in government (Food and Drug Administration, Environmental Protection Agency and National Institute of Environmental Health Sciences), and in the private sector (Tracor Jitco, Inc., Manager of Chemistry). He has over 55 scientific publications and presentations. He is presently the Director of Quality Assurance for the Toxicology Research and Testing Program at NIEHS.

ABOUT THE COVER ILLUSTRATION

The significance of defining and understanding each aspect of toxicological studies and assurance of quality cannot be disputed. The cover of this book and the poster design that preceded it were an attempt to graphically present this significance and represent hopes for achievement through this conference.

This design depicts the complexity of managing quality in toxicology studies in an environment of expanding needs for greater knowledge of toxicology. The blocks represent the various components of toxicological studies. They must be assembled much as the bricks of any building to contribute to the integrity of the structure or the toxicological study. The foundation for these blocks is not only sound science, but also good management, for it is management which sets the stage for quality. The cornerstones are the scientists and the facilities. The selection of the test substance, the test system and the preparation of the protocol define the study to be conducted. Based on these, the building blocks for animal care, analytical chemistry, pharmacokinetics, clinical chemistry, pharmacotoxic signs, environmental conditions, pathology, data collection systems, statistics and report preparation are put in place to assure the quality of toxicology research. The regulatory agencies act as inspectors, much as a building inspector does for the building trade, with their primary purpose being the protection of the public.

In addition to these defined building blocks, there are those floating blocks in space representing the smaller undefined or uncontrolled aspects of animal studies. In many ways they are as poorly defined as the outer reaches of our universe. Space explorations act as a means of sharing perspectives, which leads to expanding horizons, as does this conference for the assurance of toxicological quality. These areas of study conduct become defined as a better understanding of the intricate aspects of toxic effects is achieved. The floaters become additional building blocks and quality evaluation occurs. The elusive nature of assuring quality becomes better defined through the sharing of perspective, thus expanding our horizons.

The committee is deeply indebted to Alfred C. Laoang, National Institutes of Health, Bethesda, Maryland, for his ability to understand the problems related to quality and develop the poster for this conference. The "Award of Merit" was given to the Globe Screen Printing Corporation in recognition of printing the poster "Managing Conduct and Data Quality of Toxicology Studies," which was adjudged to be of superior quality in the 1985 Maryland Print Quality Awards Competition. This competition was held by Printing Industries of Maryland, Inc. The poster was well received and helped us present the salient goals of managing conduct and data quality of toxicology studies.

bio-research monitoring, 140
biotechnology, 5, 329
bleeding site, significance of, 200
blood cell counts, 200
blood sampling, methods of, 219
Board of Scientific Counselors, 57
bone marrow preparations, 204
British Standards 6000 and 6001,
   223, 225
budgeting processes, 21, 24, 25
Business Roundtable's Task Force
   on Corporate Responsibility, 22

caging procedures, 183–84
calibration of instruments, 198
Canadian Council on Animal Care,
   176
cannibalism, 73, 265
capability assessment, 125–37
carbon dioxide, 200
carcinogenesis, 60
Carcinogenesis and Toxicology Evaluation Branch (CTEB), 82, 83,
   84, 85, 93, 94
Carcinogenesis Bioassay Data System (CBDS), 68
carcinogenesis studies, 59
Carcinogenesis Testing Program,
   National Cancer Institute, 264,
   272
carcinogenicity tests, 24
carcinogens, potential, 8
cardiac hypertrophy, 181
C-cell tumors, 273
cedar bedding, 182
cedrene, 182
cell type interpretation, 274
Centers for Disease Control, 330
Center for Drugs, 142
certification of laboratories, 293
cesarean derivation, 155-71
chemical
   analysis, 195
   contaminants and diet, 182
   exposure, developmental effects
      of, 6

exposure, reproductive effects of,
   6
monitoring results, 66
selection, 9
-specific health and safety, 66
spills and releases, 66
stability determinations, 58
quality, 57–58
vehicle mixture, 67
Chemical Carcinogenesis Testing
   and Evaluation, 60
Chemical Manager (CM), 57, 60, 61,
   79, 80, 82, 83, 84, 85, 94
Chemical Pathology Branch (CPB),
   281
Chemical Status Report, 91, 92
Chemikaliengesetz ("Chemical Act"),
   305, 307
chemistry, 60
chemotherapeutic agents, 162
CHEMTRACK, 89, 91
chlorpromazine, 179
choline, 182
Chronic Inhalation Unleaded Gasoline Study, 232
chronic mammalian studies, 233
circadian rhythms, 173
Clean Air Act Amendments, 5
"clean conventional" animals, 158
clean corridor-dirty corridor design,
   156
clinical
   chemistry, 199–206
   chemistry capabilities, 65
   chemistry proficiency testing, 68
   disqualification procedures, 142
   laboratory data, 199
   observations, 251
   pathology data, 251
CNS depression, 179
coagulation, 203, 204
Collaborative Services Section, 84
commensals, 158
commercial breeding facilities, 161
compliance
   documentation, and industrial

342

minute virus of mice (MVM), 161
mite infestations, 162
model programs for animal health, 155–71
molecular biology, 6
"monitored" animals, 158
monitoring study performance, 79–97
monoclonal antibodies, 5
Monthly Progress Report, 92, 93
Moore, John, 30
moribund animals, 74, 251
morphologic diagnosis, 271–72
mortality verification, 74
mouse hepatitis virus, 161
mouse uterine tumor, 274
multi-generation reproduction studies, 233
multipurpose research facility, 164–65
multistage QA program of National Toxicology Program, 263–69
murine respiratory mycoplasma, 163
mutagenic chemicals, 329
mutagenicity assays, 77
mutual GLP recognition, 297
Mycoplasma arthriditis, 162
Mycoplasma ELISA, 159, 162
Mycoplasma pulmonis, 161, 163
mycoplasmal infections, 184

nasal cavity lesions, 275
National Academy of Sciences, 209, 377
National Cancer Institute Bioassay Program, 58, 62, 70, 264, 272
National Center for Drugs and Biologics, 297
National Center for Toxicology Research (NCTR), 59, 80, 278, 300
National Institute of Environmental Health Sciences (NIEHS), 6, 57, 59, 60, 79, 80, 92, 200, 278, 327
National Institute of Occupational Health and Safety (NIOSH), 59, 80

National Institutes of Health (NIH), 60, 176, 209, 307
National Research Council, 3, 6, 8
National Toxicology Program (NTP), 4, 9–12, 27, 57–70, 79–97, 159, 200, 263–69, 272, 277, 284, 327, 333
and data audits, 99–101
Annual Plan, 59
Archives, 95
Board of Scientific Counselors, 59, 60, 99
Chemical Evaluation Committee (CEC), 59
Chemical Manager, 11
Contract Laboratories, selection of, 63–64
data flow, 280–81
Executive Committee, 57, 59
General Statement of Work, 80, 84, 93
Master Agreement Statement of Work, 62–63
Monitoring System, 58, 66–70
role of, 58
Steering Committee, 59
studies, 284
Study Manager, 11
toxicology studies, review process for, 60
necropsy, 121, 249–55, 283, 284, 328
negative control groups, 75
nematodes, 158
neurobehavioral toxicology, 63, 65
ninety-day subchronic studies, 80
nodules, 253
noise, effects of, 181–82
nonclinical testing, enforcement of, 139–44
nuclear magnetic resonance, 8

observations and good toxicology practices, 51
Office of Administrative Management (OAM), 81
Office of Compliance Monitoring (OCM), 293

DATE DUE